MEDICAL DEVICE DESIGN FOR SIX SIGMA

A Road Map for Safety and Effectiveness

BASEM S. EL-HAIK
KHALID S. MEKKI

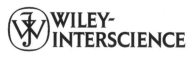

A JOHN WILEY & SONS, INC., PUBLICATION

Published by John Wiley & Sons, Inc.
Published simultaneously in Canada.

For general information on our other products and services or for technical support, please contact our Customer Care Department within the United States at (800) 762-2974, outside the United States at (317) 572-3993 or fax (317) 572-4002.

Wiley also publishes its books in a variety of electronic formats. Some content that appears in print may not be available in electronic formats. For more information about Wiley products, visit our web site at www.wiley.com.

Library of Congress Cataloging-in-Publication Data:

El-Haik, Basem.
  Medical device design for six sigma : a road map for safety and effectiveness /
Basem S. El-Haik, Khalid S. Mekki.
       p. ; cm.
  "A Wiley-Interscience publication."
  Includes bibliographical references.
  ISBN 978-0-470-16861-5
  1. Medical instruments and apparatus—Quality control.   2. Medical instruments and apparatus—Safety measures.   3. Six sigma (Quality control standard)   I. Mekki, Khalid.   II. Title.
  [DNLM: 1. Equipment and Supplies—standards.   2. Equipment Design—methods.   3. Equipment Safety—standards.   4. Quality Control. W 26 E375d 2008]
  R856.6.E44 2008
  610.284—dc22

                                                                    2007038229

Printed in the United States of America

10 9 8 7 6 5 4 3 2 1

To my parents, wife, and children for their continuous support.
—Basem El-Haik

To those that bring light to my life: my dear parents; my loving wife, Sara;
my precious children, Subhi and Talah; my sisters and brothers; and last but
not least, Dr. Basem Haik, who has been a great mentor to me.
—Khalid S. Mekki

CONTENTS

FOREWORD

The world of complex machine design has evolved steadily for many years. The techniques used to design new products have evolved from the world of one-off designs, with a unique set of characteristics in each new design, to a place today where it is understood that most design efforts are bundled into innovations that are primarily existing or known solutions repackaged for the industry or a specific niche. The theory of inventive problem solving (TRIZ) tells us that 95% of each new design falls into that category.

If this is the case, why do we see the types of quality issues in the medical device industry that we do today? I believe it is because we often confuse the creative process with the robust engineering process. While there are many books that describe the use of specific designs for six sigma (DFSS) tools, there are no texts that help the design professional with the combination of all the DFSS tools necessary to produce a safe, efficacious medical device.

This book by Dr. El-Haik and his team serves as a guide to the design of such devices using the complete tool kit at a designer's disposal. It is meant to point out the attributes and applications of a multitude of tools that have long been known to contribute to better, more robust designs in a way that brings all of these tools together in one place. Clearly, this is "the right tool at the right time."

Imagine a design based on the clarity of customer expectations born from a well-executed house of quality, design concepts conceived using axiomatic design and TRIZ, design outputs optimized using a solidly robust design of experiments, a robust failure modes effects analysis to guide risk management, and a state-of-the-art verification and validation process latched to a mistake-proofed design transfer process. These tools, developed in other industries, can now be brought together in one place for the experienced designer to bring to bear for the service of the patient. The objective is to eliminate conceptual and operational design vulnerabilities and to produce an unprecedented device quality level as defined by the customer, by "doing the right things" and "doing things right."

This book is the first on this subject. This team of authors are not academics; they are design practitioners tasked with the next generation of safe and effective products. There is much for us to learn from them.

JOSEPH P. SENER

V.P. Corporate Quality Systems and Business Excellence
Baxter International

PREFACE

Attention has begun to shift from the improvement of design quality in downstream development stages to its development in early upstream stages. This shift is motivated by the fact that design decisions made during the early stages of a product development cycle have the largest impact on the total life-cycle cost and quality of a system. It has been claimed that as much as 80% of the total life-cycle cost is determined during the concept development stage (Fredrikson, 1994). Research in the design and manufacturing arenas, including product development, is currently increasingly focused on addressing industry efforts to shorten lead times, cut development and manufacturing costs, lower total life-cycle cost, and improve the quality of end products and systems. It is the authors' experience that at least 80% of a design's quality is also determined in the early design phases.

In general, *quality* can be defined as the degree to which the design vulnerabilities do not adversely affect product performance. In the context of *design for six sigma* (DFSS) methodology, the major design vulnerabilities may be categorized as:

- Conceptual vulnerabilities that are established due to the violation of design principles.
- Operational vulnerabilities that are created as a result of factors beyond the control of the designer, called *noise factors*. These factors, in general, are responsible for causing a medical device's functional characteristic or process to deviate from target values. Controlling noise factors is very costly or difficult, if not impossible. Operational vulnerability is usually addressed by robust design (Taguchi et al., 1989).

Conceptual vulnerabilities will always result in operational vulnerabilities. However, the reverse is not true. That is, it is possible for a healthy concept that is in full conformity with design principles to be operationally vulnerable. Conceptual vulnerabilities are usually overlooked during device development due to a lack of understanding of the principles of design, the absence of a compatible systemic approach to finding ideal solutions, the pressure of deadlines, and budget constraints. These vulnerabilities are usually addressed by traditional quality methods. These methods can be characterized as after-the-fact practices, since they use lagging information relative to developmental activities, such as bench tests and field data. Unfortunately, these practices drive development toward endless design–test–fix–retest cycles, creating what is broadly known in the manufacturing industry as a "firefighting" operational mode. Companies that follow these practices usually suffer from high development costs, longer time to market, lower quality levels, and a marginal competitive edge. In addition, firefighting actions to improve the conceptual vulnerabilities are not only costly but also difficult to implement, as pressure to achieve design milestones builds during the development cycle. Therefore, it should be a goal to implement quality thinking in the conceptual stages of a development cycle. This goal can be achieved when systematic design theories are integrated with quality concepts and methods up front. This book is geared toward developing an integration framework, a process, for quality in design by borrowing from quality engineering (Taguchi, 1986) and the axiomatic design principles of Suh (1990). This is the framework of DFSS. The objective of the DFSS process is to address design vulnerabilities, both conceptual and operational, by providing tools, processes, and formulations for their quantification, then elimination or reduction.

The medical device design solutions of current practices in many companies generally suffer from heightened vulnerability, such as modest quality levels, ignorance of customer wants and desires, complexity, and lack of conformity with a systematic design methodology to address those issues. Such vulnerabilities are common and generate hidden and unnecessary developmental effort in terms of non-value-added elements, and later, operational costs in the hands of the customer. Design vulnerabilities exhibit themselves by the degree of customer dissatisfaction, modest market shares, and rigid organization structure and operations complexity. Complexity in design creates operational bureaucracy that can be attributed to the lack of conformity with sound design processes. This root cause is coupled with several sources of variation in the medical device manufacturing and delivery processes, inducing variability in customer attributes, known as critical-to-satisfaction characteristics.

The success of the six sigma initiative, process, and deployment in many industries has generated enormous interest in the business world. In creating such successes, six sigma combines people power with process power. People power involves organization support and trained teams tackling specific objectives and stretched, yet feasible goals. Process power refers to effective six sigma deployment, risk mitigation, project management, and an array of statistical and system engineering–based methods. Six sigma focuses on the *whole quality* of a business, including product or medical device quality to external customers, and also the *operational quality* of all internal processes, such as accounting and billing. A whole quality business with whole quality perspectives will not only provide high-quality products or services, but will also have much lower costs and higher efficiency, because all the business processes are optimized.

Compared with retroactive six sigma, which features the DMAIC (define–measure–analysis–improve–control) process, medical device DFSS (identify–characterize–optimize–verify/validate) is proactive. The six sigma objective is to improve a process without redesigning the current process. The ultimate goal of medical device DFSS is whole quality: Do the right things; and do things right all the time. That is, achieve absolute excellence in design, whether it is a service process facing the customer or an internal business process (including product development) facing the employee. Superior medical device design will deliver superior functions to generate great customer satisfaction. Design for six sigma will generate an optimized device both conceptually and operationally within a process that delivers the medical device in a most efficient, economical, and flexible manner. A superior development process will generate a medical device that exceeds customer needs and wants, and delivers high quality at low cost. Superior business process design will generate the most efficient, effective, and economical business process. This is what we mean by whole quality. That is, not only should we have a superior device, but the design and production processes should always deliver what they are supposed to effectively and efficiently and at six sigma quality levels. It does not do a company good to develop some very superior products but some poor products as well—an inconsistent performance.

Medical device design for six sigma as described in this book proactively produces high consistency and extremely low variation in device performance. The term six sigma indicates low variation: 3.4 defectives per million opportunities (DPMO) or better, as measured by the distance between the specification limits and the mean in standard deviation units. We care about variation because customers "feel" inconsistency and variation; they do not feel averages. Nowadays, high consistency is necessary not only for reputation; it is also a matter of survival. For example, the well-known dispute between Ford Motor Company and Firestone Tires involved only an extremely small fraction of tires, but the negative publicity and litigation placed a giant company like Ford in big trouble.

Compared to six sigma (DMAIC), many new methods are introduced that add to the effectiveness of medical device DFSS. For example, axiomatic design, design for X, the theory of inventive problem solving (TRIZ), and transfer function and scorecards are really powerful methods to create superior device designs: to do the right things within our whole quality perspective.

This book also brings another class of powerful methods, Taguchi methods (robust design), into its tool box. A fundamental objective of the Taguchi methods is to create a superior product that can perform highly consistently despite the *noise factors*, the many external disturbances and uncertainties that arise: thus doing things right all the time. Because of DFSS tool sophistication, the training of DFSS operatives (black belts, green belts, etc.) is quite involved. However, this increment in investment is rewarded by better results. A main objective of this book is to provide a complete picture of medical device DFSS to readers, with a focus on development.

Objectives

The objectives of this book are:

1. To provide in-depth and clear coverage of philosophical, organizational, and technical aspects of medical device DFSS to readers.
2. To illustrate clearly all the medical device DFSS deployment and execution processes, the DFSS road map.
3. To present the know-how behind all the principal methods used in medical device DFSS, discussing the theory and background of each method clearly. Examples are provided with a detailed step-by-step implementation process for each method.
4. To help develop readers' practical skills in applying DFSS in medical device environments.

Background Needed

The background required to study this book is some familiarity with simple statistical concepts, such as normal distribution, mean, variance, and simple data analysis techniques.

Summary of the Chapters

In Chapter 1 we introduce medical device design quality, its life cycle, and touch on the effects of regulations on device development. We define device quality as the *whole quality*, starting from idea generation until use by the customer, with the whole quality concept spanning the two boundary points and all developmental activities in between. A historical scan of quality approaches is provided. We introduce the device life cycle from several perspectives: design controls (regulations); design for six sigma tools, methods, and principles; as well as governing firm qualify system. We propose a high-level business model for medical device firms based on experience from other industries.

In Chapter 2 we provide a global perspective of medical device regulations and focus on Food and Drug Administration regulations on design controls as they relate to medical device DFSS. This approach is warranted because of the similarities among the varying regulations, which indicate global harmonization.

In Chapter 3 we review some basic statistics that are used throughout the book. Statistical descriptive and inferential statistical techniques were reviewed at the basic level to ground the reader prior to tackling the heavily technical chapters.

In Chapter 4 we explain six sigma and how it has evolved over time. We explain that it is a process-based methodology and introduce the reader to process modeling with a high-level overview of process mapping. The criticality of measurement systems analysis is demystified. The DMAIC methodology and how it incorporates these concepts into a road map method are described, as is the business process management system for a medical device firm.

In Chapter 5 we offer a high-level DFSS process. The DFSS approach, as introduced, helps design teams frame their project with financial, cultural, and strategic implications to the business. In this chapter we form and integrate several strategic and tactical and synergistic methodologies to enhance medical device DFSS capabilities and to deliver a broad set of optimized solutions. We highlight and present the DFSS phases: identify, characterize, optimize, and verify/validate (ICOV).

In Chapter 6 we discuss the deployment of a medical device DFSS initiative, starting from scratch. We present the deployment plan, roles and responsibilities of deployment operatives, project sources, and other aspects of sound deployment strategy in three phases: predeployment, initial deployment, and steady-state deployment. We also discuss certain desirable design team characteristics and offer several perspectives on cultural transformation and initiative sustainability.

In Chapter 7 we present the medical device DFSS project road map. The road map highlights the ICOV phases at a high level over seven life-cycle development stages: idea creation, voice of the customer and business, concept development, preliminary design, design optimization, verification, and launch readiness. The concept of tollgate is introduced and we highlight the most appropriate DFSS tools and methods by DFSS phase, indicating where it is most appropriate to start tool use. Methods are presented in subsequent chapters. Manufacturing processes and software developments are discussed as parts of the medical device DFSS.

In Chapter 8 we present quality function deployment (QFD), used to translate customer needs and wants into focused design actions and paralleling design mappings. QFD is key tool used to prevent problems from occurring once a design has become operational. The link to the DFSS road map allows for rapid design cycle and effective utilization of resources while achieving six sigma levels of performance.

The design activity of design mapping is presented in Chapter 9. The medical device DFSS project road map recognizes two different mappings, functional mapping and process mapping. In this chapter we present functional mapping as a logical model depicting the logical and cause–effect relationships between design elements through techniques such as axiomatic design and value engineering. A process map is a visual aid for picturing work processes which shows how inputs, outputs, and tasks are linked.

The use of creativity and innovation methods such as the theory of problem solving (TIPS or TRIZ) in medical device DFSS is presented in Chapter 10. TRIZ provides design teams with a priceless toolbox for innovation to help see the true design opportunity and provide principles to resolve, improve, and optimize concepts. TRIZ is a useful innovation and problem-solving method that when applied successfully replaces the trial-and-error method in the search for vulnerability-free concepts. TRIZ-based thinking for medical devices helped to identify the technology tools that come into play, such as innovation principles, separation principles for resolving technical contradictions and conflicts, operators for revealing and utilizing system resources, and patterns of evolution of technical systems to support conceptual optimization.

In Chapter 11 we discuss the most significant aspects of building risk management into the flow of the design and medical device DFSS development process. We show how to embed the trade-off concept of risk–benefit analysis as part of the design and development process. DFSS methodology provides traceability where relationships between hazards, requirements, and verification and validation activities are identified and linked. In addition, we show that risk management itself is a process centered on understanding risks and evaluating their acceptability, reducing risks as much as possible, and then evaluating residual risk and overall device safety against the benefits derived. Integrating risk management into the medical device DFSS methodology requires keeping risk issues at the forefront of the entire process, from design planning to verification and validation testing. In this way, risk management becomes part of the product development process, evolves with the design, and provides a framework for decision making. We also discuss failure mode and effect analysis, a very important design review method used to avoid potential failures in design stages.

In Chapter 12 we introduce the concept of design for X (DFX) as it relates to medical device design, building on the work performed for generic product design. In this context we show that DFX for medical devices requires that the device content be evaluated to minimize complexity and maximize commonality. The end result will be a robust design that meets customer's needs profitably through implementation of methods such as design for serviceability, packaging, assembly and manufacturability, and reliability.

In Chapter 13 we introduce the transfer function and design scorecard tools. The use of such DFSS tools parallels the design mappings introduced in Chapter 9. The transfer function is a mathematical relationship relating a design response to design elements. A design scorecard is used to document the transfer function as well as the optimization calculations.

In Chapter 14 we present the medical device DFSS approach to design of experiments (DOE), a prime optimization tool. DOE is a structured method for determining the transfer function relationship between factors affecting and comprising a device. DOE refers to experimental methods used to quantify indeterminate measurements of factors and interactions between factors statistically through observance of forced changes made methodically as directed by systematic tables called design arrays. The main DOE data analysis tools include analysis of variance, empirical transfer function model building, and main effects and interaction charts. These are presented in Chapter 13.

In Chapter 15 we present the use of robust parameter design methodology in the medical device design environment. Robustness thinking helps the DFSS team to classify design parameters and process variables mapped into the design as controlled or uncontrolled. The objective is to desensitize the design to uncontrolled disturbance factors, also called noise factors, thus producing a consistently performing on-target design with minimal variation.

Chapter 16 deals with the problem of how, and when, to specify tightened tolerances for a medical device so that quality and performance are enhanced. Every device (or its manufacturing processes) has a number—perhaps a large number—of design parameters (or process variables). We explain here how to identify the critical parameters and variables to target when tolerances have to be tightened. The objective is to provide useful techniques allowing further robustness gains on top of parameter design if so desired.

In Chapter 17, the final aspect of DFSS methodology, which differentiates it from the prevalent "launch and learn" method, is design verification, design validation, software validation, and process validation. This chapter covers in detail the verify/validate phase of the DFSS (ICOV) project road map. Design verification, process validation, and design validation help in identifying unintended consequences and effects of the design process, in developing plans and in reducing risk for full-scale commercialization to all stakeholders, including all customer segments. There is a degree of overlap with Chapter 18, and readers are encouraged to read these chapters in sequence.

In Chapter 18 we discuss design transfer as it relates to medical device DFSS. Design transfer simply encompasses clear establishment of a relationship between design engineering and production and service during the product life cycle. In the DFSS process this is an ongoing activity that will gain more momentum as the device design matures in the DFSS process (Chapter 7). Following the FDA regulation and to avoid duplication of effort on the part of the DFSS team, we strongly advocate use of a device master record (DMR) as the documented DFSS knowledge institutionalization. Depending on the project scope, the DFSS part may partially or fully overlap with the DMR. That is, a DMR is sufficient and necessary documentation of any device or subset. In this chapter we utilize advanced product quality planning and the production part approval process.

In Chapter 19 we present design change control, design review, and the design history file for a medical device DFSS project. The change control process manages change to ensure that any changes to a device's design, labeling, packaging, device master record, or design inputs prior to or after design transfer must be identified, documented, validated, or where appropriate, verified, reviewed, and approved prior to implementation, and finally, closed and documented in the design history file. Design reviews are a key design control element in quality system regulation 21 CFR 820.30(e). They are intended to assure that the design meets the requirements definition, and they also act as a mechanism for identification of a potential development weaknesses associated with safety, reliability, efficacy, manufacturability, service, implementation, and customer misuse of the device. These reviews are not to be mistaken with the DFSS project tollgate reviews discussed in Chapter 7.

In Chapter 20 we discuss the development of an automatic dissolving and dosing devise (Auto 3D) as a case study of medical device DFSS. In showing how DFSS applies to the development of Auto 3D, we provide a high-level understanding of the project rather than documenting every step and tool application.

What Distinguishes This Book from Others in the Area

This book is the *first* to address medical device design for six sigma and to present an approach with tool application examples and a medical device DFSS case study. The book's main distinguishing feature is its completeness and comprehensiveness, beginning with a high-level overview, deployment aspects, and a medical device design tool box. The most important topics in DFSS are discussed clearly and in depth. The organizational, implementation, theoretical, and practical aspects of the DFSS road map and DFSS toolbox methods are covered carefully and in complete detail. This is the only book that discusses all medical device DFSS perspectives, such as transfer functions, axiomatic design, TRIZ, validation and verification, design transfer, and Taguchi methods in great detail. It can be used as either a complete reference book on DFSS or as comprehensive training material for DFSS teams.

Acknowledgments

In preparing this book we received advice and encouragement from Joseph P. Sener, Vice President, Corporate Quality Systems and Business Excellence, Baxter International and appreciate his continuing support. The authors appreciate the willingness of several people to review this material: Rob Gier, George Dillon, James Plucinski, Brian Schultz, and Sahar Bahrani of Baxter International, Maher Alhaj for the artwork in Chapter 20, and Dr. Abdelqader Zamamiri of Abbott Loboratories. The authors are very thankful for the efforts of George Telecki, Melissa Valentine, and Rachel Witmer of John Wiley & Sons, Inc. We are especially thankful to www.Generator.com for many excellent examples in Chapter 10.

Contacting Dr. Basem El-Haik (basem.haik@sixsigmapi.com)

Your comments and suggestions on the book will be greatly appreciated and will be given serious consideration for inclusion in a future edition. Six Sigma Professionals, Inc. (www.SixSigmaPI.com) conducts public and in-house six sigma and design for six sigma (DFSS) training and deployment workshops and provides program and project consulting services.

1

MEDICAL DEVICE DESIGN QUALITY

1.1 INTRODUCTION

Throughout the evolution of quality, there has always been a preponderance of focus on the manufacture of parts. In recent years, more applications have focused on design in general; however, the application of a full suite of tools to medical device design is rare and still considered risky or challenging. Some companies in the medical industry that have mature six sigma deployment programs see the application of design for six sigma to product and internal processes as an investment rather than a needless expense.

Attention has begun to shift from improvement of design quality in downstream development stages to early upstream stages. This shift is motivated by the fact that design decisions made during early stages of the product development cycle have the greatest impact on total life-cycle cost and system quality. It has been claimed that as much as 80% of the total life-cycle cost is determined during the concept development stage (Fredrikson, 1994). The deployment of design for six sigma in the device development and manufacturing arenas is currently experiencing an increased focus on addressing industry efforts to shorten lead times, cut development and manufacturing costs, lower total life-cycle cost, and improve device quality. It is the author's experience that at least 80% of a design's quality is also determined in the early design phases.

Medical Device Design for Six Sigma: A Road Map for Safety and Effectiveness,
By Basem S. El-Haik and Khalid S. Mekki
Copyright © 2008 John Wiley & Sons, Inc.

As mentioned in the Preface, design vulnerabilities are the result of poor quality and design engineering practices. In the context of *design for six sigma* (DFSS), the major design vulnerabilities are categorized as follows:

- Conceptual vulnerabilities based on the violation of design principles (for examples of design principles, see Chapters 9 to 12).
- Operational vulnerabilities created as a result of factors beyond the control of designers, called *noise factors*. Such factors are, in general, responsible for causing a device's functional characteristic or process to deviate from target values. Controlling noise factors is very costly or difficult, if not impossible. Operational vulnerability is usually addressed by robust design (see Chapters 15 and 16) (Taguchi et al., 1989).

In medical device design, conceptual vulnerabilities will always result in operational vulnerabilities. However, the reverse is not true. That is, it is possible for a healthy device concept that is in full obedience to design principles to be operationally vulnerable. In this book we are addressing the two categories of design vulnerability.

Profitability is one of the most important factors for any successful business enterprise. High profitability is determined by strong sales and overall low cost in all company operations. Healthy sales are determined strongly by high quality and reasonable price; as a result, improving quality and reducing cost are among the most important tasks for any business enterprise. Six sigma and DFSS are new business excellence initiatives that would effectively reduce cost and improve quality. In medical device design, quality and safety are interlinked. Most errors and inefficiencies in patient care arise from conflicting, incomplete, or suboptimal devices.

The objective of DFSS is to design and redesign medical devices to make them safer and more effective, patient centered, timely, and efficient. How does one achieve quality and safety by quality? What is quality?

1.2 THE ESSENCE OF QUALITY

Quality is a more intriguing concept than it appears to be. The meaning of the term *quality* has evolved over time as many concepts were developed to improve product or service quality, including total quality management (TQM), the Malcolm Baldrige National Quality Award, six sigma, quality circles, the theory of constraints quality management systems [ISO 9000 and ISO 13485], axiomatic quality (El-Haik, 2005), and continuous improvement. Following are various interpretations of quality:

- "Quality means the totality of features and characteristics that bear on the ability of a device to satisfy fitness-for-use, including safety and performance" [21 CFR 820.3(s)].

- "Quality: an inherent or distinguishing characteristic, a degree or grade of excellence" (*American Heritage Dictionary*, 1996).
- "Quality and the required style of management" (W. Edwards Deming).
- "Conformance to requirements" (Philip B. Crosby in the 1980s).
- "Fitness for use" (Joseph M. Juran).
- "Degree to which a set of inherent characteristic fulfills requirements" (ISO 9000).
- "Value to some person" (Gerald M. Weinberg).
- "The loss a product imposes on society after it is shipped" (Genichi Taguchi).
- "The degree to which the design vulnerabilities do not adversely affect product performance" (Basem El-Haik).

Quality is a characteristic that a product or service must have. It refers to the perception of the degree to which a product or service meets a customer's expectations. Quality has no specific meaning unless it is related to a specific function or measurable characteristic. The dimensions of quality refer to the measurable characteristics that quality achieves. For example, in the design and development of a medical device:

- Quality supports safety and performance.
- Safety and performance support durability.
- Durability supports flexibility.
- Flexibility supports speed.
- Speed supports cost.

You can easily build the interrelationship between quality and all aspects of product characteristics, as these characteristics act as the qualities of the product. However, not all qualities are equal. Some are more important than others. The most important qualities are the ones that customers want most. These are the qualities that products and services must have. So providing quality products and services is all about meeting customer requirements. It's all about meeting the needs and expectations of customers.

When the word *quality* is used, we usually think in terms of an excellent design or service that fulfils or exceeds our expectations. When a product design surpasses our expectations, we consider that its quality is good. Thus, quality is related to perception. Conceptually, quality can be quantified as follows (Yang and El-Haik, 2003):

$$Q = \frac{\sum P}{\sum E} \qquad (1.1)$$

where Q is quality, P is performance, and E is an expectation.

In a traditional manufacturing environment, conformance to specifications and delivery are the common quality items that are measured and tracked. Often, lots are rejected because they don't have the correct documentation supporting them. Quality in manufacturing, then, is conforming product, delivered on time, and having all the supporting documentation. In design, quality is measured as consistent conformance to customer expectations.

The expected performance is actually "what this design can do for me" in the eyes of customers. The American Society for Quality (ASQ) defines quality as a subjective term for which each person has his or her own definition. In technical use, *quality* can have two meanings: (1) it represents the characteristics of a product or service that bear on its ability to satisfy stated or implied needs; or (2) it describes a product or service free of deficiencies. By examining ASQ's definition, we see that "on its ability to satisfy stated or implied needs" means that a product or service should be able to deliver potential customer needs; we call it "doing the right things." And "free of deficiencies" means that the product or service can deliver customer needs consistently. We can call this "doing things right all the time." Several concepts that are associated with quality are defined below (see the *Code of Federal Regulations* Title 21 and ISO 13485).

- *Quality system:* the organizational structure, responsibilities, procedures, processes, and resources for implementing quality management.
- *Quality policy:* the overall intentions and direction of an organization with respect to quality as established by management with executive responsibility.
- *Quality management:* includes all the activities that managers carry out in an effort to implement their quality policy. These activities include quality planning, quality control, quality assurance, and quality improvement.
- *Quality audits:* a systematic independent examination of a manufacturer's quality system that is performed at defined intervals and at sufficient frequency to determine whether both quality system activities and the results of such activities comply with quality system procedures, that these procedures are implemented effectively, and that these procedures are suitable to achieve quality system objectives.
- *Quality control:* a set of activities or techniques whose purpose is to ensure that all quality requirements are being met. To achieve this purpose, processes are monitored and performance problems are solved.
- *Quality improvement:* anything that enhances an organization's ability to meet quality requirements.
- *Quality assurance:* a set of activities whose purpose is to demonstrate that an entity meets all quality requirements. Quality assurance activities

are carried out to inspire the confidence of both customers and managers, confidence that all quality requirements are being met.

- *Quality planning:* a set of activities whose purpose is to define quality system policies, objectives, and requirements, and to explain how these policies will be applied, how these objectives will be achieved, and how these requirements will be met. It is always future oriented. A quality plan explains how you intend to apply your quality policies, achieve your quality objectives, and meet your quality system requirements.
- *Quality record:* contains objective evidence which shows how well a quality requirement is being met or how well a quality process is performing. It always documents what has happened in the past.
- *Quality requirement:* a characteristic that an entity must have. For example, a customer may require that a particular product (entity) achieve a specific dependability score (characteristic).
- *Quality surveillance:* a set of activities whose purpose is to monitor an entity and review its records to prove that quality requirements are being met.

1.3 QUALITY OPERATING SYSTEM AND THE DEVICE LIFE CYCLE

To deliver a high-quality medical device, we need a system of methods and activities that can provide an overarching structure to plan and develop the product successfully. Such a system, called a *quality operating system*, includes all the planned and systematic activities performed within the system that can demonstrate with confidence that the device will fulfill the requirements for quality. Figure 1.1 depicts a graphical flow of a typical product development life cycle that encompasses the life cycle from ideation through to phaseout or retirement. Below we enumerate the life-cycle stages as vetted with some DFSS concepts. The life cycle in Figure 1.1 will later be married with the famous waterfall design process of a medical device with design control depicted in Figure 1.2.

Design controls is U.S. Food and Drug Administration (FDA) terminology for a product design and development process. Design controls comprise an interrelated set of practices and procedures that are incorporated into the medical device design and development process, a system of checks and balances. The objective is to induce a systematic approach that exhibits deficiencies in design input requirements, and discrepancies between the proposed designs and requirements are made evident and corrected earlier in the design and development process. 21 CFR 820.30 describes what is needed but stops short of defining the "how to," a gap that is well filled by this book. Design controls as expressed in the life-cycle stages depicted here together with six sigma design principles, tools, and methods (collectively known as design for

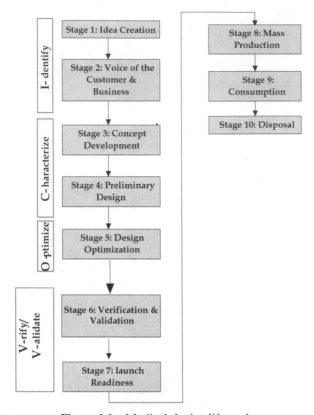

Figure 1.1   Medical device life cycle.

six sigma) constitute an insurance policy that the design transferred to production will translate into a device that exceeds user expectations while satisfying
user requirements. In practice, DFSS provides managers and designers with
improved visibility of the design process decision making. With improved visibility, managers are empowered to direct the design process more effectively:
that is, to prevent problems earlier, and if necessary, to make educated corrective decisions and adjust resource allocations. Design teams benefit both
by enhanced understanding of the degree of conformance of a design to user
and patient needs, and by improved communications and coordination among
all stakeholders of the process.

1.3.1   Stage 1: Idea Creation

The need for a new device can arise from newly emerged needs, R&D (research
and development) ideation, benchmarking, technology road maps, and/or
multigenerational plans (Chapter 6). New processes often come about because
of "revolution," not "evolution." For example, when a new management team

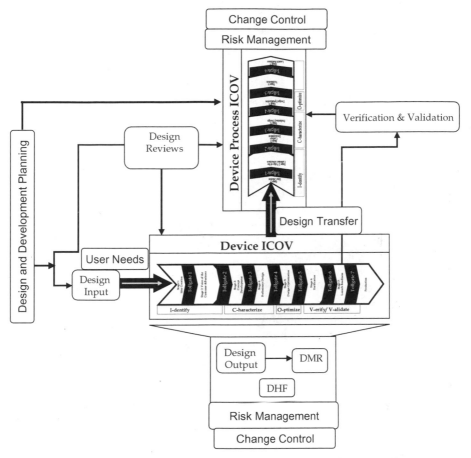

Figure 1.2 Design process with medical device design controls.

is brought in and they staff the organization with knowledgeable people to execute the new strategies and methods, often, the switching costs are huge and it takes time for the new process to start delivering benefits. If the legacy team had been able to evolve slowly, the change brought on by the new team is a revolution. It is the premise of this book that based on performance metrics and benchmarking, natural evolution via DFSS deployment can provide process redesign that is manageable and controllable.

1.3.2 Stage 2: Voice of the Customer and Business

Customer and business requirements must be studied and analyzed in the second stage even under a redesign environment. We need to understand the key functional requirements (in a solution-free environment) which will fulfill the stated or implied needs of both external and internal customers (business).

We also need to understand the relationships between the voice of the customer, the voice of regulatory bodies in the countries where the device will be sold, and the voice of the business. The quality function deployment house of quality is an ideal method for this purpose (see Chapter 8).

1.3.3   Stage 3: Concept Development

Concept development is the third stage in the medical device life cycle. In this stage, concepts are developed to fulfill the functional requirements obtained from the preceding stage. This stage of the life-cycle process is still at a high level and remains solution-free; that is, the design team is able to specify what needs to be accomplished to satisfy the customer wants, not how to accomplish these wants. The strategy of the design team is to create several innovative concepts and use selection methodologies to narrow down the choices. At this stage we can highlight the Pugh concept selection method (Pugh, 1996), summarized in Figure 1.3.

The method of controlled convergence was developed by Stuart Pugh (1991) as part of his solution selection process. Controlled convergence is a solution iterative selection process that allows alternate convergent (analytic) and divergent (synthetic) thinking to be experienced by the service design team. The method alternates between generation and convergence selection activities.

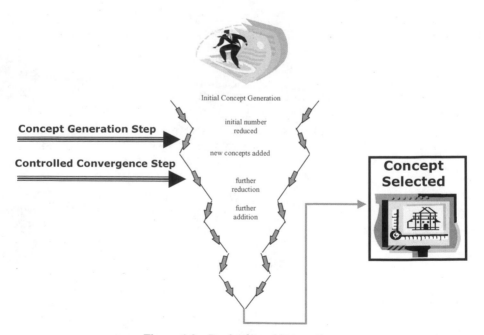

Figure 1.3   Pugh phased innovation.

Tools such as TRIZ [theory of Russian inventive science, also known as TIPS (theory of inventive problem solving)] and the morphological matrix are better suited to creativity, while the Pugh selection matrix helps with the critical selection. TRIZ is explored in Chapter 10.

1.3.4   Stage 4: Preliminary Design

In stage 4, the prioritized functional requirements must be translated into design parameters with detail specifications. Appropriate tools for this purpose are QFD (Chapter 8) or axiomatic design (Chapter 9).

A preliminary design, which could consist of a design structure (architecture or hierarchy) with subsystem requirements flow-down, should be developed in this phase. QFD (Chapter 8) and functional modeling (Chapter 9) are very beneficial in this stage. Design targets for reliability, quality, process ability, and ease are established in stage 4. When one potential design solution has been selected, the team can begin to focus on the specific failure modes of that design using a design failure modes and effects analysis. Concurrently, from all of these design requirements the first elements for inclusion on the design scorecard (Chapter 13) can be identified and recorded.

1.3.5   Stage 5: Design Optimization

In stage 5 the design team will ensure that the final design matches the customer requirements that were identified in stage 2 (capability flows up to meet the voice of the customer). There are techniques [DFX (Chapter 12), FMEA (Chapter 11)] that can be used at this point to ensure that the design cannot be used in a way that was not intended, cannot be processed or maintained incorrectly, or that if there is a mistake, it will be obvious immediately. A final test plan is generated to assure that all requirements are met at six sigma level by the pilot or prototype that is implemented or built in the next stage.

In stage 5, detailed designs are formulated and tested either physically or through simulation. Functional requirements are flowed down from system level into subsystem design parameters using transfer functions (Chapter 13), functional modeling (Chapter 9), and design of experiments (Chapter 14). Designs are made robust to withstand the noise introduced by external uncontrollable factors (Chapter 15). All of the activities in stage 5 should result in a design that can be produced in a pilot or prototype form.

1.3.6   Stage 6: Verification and Validation

Test requirements and procedures are developed and the pilot is implemented and/or the prototype is built in this stage. The pilot is run in as realistic a setting as possible, with multiple iterations and subjected to as much noise as possible in an environment that is as close as possible to its final usage conditions. The same philosophy applies to the testing of a prototype. The prototype should be tested at the extremes of its intended range and sometimes beyond. To the extent possible or allowed by regulation, simulation should replace as much testing as is feasible in order to reduce cost and risk. In the medical device industry, a distinction is made between design verification and validation. *Design verification* is a process whose purpose is to examine design outputs and to use objective evidence to confirm that outputs meet input requirements. *Design validation* is a process whose purpose is to examine devices and to use objective evidence to confirm that these products meet user needs. See Figure 1.2 for more clarification.

In general, the results of pilot or prototype testing allows the design team the opportunity to make final adjustments or changes in the design to ensure that the product, service, or business process performance is optimized to match customer expectations. In some cases only real-life testing can be performed. In this situation, design of experiments is an efficient way to determine if the desired impact is created and confirmed.

1.3.7   Stage 7: Launch Readiness

Based on successful verification and validation in a production environment, the team will assess the readiness of all the process infrastructure and resources. For instance, have all standard operating procedures been documented and personnel trained in the procedures? What is the plan for process switchover or ramp-up? What contingencies are in place? What special measures will be in place to ensure rapid discovery? Careful planning and understanding of the desired behavior are paramount to successful transition from the design world into the production environment. In Chapter 18 we describe in detail all the requirements, through best-demonstrated practices, for successful design transfer to production and service.

1.3.8   Stage 8: Mass Production

In this stage, if the team has not already begun implementation of the design solution in the production environment, the design team should do so now. The product will be produced and shipped to the market. Some parts or subassemblies might be produced by suppliers. During production it is very important that the manufacturing process be able to function consistently and free of defect, and all parts and subassemblies supplied by suppliers should be consistent with quality requirements.

For quality assurance at this stage, the key task is to ensure that the final design is in conformance with design requirements. That is, all products, together with their parts and subassemblies, should conform to their design requirements; they should be interchangeable and consistent. The quality methods used in this stage include statistical process control, quality standard and acceptance inspection for suppliers, and production troubleshooting and diagnosis methods.

1.3.9   Stage 9: Consumption

During this stage, devices are consumed by customers. This stage is really the most important to consumers, for it is the consumer who will form opinions of the design and brand name. When customers encounter problems such as defects, warranty, and service when using a design during consumption, it is important to keep the design in use and the customer satisfied.

For quality assurance in this stage, it is impossible to improve the quality level for designs already in use because they are already out of the hands of the producer. However, a good warrantee and service program will certainly help to keep the design in use by repairing defective units and providing other after-sale services. Usually, warranty and service programs are very expensive compared to doing things right the first time. Warranty and service programs can also provide valuable information for the quality improvement of future production and device design.

1.3.10   Stage 10: Disposal or Phaseout

Eventually, all products and services become obsolete, replaced by either new technologies or new methods. Also, the dynamic and cyclical nature of customer attributes dictates continuous improvement to maintain adequate market share. Usually, it is difficult to turn off the switch, as customers depend on a device differently. Just look at dialysis machines: One cannot just convert to a single new dialysis process; there must be a coordinated effort and change management is often required to convince customers to shift to the new device.

1.4   EVOLUTION OF QUALITY

The earliest Egyptian, Mayan, and Aztec societies left archeological evidence of precision and accuracy nearly unmatched today. Following these societies we entered into an extended period of apprenticeship in which we developed conformance to customer requirements with never more than one degree of separation between the producer and the customer. During the industrial revolution, societies began to separate producers from consumers, and this led to the discovery and development of quality methodologies to improve the customer experience. These practices evolved around product-based processes during this era of globalization.

There are three components that drive the evolution of quality: knowledge, technology, and resources. Basic knowledge of quality philosophy, methods, and tools precedes the automation of these tools via technology and is followed by general awareness and adoption by practitioners.

In the early days of the pioneering Walter A. Shewhart, slide rules were the prevalent technology, and even the simplest calculations were tedious. The high level of effort required for calculations resulted in simplification of statistical process control to use $\bar{X}$- and R-charts and prevented rapid adoption of statistical process control. Today, we have mature knowledge with automated data capture systems and the ability to analyze large data sets with personal computers and statistical software. Today's resources have higher math skills than the average person had in Shewhart's time, and the penetration of quality methods has expanded into customer-touching support processes as well as product-based processes. The adoption of enabling processes such as human resources, supply chain, legal, and sales, although analogous to customer-touching processes, is weak, due to the perceived cost–benefit deficit and a lack of process-focused metrics in these processes.

Let us look at an abbreviated chronological review of some of the pioneers who added notably to the knowledge of quality. Much of quality evolution has occurred in the following five disciplines: (1) statistical analysis and control, (2) root-cause analysis, (3) total quality management, (4) design quality, and (5) process simplification. The earliest evolution began with statistical analysis and control, so we start our chronology there.

1.4.1 Statistical Analysis and Control

In 1924, Walter A. Shewhart introduced the first application of control charting to monitor and control important production variables in a manufacturing process. This charting method introduced the concepts of special and common cause variation. He evolved his concepts and in 1931 published *Economic Control of Quality of Manufactured Product*, which brought together successfully the disciplines of statistics, engineering, and economics, and with this book, Shewhart became known as the father of modern quality control. Shewhart also introduced plan–do–study–act (Shewhart cycle), later made popular by Deming as the PDCA cycle.

In 1925, Sir Ronald Fisher published *Statistical Methods for Research Workers* and introduced the concepts of randomization and analysis of variance (ANOVA). Later in 1925 he published *Design of Experiments*. Frank Yates, an associate of Fisher, contributed Yates' standard order for ANOVA calculations. In 1950, Gertrude Cox and William Cochran coauthored *Experimental Design*, which became the standard of the time. In Japan, Genechi Taguchi introduced orthogonal arrays as an efficient method for conducting experimentation within the context of robust design. He followed this up in 1957 with the book *Design of Experiments*. Taguchi's robustness methods have been used in product development since the 1980s. In 1976, Douglas Montgomery published *Design and Analysis of Experiments*, followed by George

Box, William Hunter, and Stuart Hunter's *Statistics for Experimenters* in 1978.

1.4.2 Root-Cause Analysis

In 1937, Joseph Juran introduced the Pareto principle as a means of delineating root causes. In 1943, Kaoru Ishikawa developed the cause-and-effect or fishbone diagram. The use of multivariable charts was promoted first by Len Seder of Gillette Razors in 1949 and then service-marked by Dorian Shainin, who added it to his Red X tool box, which became known as the Shainin techniques in the period 1951 through 1975. Root-cause analysis as known today relies on seven basic tools: the cause-and-effect diagram, check sheet, control chart (special cause versus common cause), flowchart, histogram, Pareto chart, and scatterplot (Figure 1.4).

1.4.3 Total Quality Management

The integrated philosophy and organizational alignment for pursuing the deployment of quality methodologies is often referred to as total quality management (TQM). Its level of adoption has often been related directly to the tools and methodologies referenced by the leaders who created the methods and tools as well as the perceived value of adopting them. Armand V. Feigenbaum published *Total Quality Control* in 1951 while at MIT pursuing his doctorate. He later became head of quality for General Electric and interacted with Hitachi and Toshiba. His pioneering effort was associated with the translation into Japanese of his 1951 book *Quality Control: Principles, Practices and Administration* and his articles on total quality control.

Joseph Juran followed closely in 1951 with the *Quality Control Handbook*, the most comprehensive "how-to" book on quality ever published. At this time, W. Edwards Deming was gaining fame in Japan following work for the U.S. government in the Census Bureau developing survey statistics, and pub-

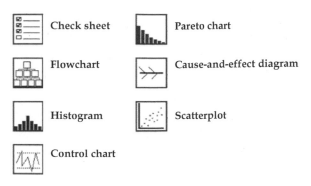

Figure 1.4 Seven basic quality tools.

lished his most famous work, *Out of the Crisis*, in 1986. Deming had associations with Walter Shewhart and Sir Ronald Fisher and has become the most notable TQM proponent. Deming's basic quality philosophy is that productivity improves as variability decreases and that statistical methods are needed to control quality. He advocated the use of statistics to measure performance in all areas, not just conformance to design specifications. Furthermore, he thought that it is not enough to meet specifications; one has to keep working to reduce the variations as well. Deming was extremely critical of the U.S. approach to business management and was an advocate of worker participation in decision making. Kaoru Ishikawa then became noticed for his development of quality circles in Japan and published the *Guide to Quality Control* in 1968. The last outstanding pioneer is Philip Crosby, who in 1979 published *Quality Is Free*, in which he focused on the "absolutes" of quality and the basic elements of improvement and the pursuit of "zero defects."

1.4.4 Design Quality

From a regulatory perspective, 21 CFR Part 820 is a high-level description of design controls that will assure design quality. However, adherence to regulations implies only the bare minimum of what needs to be done. The quality of work and how to do it can be assured only via a rigorous process such as design for six sigma, the subject of this book.

Design quality includes philosophy and methodology. The earliest contributor in this field was the Russian Genrich Altshuller, who provided us with the theory of inventive problem solving (TRIZ or TIPS) in 1950. TRIZ is based on inventive principles derived from a study of over 3.5 million of the world's most innovative patents and inventions. TRIZ is a revolutionary way of solving problems systematically based on science and technology. TRIZ helps organizations use the knowledge embodied in the world's inventions to develop elegant solutions to the most difficult design and engineering problems quickly, efficiently, and creatively. The next major development was quality function deployment (QFD), promoted in Japan by Yoji Akao and Shigeru Mizuno in 1966 but not Westernized until the 1980s. Their purpose was to develop a quality assurance method that would design customer satisfaction into a product before it was manufactured. Prior quality control methods were aimed primarily at fixing a problem during or after manufacturing. QFD is a structured approach to defining customer needs or requirements and translating them into specific plans to produce products or services to meet those needs. The *voice of the customer* is the term used to describe these stated and unstated customer needs or requirements.

In the 1970s Taguchi promoted the concept of the quality loss function, which stated that any deviation from nominal was costly and that by designing with the noise of the system the product would operate within, one could optimize designs. Taguchi packaged his concepts in the methods named after him: robust design and quality engineering.

The last major development in design quality was that of Nam P. Suh and his axiomatic design approach. Axiomatic design is a principle-based method that provides a designer with a structured approach to design tasks. In this approach, design is modeled as mapping between different domains. For example, in the concept design stage, it could be a mapping between customer attribute domain and the design function domain; in the product design stage, it is a mapping from the function domain to the design parameter domain. There are many possible design solutions for the same design task. However, based on its two fundamental axioms, axiomatic design method developed many design principles to evaluate and analyze design solutions and gave designers directions by which to improve designs. The axiomatic design approach can be applied not only in engineering design but also in other design tasks, such as in organization systems. El-Haik (2005) integrated robust design and axiomatic design in a framework called *axiomatic quality*. Design quality is the focus of this book.

1.4.5 Process Simplification

Lately, "lean" has become a topic of great interest. The pursuit of the elimination of waste has led to several quality improvements. The earliest development was poka-yoke (mistake-proofing), developed by Shigeo Shingo in Japan in 1961. The essential idea of poka-yoke is to design processes such that mistakes are impossible to make or at least are easily detected and corrected. Poka-yoke devices fall into two major categories: prevention and detection. A prevention device affects a process such that it is impossible to make a mistake. A detection device signals the user when a mistake has been made so that the problem can be corrected quickly. In 1970, Shingo, developed single minute exchange of die (SMED). This trend toward "lean" has also seen more systemwide process mapping and value analysis, which has evolved into value stream maps.

1.4.6 Six Sigma and Design for Six Sigma

The initiative known as six sigma[1] follows in the footsteps of all the techniques described above. Six sigma was conceptualized and introduced by Motorola in the early 1980s. It spread to Texas Instruments and Asea Brown Boveri, then to Allied Signal and to General Electric in 1995. It has been enabled by the emergence of the personal computer and by statistical software packages such as Minitab, SAS, BMDP, and SPSS. It combines each of the elements of process management and design: define–measure–analyze–improve–control and design for six sigma. We discuss these in detail in later chapters.

[1]The word *sigma* refers to the Greek letter σ, used by statisticians to measure variability. As the numerical levels of σ increase, the number of defects in a process fall exponentially. Six sigma design is the ultimate goal since it means that if the same task were performed 1 million times, there would be only 3.4 defects, assuming normality.

Design for six sigma (DFSS; see Chapters 5 to 7) is a disciplined methodology that embeds customer expectations into the design, applies the transfer function approach to ensure that customer expectations are met, predicts design performance prior to the pilot phase, builds into the design performance measurement systems with scorecards to ensure effective ongoing process management, leverages a common language for design, and uses tollgate reviews to ensure accountability.

DFSS is a disciplined and rigorous approach to service, process, and product design through ensuring that new designs meet customer requirements prior to launch. It is a design approach that ensures complete understanding of development steps, capabilities, and performance measurements by using scorecards and tollgate reviews to ensure accountability of design stakeholders, black belts, project champions, deployment champions, and the rest of an organization.

DFSS may be used to design or redesign a product or service. The expected process sigma level for a DFSS product or service is at least 4.5 but can be 6 sigma or higher, depending on the designed entity. The production of such a low defect level from product or service launch means that customer expectations and needs must be understood completely before a design can be operationalized. That is, quality is defined by the customer. Our DFSS approach has the following four phases:

1. Identify customer wants and design inputs and map them to design outputs.
2. Characterize the medical design entity and develop its conceptual structure.
3. Optimize the medical device entity in its environment of use.
4. Verify/validate the medical device entity that delivers its functional outputs. This includes validation to customer wants.

Figure 1.5 illustrates the the DFSS *Identify–characterize–optimize–verify/ validate* (ICOV) *process* over the device life cycle shown in Figure 1.1.

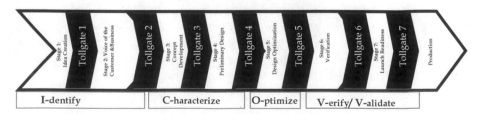

Figure 1.5   DFSS ICOV process.

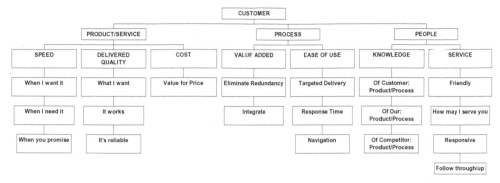

Figure 1.6 Customer experience channels.

1.5 BUSINESS EXCELLENCE: A VALUE PROPOSITION

At the highest level, business excellence is featured by good profitability, business viability, and growth in sales and market share based on quality (Peters and Waterman, 1980). Achieving design excellence is the common goal for all business leaders and their employees. To achieve design excellence, design quality itself is not sufficient; *quality* has to be replaced by *whole quality*, which includes quality in business operations as well, as shown in Figure 1.6. To understand business excellence, we need to understand business operation and other metrics in business operation, which we cover in the next section.

1.5.1 Business Operation Model

Figure 1.7 shows a typical high-level business operation model for a manufacturing company. For companies that are service-oriented, the business model

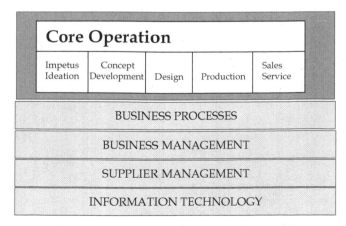

Figure 1.7 Typical business operation model.

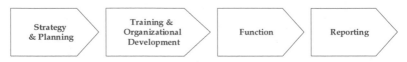

Figure 1.8 Business functional core operation and auxiliary requirements model.

could look somewhat different. However, for every company there is always a *core operation* and a number of other enabling business elements. The core operation is the collection of all activities (processes and actions) that provide service designs to customers. For example, the core operation of Federal Express is to deliver packages around the world, and the core operation of Starbucks is to provide coffee service all over the world. Core operations extend across all activities in the design life cycle.

For a company to operate, the core operation alone is not enough. Figure 1.7 listed several other typical elements that are needed to make a company fully operational, such as business process and business management. The success of a company depends on the success of all aspects of business operation. In addition to the structure depicted in Figure 1.7, each function also has a life cycle of its own, as shown in Figure 1.8. Each of the blocks from Figure 1.7 can be dropped into the function chevron of Figure 1.8, and then each function requires strategy and planning, training and organizational development, and reporting to support its core function.

Before six sigma, quality was narrowly defined as the quality of the design that a company provided to external customers; therefore, it relates to the core operation only. Clearly, from the point of view of a business leader, this "quality" is only part of the story, because other critical factors of business success, such as cost, profit, time to market, and capital acquisition, are also related to other aspects of business operation.

The key difference between six sigma and all quality systems and methods developed previously is that six sigma is a strategy for the *whole quality* (every quality dimension concurrently), which is a dramatic improvement for the *whole business operation*. Notice that although we focus on the first seven stages of the medical device life cycle, the concepts are applicable to the remaining stages as well.

In the following sections we show that improving the whole quality will lead to business excellence because that involves improving all major performance metrics of business excellence, such as profit, cost, and time to market.

1.5.2 Structure of the Medical Device Quality Function

In this section we provide a current-state critique of the medical device industry's quality, regulatory, and compliance functional requirements and provide suggestions for improvement. We open with a definition of ideal functional structure to help companies to set up their internal functions and organization architecture for design excellence and regulatory compliance based on best practices. We believe that an ideal organization should have the following structure:

1. If a medical device company has many divisions and a corporate headquarters, the corporate staff should have oversight of the quality and regulatory compliance activities of the divisions. The FDA will hold all of the divisions accountable for fixing discrepancies found at any location. Corporate staff needs the authority to institute corrective and preventive actions throughout the company. Many companies have organized their quality, regulatory, and compliance functions locally by manufacturing site, whereas others have corporate oversight for these functions. In large companies, the quality system used at any manufacturing site should have a definite mechanism for assuring that the site complies with corporate quality policies. The FDA will hold headquarters management responsible and accountable for site failures. Corporate management reviews should include assessments of site quality functions. The most effective quality assurance and regulation assurance groups have a major role in establishing, maintaining, and continuously improving metrics and for monitoring and reporting quality data. The key areas are corrective action/preventive action (CAPA), complaints, regulations, field actions, change management, risk management, and assurance of management functions. Quality engineering for research and development should also be extended beyond the traditional assurance function, a gap that is nicely filled by design for six sigma.

2. The most common functional responsibilities are:
   - Quality personnel have responsibility for CAPA management, document control, equipment calibration, external audits, final inspection, incoming inspection of raw material, in-process inspection, internal quality audits, management representative, product and GMP (good manufacturing practice) audits, product complaint management, product releases, process validation, risk management, sterilization, supplier program management, and supplier qualification.
   - Regulatory personnel have responsibility for adverse-event reporting, annual product releases, facility registration and licenses, production registration and certification, product regulatory submissions, and recalls.
   - Compliance personnel have responsibility for the business code of conduct, environmental program management, health and safety program management, preventive maintenance, and training.

3. The top officials for quality, regulatory, and compliance concerns should be at the vice presidential level, equal in seniority to other officials in staff positions. There is a wide variation as to the title of the top official for the quality, regulatory, and compliance functions. The most common

title is vice president or senior vice president. The major issue here is that the top quality assurance, regulatory assurance, and compliance person is at the same level as the top finance, marketing, R&D, and other executives. It is important that the quality organization have titles similar to those used in production and manufacturing. These groups should be viewed as peers. Senior vice president is appropriate in larger companies.

4. All companies need to measure the *cost of poor quality* (the cost of internal and external failures, appraisal, and preventive action) and invest sufficient resources in preventive action, but the majority of companies are not doing so. The cost of poor quality is a metric that all good companies should utilize. Companies could not measure effectiveness and efficiency without it. It must include both the price of conformance and the price of nonconformance. It can be just as important to lower the price of conformance as to lower the price of nonconformance. The price of nonconformance was one of the four absolutes that Phil Crosby promoted in his fundamental overview of quality, which is still relevant today. When nothing bad is happening, how do responsible functions convince management that it is because of the good quality system that is in Hace? They need to show how good quality has increased market share, decreased inspection times, reduced nonconformities, increased yields, and reduced the cost of products purchased.

5. Companies need to embrace risk management and utilize its concepts throughout their quality, regulatory, and decision-making processes. The majority of companies use risk management principles throughout their quality system: design control, CAPA, complaint management, management review, and process control. Risk management principles need to be utilized throughout the life cycle of a device (Figure 1.1), as it is a dynamic process, not simply a design control tool. Using risk to help make better decisions will assure that resources are spent wisely—but only if quality is part of our risk decisions, not just cost–benefit issues.

    Risk management is huge. Clearly, it is not just needed simply for design control. The FDA stated in the QSR preamble that risk management should also be used in CAPA. It is also essential in production and process control. It is worth noting that the FDA used the word *risk* close to 50 times in the QSR preamble.

Having separate functions for the quality, regulatory, and compliance functions is normal. The management representative should have a mechanism to be informed of all quality issues, no matter what department he or she is part of. It is also important to assure that quality remains independent of production (or R&D in design-only) facilities. From a reporting structure point of view, variant forms are noted. Many companies have a reporting structure with quality, regulatory, and compliance groups reporting to a single point of control. Others have independent quality, regulatory, and compliance groups reporting structures. There are as many ways to develop a reporting structure as there are companies. The goal is to have a structure that allows effective, efficient, and timely oversight and control. The most effective companies have an independent facility for quality, regulatory, and compliance groups, with a common corporate oversight group that establishes and maintains consistency and tackles common issues when they arise. Most companies have their quality, regulatory, and compliance officials report directly to the president. Companies whose quality and compliance functions do not report to the president are often companies that face compliance actions by the FDA. It is essential that quality personnel report to the CEO or president. This assures independence as well as access to resources. A majority of firms had their senior quality, regulatory, and compliance functions report periodically to the board of directors with regular updates. Since the board of directors can also be held responsible for quality system deficiencies, they should be aware through management reviews of quality problems.

All world-class quality companies empower the quality and regulatory functions to stop production or initiate a recall. This is a positive trend that should be reinforced. From an authority perspective, some medical device companies have their regulatory personnel responsible for product submissions, compliance to QSR, and ISO 13485; others have their regulatory personnel responsible only for product registrations and licenses. Depending on the size and structure of the organization, this can be combined or separated. In either case, personnel must communicate and coordinate their activities. In our view, to be effective, regulatory and quality responsibility arc almost inseparable functions that need to be tightly coordinated. We are seeing more and more separation of the quality and regulatory functions. Unless a company is quite small, we would not recommend combining responsibilities as it spreads management too thin.

Commitment to quality varies by company. A few strive to be the best in an industry, others wants to assure product safety and cfficacy and essential quality system compliance, and some want only to meet the requirements minimally. But for the very best outcome, all companies should strive to be "state of the art," which starts with design and product development.

Best-in-class and world-class efforts should not be fell to be beyond many companies' ability to achieve. The investment is small to moderate in terms of people, resources, and capital. Focus is critical. To be the best in the business and an attractive place to work are attractive goals for both employees and managers. The goal for products, processes, and systems should be six sigma perfection. A company that strives to be the best in quality shows a true understanding of the reason for having a quality system. Six sigma perfection may be a long-term objective, but moving in that direction is why companies control design, manufacturing and changes, and utilize a feedback loop (CAPA). In the medical device business, laggards who strive only to meet minimal requirements often suffer regulatory violations and customer dissatisfaction.

The brutal facts are that only a small percentage if companies are among the best. Most are in the average competently range, and a few are not effective at all. The problem is that many of the average competent companies fail to recognize and accept their true status and therefore fail to make the investments (in people, infrastructure, systems) required to reach and maintain the state of the art, let alone continuous improvement. If you believe that your quality system needs an overhaul, take the time to look at your policies, procedures, and actual practices as part of a failure investigation. Process-map your systems and your processes. Use technical writers to write your procedures to assure that they are concise, well written, and not ambiguous. Make sure that your mapping for each process or subsystem flows together to form a complete quality system. Time spent in developing systems and processes that are complete and easy to follow, implement, and comply with is time well spent.

1.5.3 Quality and Cost

Given that you have a salable product or service, low cost is related directly to high profitability. Cost can be divided roughly into two parts: life-cycle costs related to all designs offered by the company, and the cost of running the supporting functions within the company, such as various enabling operations-related departments. For a particular product or service, life-cycle cost includes production and service cost, plus the cost for design development.

The relationship between quality and cost is rather complex; in this context the quality referred to is the design quality, not the *whole quality*. This relationship is very dependent on what type of quality strategy is adopted by a particular company. If a company adopted a quality strategy focused heavily on the downstream end of the design life cycle (i.e., firefighting, rework, and error corrections), that quality is going to be very costly. If a company adopts a strategy emphasizing upstream improvement and problem prevention, improving quality could actually reduce the life-cycle cost because there will be less rework, less recall, less firefighting, and therefore less design development cost. In a service-based company, it may also mean fewer complaints, higher throughput, and higher productivity. For more discussion of this topic, see Chapter 3 of Yang and El-Haik (2003).

If we define quality as whole quality, higher whole quality will definitely mean lower total cost. Because whole quality means higher performance levels of all aspects of business operation, it means high performance of all supporting functions, high performance of production system, less waste and higher efficiency. Therefore, it will definitely reduce business operation cost, production cost, and service cost without diminishing the service level to the customer.

1.5.4   Quality and Time to Market

Time to market is the speed in introducing new or improved products and services to the market. It is a very important measure for competitiveness in today's marketplace. For two companies that provide similar designs with comparable functions and price, the company with the faster time to market will achieve a tremendous competitive position. The first provider sets a psychological effect that will be very difficult for latecomers to overcome.

Many techniques are available to reduce time to market, such as:

- *Concurrency:* encouraging multitasking and parallel working
- *Complexity reduction* (Suh, 2001; El-Haik, 2005)
- *Project management:* tuned for design development and life-cycle management

In the six sigma approach and whole quality concept, improving the quality of managing the design development cycle is a part of the strategy. Therefore, improving whole quality will certainly help to reduce time to market.

1.6   SUMMARY

Quality as a characteristic refers to the perception of the degree to which the product or service will meet customers' expectations. Quality has no specific meaning unless related to a specific function or measurable characteristic. The best quality assurance strategy is "do the right things, and do things right all the time." "Do the right things" means that we have to design the best product or service for customers' needs at a cost that represents value to them. "Do things right all the time" means that products and services are performing consistently and customers are satisfied at all times. If we miss any of that, quality will be missed as well.

Quality has evolved over time from the early 1920s, when Shewhart introduced the first control chart, through the transformation of Japan from the 1950s to the late 1980s, when six sigma came on the scene. Six sigma, design for six sigma (DFSS), and lean have now been merged and enabled by personal computers and statistical software to provide easy-to-use and high-value methodologies to attack waste and reduce variation on both new designs and existing processes in order to fulfill customer requirements.

Six sigma design principles, tools, and methods (collectively known as design for six sigma) provide an insurance policy for the design transferred to production, which will be translated into a device that exceeds user expectations while satisfying user requirements. In other words, DFSS as a design quality tool kit provides managers and designers with improved visibility of design process decision making. With improved visibility, managers are empowered to direct the design process more effectively: that is, to prevent problems earlier, and if necessary, to make educated corrective decisions and adjust resource allocations.

2

DESIGN FOR SIX SIGMA AND MEDICAL DEVICE REGULATION

2.1 INTRODUCTION

The regulation of medical devices is an immense and rapidly evolving field that is often complicated by legal technicalities. As a legal term, a *regulation* is a rule created by an administration or administrative agency or body that interprets the statutes setting out the agency's purpose and powers or the circumstances of applying the statute. Regulations have costs for some and benefits for others. Typically, efficient regulations live where the total benefits to some people exceed the total costs to others. In this context, this chapter is written to promote a general understanding of medical device regulations as related to design for six sigma (DFSS). First, we give a global perspective on regulation and then zoom in on peculiarities that we feel have the greatest impact on the deployment and technical aspects of DFSS, taking the Food and Drug Administration as a case. We believe that overwhelming similarities are appealing for international readers who have some knowledge of European, Japanese, Canadian, Australian, and global regulations.

2.2 GLOBAL PERSPECTIVE ON MEDICAL DEVICE REGULATIONS

The term *medical devices* covers a vast range of equipment. Medical devices range from simple tongue depressors, syringes, and bandages to pacemakers,

Medical Device Design for Six Sigma: A Road Map for Safety and Effectiveness,
By Basem S. El-Haik and Khalid S. Mekki

dialysis equipment, baby incubators, heart valves, and laser surgical devices. In addition, medical devices include in vitro diagnostic products such as general-purpose lab equipment, reagents, and test kits.

The Global Harmonization Task Force[1] (GHTF) has proposed the following harmonized definition for medical devices: A *medical device* (GHTF document SG1/N029R11) means any instrument, apparatus, implement, machine, appliance, implant, in vitro reagent or calibrator, software, material, or similar or related article:

(a) Intended by the manufacturer to be used, alone or in combination, for human beings for one or more of the specific purpose(s) of:
- Diagnosis, prevention, monitoring, treatment, or alleviation of disease
- Diagnosis, monitoring, treatment, alleviation of, or compensation for an injury
- Investigation, replacement, modification, or support of the anatomy or of a physiological process
- Supporting or sustaining life
- Control of conception
- Disinfection of medical devices
- Providing information for medical or diagnostic purposes by means of in vitro examination of specimens derived from the human body
(b) Which does not achieve its primary intended action in or on the human body by pharmacological, immunological, or metabolic means but which may be assisted in its intended function by such means.

Following are some important notes:

Note 1: The definition of a device for in vitro examination includes, for example, reagents, calibrators, sample collection and storage devices, control materials, and related instruments or apparatus. The information provided by such an in vitro diagnostic device may be for diagnostic, monitoring, or compatibility purposes. In some jurisdictions, some in vitro diagnostic devices, including reagents and the like, may be covered by separate regulations.

Note 2: Products that may be considered as medical devices in some jurisdictions but for which there is not yet a harmonized approach are:

- Aids for disabled or handicapped people
- Devices for the treatment or diagnosis of diseases and injuries in animals

[1]The Global Harmonization Task Force was conceived in 1992 in an effort to respond to the growing need for international harmonization in the regulation of medical devices. You can visit the GHTF Web site at www.GHTF.org.

- Accessories for medical devices (see Note 3)
- Disinfection substances
- Devices incorporating animal and human tissues which may meet the requirements of the definition above but are subject to different controls

Note 3: Accessories intended specifically by manufacturers to be used together with a "parent" medical device to enable that device to achieve its intended purpose should be subject to the same GHTF procedures as those that apply to the device itself. For example, an accessory will be classified as though it is a medical device in its own right. This may result in the accessory having a different classification from that of the parent device.

Note 4: Components used in medical devices are generally controlled through the manufacturer's quality management system and the conformity assessment procedures for the device. In some jurisdictions, components are included in the definition of a medical device.

In former times, many medical device manufacturers were regulated under pharmaceutical legislation, which required fulfillment of good manufacturing practice (GMP) regulations, later revised to *current* good manufacturing practice (cGMP). According to global statistics, 85% of medical devices are manufactured in the United States, the European Union, Canada, Japan, and Australia. Therefore, the information hereafter pertains primarily to these five jurisdictions. Quality management system requirements and guidance were created by local, regional, national, and/or international organizations or regulatory authorities. An example of a medical device international standard is ISO 13485:2003, the quality management system (QSM). This standard is based on, but is clearly more extensive than, the ISO 9001:2000 process model approach. Many countries require medical device manufacturers to have their quality management systems registered to ISO 13485:2003.

Authorities acknowledge product clearance for the market in various ways. In the United States, the manufacturer of the device receives a marketing clearance [510(k)] or an approval letter (PMA) from the Food and Drug Administration. In Canada, a device license is awarded by the Therapeutic Products Directorate. In the European Union, after receiving an *EC certificate* from the notifying body, the manufacturer places the *CE mark* on or with the device. In Japan, a *shounin* is issued by the Pharmaceutical and Medical Safety Bureau of the Ministry of Health, Labor and Welfare. In Australia, the Therapeutic Goods Administration issues an *ARTG* (Australian Register of Therapeutic Goods) *number* to devices cleared for the market.

In an attempt to make this complex subject easier to grasp, we present a quick overview of the framework that integrates the regulatory systems of the five countries or regions with the best established medical device regulations: United States, European Union, Canada, Japan, and Australia.

1. *United States.* The Food and Drug Administration (FDA) is an agency of the U.S. Department of Health and Human Services responsible for regulating food, dietary supplements, drugs, cosmetics, medical devices, radiation-emitting devices, biologics, and blood products. The FDA is a public health agency, charged with protecting American consumers by enforcing the Federal Food, Drug, and Cosmetic Act and related public health laws. It is the FDA's job to ensure that the medical devices we use are safe and effective. The FDA also ensures that all of these products are labeled truthfully with the information that people need to use them properly.

2. *European Union.* Medical devices in the European Union (EU) are regulated by three main directives: the active implantable medical devices directive, medical devices directive, and (in vitro) diagnostic medical devices directive. These three directives define the essential requirements that medical devices must meet before being placed on the market.

3. *Canada.* Health Canada is the Canadian federal department responsible for helping the people of Canada maintain and improve their health. Under the Canadian Medical Devices Conformity Assessment System, Health Canada assesses all medical devices for safety, effectiveness, and quality before authorizing them for sale in Canada.

4. *Australia.* The Australian Therapeutic Goods Administration carries out a range of assessment and monitoring activities to ensure that medical devices available in Australia are of an acceptable standard. The Therapeutic Goods Act of 1989 provides a legislative basis for uniform national controls over goods used in the prevention, diagnosis, curing, or alleviation of a disease, ailment, defect, or injury. The Medical Devices Evaluation Committee provides advice on the policies, procedures, and priorities that should be applied to the administration of medical devices legislation.

5. *Japan.* The Japanese National Institute of Health Sciences conducts testing, research, and studies toward proper evaluation of the quality, safety, and efficacy of pharmaceutical products, foods, and the numerous chemicals in the living environment. However, the requirements predetermined from the Ministry of Health, Labor and Welfare come from Ministerial Ordinance 169 and are based on ISO 13485:2003. The medical device manufacturer and their market authorization holder have the responsibility for product certification under Japan's Pharmaceutical Affairs Law.

2.3 MEDICAL DEVICE CLASSIFICATION

According to U.S. regulation 21 CFR 820 and Directive 93/42/CEE, the medical device classification entails the type of procedure necessary to obtain accreditation. Medical devices are divided into different classes according to the potential risk associated with the design, manufacture, and use of these devices. Several criteria are considered to evaluate potential risks associated

TABLE 2.1 Medical Device Classification and Examples

USA	Europe	GHTF	Examples of Medical Devices
Class I	Class I	Class A	Stethoscopes, examination gloves
Class II	Class IIa	Class B	Intravenons sets, sterile surgical gloves
	Class IIb	Class C	Blood bags, orthopedic implants
Class III	Class III	Class D	Heart valves, implantable defibrillators

TABLE 2.2 FDA Medical Device Classification

U.S. Classification	Description
Class I	Most class I devices are exempted from clearance, but they are subject to general inspection requirements.
Class II	Most class II and some class I devices require premarket notification submission in accord with Section 510(k), which requires the manufacturer to submit an information pack to show that the device proposed is substantially equivalent to an already existing device on the U.S. market.
Class III	Most class III devices require premarket approval in accord with Section 515 of the act. These devices are more rigorous than devices that require a 510(k).

with a medical device, such as the duration of device contact with the body, the degree of invasiveness, and whether the device delivers medicines or energy to the patient. Table 2.1 lists the various classification criteria in the United States and the EU. Also included are the work-in-progress GHTF global system criteria, with regulatory authorities working toward the establishment of a global classification system. Such a system is based on common features of existing national requirements, with the aim of future convergence.

In the United States, the marketing of a medical device is subject to FDA inspection and, unless exempt, requires marketing clearance. Table 2.2 describes the FDA medical device classification.

In Europe, the marketing of a medical device requires a conformity certification, for which the procedures differ according to the classification. It is the manufacturer who decides on the classification of his product. Table 2.3 describes the EU directive classification.

The GHTF medical device classification is shown in Table 2.4.

2.4 MEDICAL DEVICE SAFETY

Regulatory controls are intended to safeguard the health and safety of patients, users, and other persons by ensuring that manufacturers of medical devices follow specified procedures during design, manufacturing, and marketing.

TABLE 2.3   EU Directive Medical Device Classification

EU Classification	Description
Class I	The conformity assessment procedures can be carried out under the responsibility of the manufacturer (low potential risk), except for sterile devices or devices with a measuring function. In the latter case, the intervention of a notified body is necessary.
Class IIa	The intervention of a notified body is compulsory at the production stage.
Class IIb	The intervention of a notified body is compulsory to control the design and manufacture.
Class III	The intervention of a notified body is compulsory to control the design and manufacture. An explicit prior authorization with regard to conformity is also required.

TABLE 2.4   GHTF Medical Device Classification

GHTF Classification	Description
Class A	Low risk
Class B	Low–moderate risk
Class C	Moderate–high risk
Class D	High risk

Source: GHTF study group 1, SG1-N15-2006.

Safety can only be considered in relative terms. All devices carry a certain degree of risk and could fail under certain conditions. Many medical device problems cannot be detected until extensive market experience is gained. For example, an implantable device may fail in a manner that was not predictable at the time of implantation; the failure may reflect conditions unique to certain patients. For other devices, component failure can also be unpredictable or random. One approach to device safety is to estimate the potential of a device becoming hazardous, which may result in safety problems and harm. This estimate is often referred to as *risk assessment* (Chapter 11). A *hazard* is a potential for an adverse event, a source of danger. *Risk* is a measure of a combination of (1) the severity of hazard or overall impact and (2) the likelihood of occurrence of the adverse event. Risk assessment begins with risk analysis to identify all possible hazards, followed by risk evaluation to estimate the risk of each hazard. In general, risk assessment is based on experience, evidence, computation, or even guesswork.

Risk assessment is complex, as it can be influenced by personal perception and other factors, such as cultural background, economic conditions, and political climate. In practice, risk assessment of medical devices is based on the experience of health care professionals and on safety design engineering.

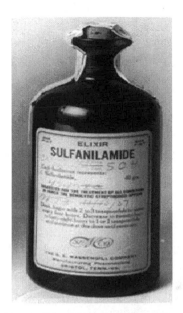

Figure 2.1   Elixir Sulfanilamide.

Refer to Chapter 11 for more details on risk assessment and risk management.

2.5 MEDICAL DEVICE QUALITY MANAGEMENT SYSTEMS REQUIREMENTS

Quality management systems regulation (QMSR) requires that each manufacturer establish and maintain a quality system that is appropriate for the specific device(s) designed or manufactured. The quality system should be an integrated effort, a total systems approach, to satisfy the particular safety and performance needs of a specific manufacturer, product, and user market.

In the United States, federal regulations were first applied to drug supplies in 1848 with the inspection of imported drugs. The most significant milestone in U.S. medical device quality management systems regulations history was the Food, Drug, and Cosmetic Act[2] signed on June 25, 1938. This law was crafted in response to a terrible tragedy in which a Tennessee drug company marketed Elixir Sulfanilamide, a form of a "new sulfa wonder drug" that would appeal to pediatric patients (Figure 2.1). However, the solvent in this untested product was a highly toxic chemical analog of antifreeze. Over 100 people died, including many children. Prior to this incident there were no clear

[2]The U.S. Federal Food, Drug, and Cosmetic Act (abbreviated as FFDCA, FDCA, or FD&C) is a set of laws passed by Congress in 1938 giving authority to the Food and Drug Administration to oversee the safety of food, drugs, and cosmetics.

standards for drug products and medical devices. It was not an offense to make false medical claims, and products did not have to be tested for safety or effectiveness. Today, these requirements seem very obvious and they became the foundation for good manufacturing practices (GMP) requirements in the quality system regulation.

Part 211, Current Good Manufacturing Practice Regulations for Finished Pharmaceuticals, of Title 21 of the *U.S. Code of Federal Regulations* (CFR) contains the minimum current good manufacturing practice for preparation of drug products for administration to humans or animals. Part 820, Quality System Regulation, of Title 21 of the CFR contains basic requirements applicable to manufacturers of finished medical devices.[3] The main requirements in each regulation are listed in Table 2.5.

The International Organization for Standardization[4] (ISO) document ISO 13485[5] is a prime reference for quality management systems for medical devices. ISO member bodies currently come from 146 countries. ISO standards are developed by technical committees. The people who serve on these technical committees come from many national standards organizations. Consequently, ISO standards tend to have worldwide support. ISO 13485 was developed by ISO Technical Committee 210, which is responsible for quality management and corresponding general aspects for medical devices.

ISO 13485 establishes a quality management system guideline that is oriented toward the design, development, production, and installation of medical devices and related services to (1) demonstrate the ability to supply medical devices and related services that meet customer expectations and comply with regulatory requirements, and (2) evaluate how well organizations are able to meet customer expectations and comply with regulatory requirements.

ISO 13485 is *not* a product standard. It is a *process* standard. Therefore, it is not adequate to establish a quality management system that complies with the ISO 13485 standard alone; companies also need to comply with technical standards and regulations as well as all relevant product and service best practices—hence this book. Table 2.6 shows the quality system standards used by various international authorities.

The model of a process-based quality management system based on the ISO 13485 deliverable structure is shown in Figure 2.2. This model illustrates the process linkage among the various quality management systems elements or parts. It also shows that customers play a significant role in defining requirements as inputs where continuous monitoring and analyses of customer satisfaction evaluates their perception as to whether it has been met. Management responsibility provides a commitment to development and implementation of

---

[3]FDA publications are available on their Web site, www.fda.gov.
[4]The ISO was set up in 1947 and is located in Geneva, Switzerland. Its purpose is to facilitate and support international trade by developing standards that people everywhere recognize and respect.
[5]The new ISO 13485:2003 standard of July 15, 2003 replaces the ISO 13485:1996 and ISO 13488:1996 standards.

TABLE 2.5   Requirements for 21 CFR Part 820 Versus Part 211

Part 820: Quality System Regulation		Part 211: Current Good Manufacturing Practice for Finished Pharmaceuticals	
Section No.	Section Name	Section No.	Section Name
820.1,3,5	General Provisions	211.1,3	General Provisions
820.20,22,25	Quality System Requirements	211.22,25,28,34	Organization and Personnel
820.30	Design Controls	211.42,44,46,48,50,52,	Buildings and
820.40	Document Controls	56,58	Facilities
820.50	Purchasing Controls	211.63,65,67,68,72	Equipment
820.60,65	Identification and Traceability	211.80,82,84,86,87,89,94	Control of Components and
820.70,72,75	Production and Process Controls		Drug Product Containers and Closures
820.80,86	Acceptance Activities	211.100,101,103,105, 110,111,113,115	Production and Process Controls
820.90	Nonconforming Product	211.122,125,130,132, 134,137	Packaging and Labeling Control
820.100	Corrective and Preventive Action	211.142,150	Holding and Distribution
820.120,130	Labeling and Packaging Control	211.160,165,166,167, 170,173,176	Laboratory Controls
820.140,150, 160,170	Handling, Storage, Distribution,	211.180,182,184,186, 188,192,194,196,198	Records and Reports
820.180,181, 184,186,198	and Installation Records	211.204,208	Returned and Salvaged Drug Products
820.200	Servicing		
820.250	Statistical Techniques		

the quality management system and continuous maintenance of its effectiveness. Under resource management, the selection of personnel selected to perform work affecting product quality must be competent on the basis of appropriate education, training, skills, and experience. The model also illustrates DFSS as a hub of the various quality management system sections, as the DFSS tool kit can provide a great deal of aid to all elements of a quality management system. Our focus in this chapter will be on mapping the DFSS tool kit to product development, to a section under product realization in ISO

TABLE 2.6   Quality System Standards Used by Various Authorities

Country	Standards/Regulations	Conformity Assessment
Australia	ISO 13485	Government and third party
Canada	ISO 13485	Third party
European Union	ISO 13485	Third party
Japan	GMP 40 ordinance	Government
	GMPI 63 ordinance	
	QS standard for medical device	
	1128 notice	
United States	QS (21 CFR part 820)	Government

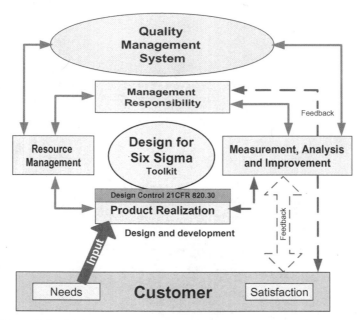

Figure 2.2   DFSS process-based quality management systems model.

13485, and to 21 CFR 820.30 design controls (see Chapter 7 for comprehensive DFSS project road map coverage). Figure 2.3 represents our DFSS ICOV (identify–characterize–optimize–verify/validate) process. In Section 2.6 we map device regulation to life cycle and the DFSS tool kit, and expand, where appropriate, on the 21 CFR 820.30 design control elements.

2.6 MEDICAL DEVICE REGULATION THROUGHOUT THE PRODUCT DEVELOPMENT LIFE CYCLE

For medical devices, the design control section of 21 CFR 820.30 of the U.S. regulations as well as the product realization section of ISO 13485 apply to

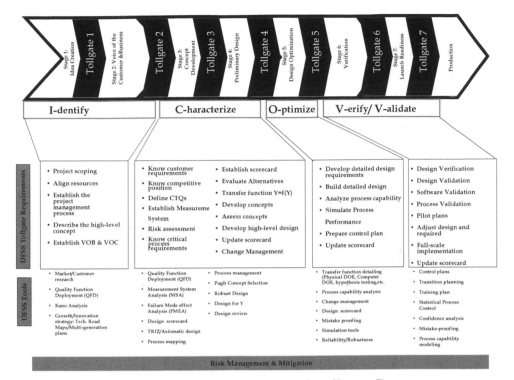

Figure 2.3 DFSS ICOV process (see Chapter 7).

the design and development of products and processes, as well as to any changes to existing designs and processes. Changes to an existing design or process must be made according to the requirements even if the original design was not subject to these requirements. Figure 2.4 depicts the graphical flow of a typical product development life cycle that encompasses the medical device life cycle. Refer to Chapter 1 for a detailed description of each life-cycle stage.

Table 2.7 describes each life-cycle stage in the context of 21 CFR Part 820, quality system regulation, and ISO 13485, quality management system.

Medical device companies need to establish and maintain procedures to control the design of a device, according to its classification, to make sure that the design requirements specified are met. The details of design control systems will vary depending on the complexity of the product or process being designed.

Some of the regulatory design requirements are in standards. For example, some parameters for medical gloves are in standards of the American Society for Testing and Materials (ASTM). Medical gloves are required to meet these standards to be substantially equivalent to gloves already in commercial distribution.

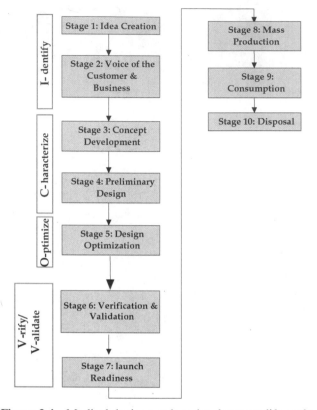

Figure 2.4   Medical device product development life cycle.

In the remaining part of this section we summarize a brief description of the 21 CFR 820.30 design controls elements. More information can be found at the FDA Web site at www.fda.gov.

2.6.1   Design and Development Plan

The design and development plan[6] requires that:

- "Each manufacturer shall establish and maintain plans that describe or reference the design and development activities and define responsibility for implementation.
- The plans shall identify and describe the interfaces with different groups or activities that provide, or result in, input to the design and development process.
- The plans shall be reviewed, updated, and approved as design and development evolves."

[6]The design and development plan is defined under 21 CFR 820.30(b).

TABLE 2.7 Life-Cycle Key DFSS Objectives and Methods

ISO 13485: Quality Management System	Part 820: Quality System Regulation	DFSS Phase	Product Life-Cycle Stage	Stage Objective	Key DFSS Methods/Tools
7.1 Planning of Product Realization	820.30(a) General Planning	Identify	Stage 1: ideation creation	Exploration of business case Invention that capture's the market Ensure that the new technology/ideas are robust for downstream development	Voice-of-the-customer analysis Elementary market analysis Business risk Market and customer research Technology road maps Growth strategy
7.3.1 Design and development planning	820.30(b) Design and Development Plan	Identify	Stage 2: voice of the customer and business	Ensure that the new design concept comes up with the right functional requirements	Quality function deployment (QFD) Kano analysis Customer engagement methods (survey, interview, etc.) Multigeneration plan Risk management
7.3.2 Design and development input	820.30(c) Design Input				
7.3.4 Design and development review	820.30(e) Design Review 820.30(j) Design History File				

TABLE 2.7 *Continued*

ISO 13485: Quality Management System	Part 820: Quality System Regulation	DFSS Phase	Product Life-Cycle Stage	Stage Objective	Key DFSS Methods/Tools
7.3.2 Design and development input	(Design Process) 820.30(c) Design Input	Characterize	Stage 3: concept development	Ensure that the new concept can lead to sound design free of design vulnerabilities	QFD
7.3.4 Design and development review	820.30(e) Design Review			Ensure that the new concept is robust for downstream development	Theory of inventive problem solving (TRIZ)
7.3.7 Control of design and development changes	820.30(i) Design Changes				Design mapping (process and functional mappings)
	820.30(j) Design History File				Design reviews
					Failure mode and effect analysis (FMEA)
					Design for serviceability
					Simulation/optimization
					Design scorecard
					Design reviews
					Risk management

ISO 13485	Design Process (21 CFR 820.30)		Stage	Deliverables	Tools
7.3.2 Design and development input	(Design Process) 820.30(c) Design Input	Characterize	Stage 4: preliminary design	Design parameters with detailed specifications	Design mapping (process and functional mappings)
7.3.3 Design and development output	820.30(d) Design Output			Design targets for reliability, quality, process-ability, and ease of use	Creativity tools: TRIZ and axiomatic design
7.3.4 Design and development review	820.30(e) Design Review				FMEA
7.3.7 Control of design and development changes	820.30(i) Design Changes				Pugh concept selection
	820.30(j) Design History File				Robust design
					Design reviews
					Risk management
					Process management
7.3.3 Design and development output	(Design Process) 820.30(d) Design Output	Optimize	Stage 5: design optimization	Capability flow up to prove that customer needs are met	Transfer functions detailing (DOE, simulation, etc.)
7.3.4 Design and development review	820.30(e) Design Review			Final test plan	Taguchi
7.3.7 Control of design and development changes	820.30(h) Design Transfer				Robust design
	820.30(i) Design Changes				Reliability
	820.30(j) Design History File				Simulation
					Change management
					Process capability
					Design scorecard
					Mistake-proofing
					Hypothesis testing
					Design reviews
					Risk management

TABLE 2.7 *Continued*

ISO 13485: Quality Management System	Part 820: Quality System Regulation	DFSS Phase	Product Life-Cycle Stage	Stage Objective	Key DFSS Methods/Tools
7.3.4 Design and development verification	820.30(f) Design Verification	Verify/validate	Stage 6: verification and validation	Ensure that the product designed (i.e., the design parameters) deliver the desired product functions over the product's useful life	Design verification
7.3.5 Design and development validation	820.30(g) Design Validation				Design validation
7.3.6 Design and development review	820.30(e) Design Review			Ensure that the process/service design is robust for variations from production, consumption, and disposal stages	Software validation
7.3.7 Control of design and development changes	820.30(h) Design Transfer				Process validation
	820.30(i) Design Changes			Ensure that the customer confirms that the right product was built	Piloting/prototyping
	820.30(j) Design History File				DOE
					Simulation
					Process capability
					Confidence intervals
					Sample size
					Hypothesis testing
					Design reviews
					Risk management

7.5 Production and Service Provision 7.3.6 Design and development review 7.3.7 Control of design and development changes	820.30(f) Design Verification 820.30(g) Design Validation 820.30(h) Design Transfer 820.30 (e) Design Review 820.30(i) Design Changes 820.30(j) Design History File	Verify/validate	Stage 7: launch readiness	Ensure that the process is able to deliver the service designed consistently Ensure that the customer confirms that the right product was built	Control plans Statistical process control Transition planning Mistake-proofing Troubleshooting and diagnosis Training plans Design reviews Risk management
7.5 Production and Service Provision	820.70 Production and Process Controls 820.200 Servicing	Verify/validate	Stage 8: production	Produce the service designed with a high degree of consistency and free of defects	Statistical process control Inspection Mistake-proofing Risk management
Out of scope of this book	Out of scope of this chapter		Stage 9: consumption	Ensure that customers have a satisfactory experience in consumption	Quality in after-sale service Risk management
Out of scope of this book	Out of scope of this chapter		Stage 10: phaseout	Ensure that customers have troublefree disposal of used designs	Service quality Risk management

The design and development plan must summarize product, medical device, goals, and objectives and should include information on the chronology of the development strategy as well as defining the roles and responsibility of completing the deliverables outlined in the plan.

The scope of the design and development plan depends on the size, scope, and complexity of the product under development. The following activities are performed in the design of a medical device:

- Design input
- Design output
- Design review
- Design verification (see Chapter 17)
- Design validation (see Chapter 17)
- Design transfer (see Chapter 18)
- Design changes (see Chapter 19)
- Design history file
- Risk management (see Chapter 11)

2.6.2 Design Input

Design input[7] means the physical and performance requirements of a device used as a basis for device design [21 CFR 820.3(f)]. Section 820.30(c), Design Input, requires that:

- "Each manufacturer shall establish and maintain procedures to ensure that the design requirements relating to a device are appropriate and address the intended use of the device, including the needs of the user and patient.
- The procedures shall include a mechanism for addressing incomplete, ambiguous, or conflicting requirements.
- The design input requirements shall be documented and shall be reviewed and approved by designated individual(s).
- The approval, including the date and signature of the individual(s) approving the requirements, shall be documented."

Under a design control system, manufacturers should identify device requirements during the design input phase or beginning of design activity. Design input includes determining customer needs, expectations, and requirements plus determining regulatory, standards, and other appropriate requirements. These various requirements are documented by the manufacturer in a set of device requirements. When converted to engineering terminology, a set

---

[7]Design input is defined under 21 CFR 820.30(c).

of design input requirements, finalized and accepted as part of the device master record (DMR), is called a device or product specification.

The design input phase is usually a continuum because intensive and formal input requirements activities usually occur near the beginning of the identify phase and continue to the early characterize design activities phase (Chapter 7). After the initial design input phase there are also intensive and formal activities to translate the input requirements to engineering-type input specifications, usually called a product or device requirement. The DFSS methodology uses high-level functional requirements as terminology. Quality function deployment (QFD; see Chapter 8) is a prime translation tool between design inputs and high-level functional requirements (FRs; see Chapter 9), shown in Table 2.7.

Product or device requirements, as translated from user and patient needs, should identify all of the desired performance, physical, safety, and compatibility characteristics of the device proposed and, ultimately, the finished device. Design input also includes requirements for labeling, packaging, manufacturing, installation, reliability, maintenance, servicing, and others, as appropriate. The product or device requirements may incorporate other requirements by reference, such as a reference to the manufacturer's list of requirements for a type of device, to specific paragraphs in standards, or to all of a standard, and so on, where it should be very clear exactly what is going to be met. It is possible to develop device requirements diligently and still forget one or more elements. Hopefully, no key factors will be left out. To reduce the probability of a requirement or characteristic being left out, the needs, wants, and desires of the customer segments, business interests, and regulatory bodies should be understood.

This input will be that in room 1 of the house of quality (Figure 2.5), quality function deployment in the DFSS methodology, presented throughout this book. Potential sources of information for the design inputs can come from a collection of sources, such as customer complaint data, field failure analysis, warranty and service failures, corrective and preventive actions, voice of the customers and user needs analysis, market research studies, clinical and regulatory needs analysis, and others as appropriate. The input requirements should cover any standards that the manufacturer plans for the device to meet. In the United States, information about essentially all national and international standards may be obtained from the American National Standards Institute (ANSI), 11 West 42nd Street, New York, NY 10036. ANSI is a private organization that monitors most of the standards activity in the United States and foreign activity in which U.S. citizens "officially" participate. Thus, ANSI can supply addresses and other information about all well-established standards-writing groups. Also, ANSI has for sale many different types of standards, including quality system standards.

The quality system regulation requires that the input procedures address incomplete, ambiguous, or conflicting requirements. Thus, every reasonable effort should be made to collect all of the requirements from which designers

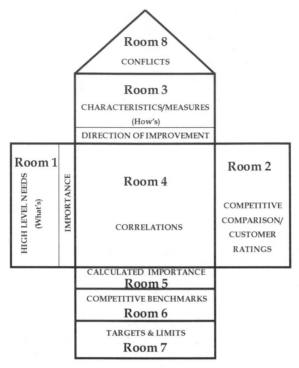

Figure 2.5   QFD house of quality rooms.

can generate detailed design specifications that are clear, correct, and complete. Room 8 of the house of quality, quality function deployment in the DFSS methodology, can help in pointing out if any conflicting requirements exist. See Chapter 8 for detailed information on how to use quality function deployment. At the end of the major aspects of the design input stage, the design input requirements must be reviewed and approved by one or more designated persons and documented in the design history file.

2.6.3 Design Output

Design output[8] means the results of a design effort at each design phase and at the end of the total design effort. Section 820.30(d), Design Output, requires that:

- "Each manufacturer shall establish and maintain procedures for defining and documenting design output in terms that allow an adequate evaluation of conformance to design input requirements.

[8]Design output is defined under 21 CFR 820.30(d).

- Design output procedures shall contain or make reference to acceptance criteria and shall ensure that those design outputs that are essential for the proper functioning of the device are identified.
- Design output shall be documented, reviewed, and approved before release.
- The approval, including the date and signature of the individual(s) approving the output, shall be documented."

The finished design output is the basis for the device master record[9] (DMR). The total finished design output consists of the device, its packaging and labeling, and the DMR.

The design output at each phase are documents and physical design elements that are either complete or are used to move the design effort into the next stage. For example, the first design output will usually be the design requirements document, here documented in a QFD house of quality matrix. From the requirements and their engineering knowledge, the design team will derive the preliminary design specifications, the translated minimum set of high-level functional requirements that deliver design core goals completely. Then the characterize phase (Figure 2.3) of the conceptual design begins. For example, the designers may begin the selection of known routine components that are part of legacy design and documenting their purchasing and acceptance requirements documented to meet Section 820.50(b), Purchasing Controls, Purchasing Data, which requires that "each manufacturer shall establish and maintain data that clearly describe or reference the specified requirements, including quality requirements, for purchased or otherwise received product and services." Other components will be selected as the design evolves in the DFSS characterize phase. The design output for some special or new components, or components in unusual applications, will include verification protocols and purchasing and acceptance requirements.

Many of the design output are documents that form part of the DMR directly. The remaining DMR documents are created by quality assurance, production engineering, process engineering, technical writing, installation, and servicing using design output data and information. For example, the finished device final test methods and some installation and servicing test methods and data forms may be derived from the design verification protocol(s). When all of these design and documentation activities are completed, the DMR is complete. When the DMR is complete and initial production units, including packaging, meets all specifications, the total finished design output exists.

Documenting design output in terms that allow an adequate evaluation of conformance to design input requirements is a significant design activity. The DFSS technique for achieving this conformance is listed in Table 2.7 and demystified throughout the book. Generation of verification requirement

[9]A compilation of records containing the procedures and specifications for a finished device (see Chapter 19).

documents and test methods for the design requires that each functional requirement, design parameter, and in many cases, process variables are referenced by the same line or paragraph number that it has in the design engineering specification where the functional requirements are listed.

The verification documents and data contain more information than is typically needed for production evaluation and acceptance of components, in-process items, and finished devices. For legacy devices, it is easy to copy and modify verification documents to meet the quality system requirement that design output procedures must contain or make reference to acceptance criteria and ensure that those design outputs that are essential for the safety, quality, and proper functioning of the device are identified. As a practice, this technique of deriving test procedures from the verification protocols also yields the test method(s) and data form(s) needed to meet the DMR requirements for quality assurance procedures and acceptance criteria in 21 CFR 820.181(c).

In addition, design output must be reviewed and approved before release and documented in the design history file. The approval, including the date and signature of the person(s) approving the output, must be documented. Manufacturers may choose to have a group review certain documents and have individuals review other documents. Output documents that are directly part of the DMR are reviewed, dated, and signed by the author, a DFSS team, which is current practice; and reviewed, dated, and approved by a person or persons designated by the manufacturer. As appropriate, these reviews should cover technical issues as well as adequacy for use in production, purchasing, servicing, and so on. DMR documents that are generated and approved under 21 CFR 820.30 automatically meet the approval requirements of 21 CFR 820.40, Document Controls, and do not have to be reapproved.

Design output reports, data, and any other document that will be used to create documents in the DMR are reviewed, dated, and signed by the author, which is current practice; and reviewed, dated, and approved by a person or persons designated by the manufacturer. Design output includes the physical device, which, of course, is not intended to be signed or dated. Approval of the device design consists of the validation that is done on initial production units.

2.6.4 Design Review

Design review is a key design control element in quality systems. The objectives of design review are stated in the definition of design review in 21 CFR 820.30(h) as follows: Design review comprises a documented, comprehensive, systematic examination of a design to evaluate the adequacy of the design requirements, to evaluate the capability of the design to meet these requirements, and to identify problems. Section 820.30(e), Design Review, requires that:

- "Each manufacturer shall establish and maintain procedures to ensure that formal documented reviews of the design results are planned and conducted at appropriate stages of the device's design development.
- The procedures shall ensure that participants at each design review include representatives of all functions concerned with the design stage being reviewed and an individual(s) who does not have direct responsibility for the design stage being reviewed, as well as any specialists needed.
- The results of a design review, including identification of the design, the date, and the individual(s) performing the review, shall be documented in the design history file (the DHF)."

To meet the systematic design review requirement for product design, tollgate reviews (see Chapter 7) and design reviews should progress through defined and planned phases, starting with the design input phase and continuing through validation of initial production units or lots. Whereas the regulation is generic, DFSS is not. Table 2.7 has a mapping between design controls and DFSS stages and phases (see Chapter 7 for more details).

Subsequent activities are usually design changes. Assessments should include a formal review of the main device functionality and subsystems, including accessories, components, software, labeling, and packaging; production and resource needs; and installation and service, if needed. The scope includes performance, physical safety, compatibility with other devices, overall device system requirements, human factors, and environmental compatibility.

The design review of the initial requirements and DFSS tollgate reviews (Chapter 7) allow input from all parties while making sure that the right decisions are made. As the design input and review activities progress, any conflicts are resolved and the preliminary specifications for the device, accessories, labeling, and packaging are established. As the development progresses and the design and production processes evolve, design reviews reduce errors, help avoid problems, help find existing problems, help propose solutions, increase produceability, and reduce design transfer problems. Throughout the design program, and particularly toward the end of the development cycle, design reviews help assure that the final design of the device meets the current design requirements and specifications.

In reference to Table 2.7, design review can be initiated as early as the identify phase of the DFSS ICOV process. Chapter 19 covers a best demonstrated practice in conducting a formal design review.

2.6.5 Design Verification and Validation

Verification (see Chapter 17) per 21 CFR 820.3(a) means confirmation by examination and provision of objective evidence that specified requirements have been fulfilled. *Validation* (see Chapter 17) per 21 CFR 820.3(z) means confirmation by examination and provision of objective evidence that the particular requirements for a specific intended use can be fulfilled consistently.

Section 820.30(f), Design Verification, requires that:

- "Each manufacturer shall establish and maintain procedures for verifying the device design.
- Design verification shall confirm that the design output meets the design input requirements.
- The results of the design verification, including identification of the design, method(s), the date, and the individual(s) performing the verification, shall be documented in the Design History File."

Section 820.30(g), Design Validation, requires that:

- "Each manufacturer shall establish and maintain procedures for validating the device design.
- Design validation shall be performed under defined operating conditions on initial production units, lots, or batches, or their equivalents.
- Design validation shall ensure that devices conform to defined user needs and intended uses and shall include testing of production units under actual or simulated use conditions.
- Design validation shall include software validation and risk analysis, where appropriate.
- The results of the design validation, including identification of the design, method(s), the date, and the individual(s) performing the validation, shall be documented in the Design History File."

Design verification is always done versus specifications, the high-level functional requirements, or design output. Therefore, to control the specifications and increase the probability of achieving desired safety and performance characteristics, device, software, labeling, packaging, and any other specifications should be complete and reviewed thoroughly before development begins. As the hardware and software designs evolve, they should be evaluated versus their current specifications.

Design verification and validation should be done with test equipment calibrated and controlled according to quality system requirements. Otherwise, there is limited confidence in the data. Verification and validation should also be done according to a written protocol(s). The protocol(s) should include defined conditions for the testing and should be approved before being used. Test protocol(s) are not perfect for a design, particularly a new design. Therefore, the design team and other verification personnel carefully annotate any ongoing changes in a protocol. Similarly, the verification personnel should record technical comments about any deviations or other events that occurred during testing. The slightest problem should not be ignored. During design reviews, comments, notes, and deviations may be as important as test data from the formal protocol(s).

Software is evaluated and reviewed versus the software specifications during ongoing development of the device design. When a "final" prototype is available, the software and hardware are validated to make certain that manufacturer specifications for the device and process are met. Before testing the software in actual use, the detailed code should be reviewed visually versus flowcharts and specifications. All cases should be reviewed and the results documented.

The validation program is planned and executed such that all relevant elements of the software and hardware are exercised and evaluated. The testing of software usually involves the use of an emulator and should include testing of the software in the finished device. The testing includes normal operation of the complete device; and this phase of the validation program may be completed first to make certain that the device meets the fundamental performance, safety, and labeling specifications. Concurrently or afterward, the combined system of hardware and software should be challenged with abnormal inputs and conditions. We cover DFSS design verification and validation in great detail in Chapter 17.

2.6.6 Design Transfer

Design controls section 820.30(h), Design Transfer (see Chapter 18), requires that:

- "Each manufacturer shall establish and maintain procedures to ensure that the device design is correctly translated into production specifications."

It is common practice for sections of a design to be transferred to manufacturing personnel before the entire design is completed. Quality system regulation does not prevent such split or multiple transfers. Transfer is to be performed only for completed elements of the design; multiple transfers may not be used to bypass any design, labeling, or other good manufacturing practice requirements.

A significant part of the transfer requirement is met when the design output is being created. That is, some of the design output documents are part of the DMR (see Chapter 18) and are used directly for production. The remaining DMR documents are based on design output information. A procedure is needed to cover generation of the remaining device master record documents based on information in the design output documents. Design transfer should assure that the section of the design being transferred:

- Meets input requirements
- Contains acceptance criteria, where needed
- Contains design parameters that have been verified appropriately
- Is complete and approved for use
- Is fully documented in the DMR or contains sufficient design output information to support generation of the remaining DMR documents
- Is placed under change control, if not already done

Design transfer may include training of production, installation, and service employees, and such training should be covered by or referenced by the transfer procedure. We cover the DFSS design transfer processes in great detail in Chapter 18.

2.6.7 Design Changes

Design changes to a design element are controlled under 21 CFR 820.30(i), Design Changes, which requires that:

- "Each manufacturer shall establish and maintain procedures for the identification, documentation, validation or where appropriate verification, review, and approval of design changes before their implementation."

As the design activity progresses toward the final production stage, it is expected that the degree of change control will increase. Those elements of the design that have been verified and accepted obviously should be under change control. A design that has been submitted to the FDA for marketing clearance should be under change control. A design undergoing clinical trials should be under change control, or the clinical data may not be accepted by the FDA. A design that is released for production should be under design and general change control.

After design activities are begun and the physical design evolves into an accepted entity, subsequent changes to the device specification(s) are proposed, evaluated, reviewed, approved, and documented through all of 21 CFR 820.30. The revised specification(s) becomes the current design goal in accord with the manufacturer procedures for design control, design change control, and document control. As is clear from Table 2.7, the design change control process can be initiated as early as the identify phase (see Chapter 7) of the DFSS ICOV process. Chapter 19 covers DFSS best demonstrated practice in conducting a pre- and postdesign transfer change control process.

2.6.8 Design History File

A design history file (DHF) is a compilation of records that describes the design history of a finished device [21 CFR 820.3(e)]. Section 820.30(j), Design History File, requires that:

- "Each manufacturer shall establish and maintain a DHF for each type of device.
- The DHF shall contain or reference the records necessary to demonstrate that the design was developed in accordance with the approved design plan and the requirements of this part."

Each type of device represents a device or family of devices that are manufactured according to one DMR. That is, if the variations in the family of devices are simple enough that they can be handled by minor variations on the drawings, only one DMR exists. It is common practice to identify device variations on drawings by dashed numbers. For this case, only one DHF could exist because only one set of related design documentation exists. Documents are never created just to go into the DHF.

The quality system regulation also requires that the DHF contain or reference the records necessary to demonstrate that the design was developed in accord with the approved design plan and the requirements of this part. As noted, this requirement cannot be met unless the manufacturer develops and maintains plans that meet the design control requirements. The plans and subsequent updates should be part of the DHF. Chapter 19 covers the design history file aspects.

2.6.9 QSIT Design Control Inspectional Objectives

The following guidelines to a new inspectional process[10] may be used by the FDA field staff to assess a medical device manufacturer's compliance with the regulations related to Quality System Regulation–Design Controls. The new inspectional process is known as the *quality system inspection technique* (QSIT). Field investigators may conduct an efficient and effective comprehensive inspection using this guidance material, which will help them focus on key elements of a firm's quality system.

1. Select a single design project. (*Note:* If the project selected involves a device that contains software, consider reviewing the software's validation while proceeding through the assessment of the firm's design control system.)
2. For the design project selected, verify that design control procedures that address the requirements of Section 820.30 have been defined and documented.
3. Review the design plan for the project selected to understand the layout of the design and development activities, including assigned responsibilities and interfaces. (*Note:* Evaluate the firm's conduct of risk analysis while proceeding through assessment of the firm's design control system.)

[10]The guide was released in August 1999.

4. Confirm that design inputs were established.
5. Verify that the design outputs that are essential for proper functioning of the device were identified.
6. Confirm that acceptance criteria were established prior to the performance of verification and validation activities.
7. Determine if design verification confirmed that design outputs met the design input requirements.
8. Confirm that design validation data show that the approved design met predetermined user needs and intended uses.
9. Confirm that the completed design validation did not leave any discrepancies unresolved.
10. If the device contains software, confirm that the software was validated.
11. Confirm that risk analysis was performed.
12. Determine if design validation was accomplished using initial production devices or their equivalents.
13. Confirm that changes were controlled, including validation or, where appropriate, verification.
14. Determine if design reviews were conducted.
15. Determine if the design was transferred correctly.

2.7 SUMMARY

In this chapter we provide a high-level scan of the information needed to meet the regulations required by ISO standards, FDA QSR, and European medical device directives. Readers will gain a thorough understanding of the need for design control; similarities and differences between ISO 13485 and QSR; documentation and records required; and a knowledge of our simple life-cycle model linking DFSS and regulation for device design development; and technical file and risk analysis.

3

BASIC STATISTICS

3.1 INTRODUCTION

A working knowledge of statistics is necessary for an understanding of medical device six sigma, design for six sigma, and lean six sigma. In this chapter we provide a very basic review of appropriate terms and statistical methods that are encountered in this book.[1]

Statistics is the science of data: It involves collecting, classifying, summarizing, organizing, analyzing, and interpreting data. The purpose is to extract information to aid decision making. Statistical methods can be categorized as descriptive or inferential. *Descriptive statistics* involves collecting, presenting, and characterizing data. The purpose is to describe the data graphically and numerically. *Inferential statistics* involves estimation and hypothesis testing in order to make decisions about population characteristics. The statistical analysis presented here is applicable to all analytical data that involve counting or multiple measurements.

3.2 COMMON PROBABILITY DISTRIBUTIONS

Table 3.1 is a description of common probability distributions see also associated statistical tables in the Appendix.

[1]This chapter barely touches the surface and we encourage the reader to consult other resources for further reference.

Medical Device Design for Six Sigma: A Road Map for Safety and Effectiveness,
By Basem S. El-Haik and Khalid S. Mekki
Copyright © 2008 John Wiley & Sons, Inc.

TABLE 3.1   Common Probability Distributions

Density Function	Graph

Bernoulli distribution:

$$p(x) = \begin{cases} 1-p & \text{if } x=0 \\ p & \text{if } x=1 \\ 0 & \text{otherwise} \end{cases}$$

  Generalized random
  experiment of two
  outcomes

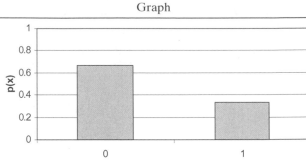

Binomial distribution:

$$p(x) = \binom{n}{x} p^x (1-p)^{n-x}$$

  Number of successes in
  n experiments (number
  of defective items in a
  batch)

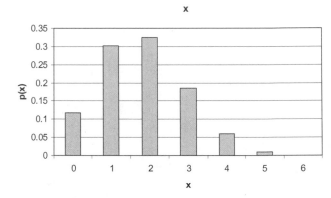

Poisson distribution:

$$p(x) = \frac{e^{-\lambda}\lambda^x}{x!}, \quad x = 0, 1, \ldots$$

  Stochastic arrival processes
  λ: average number of
  arrivals per time unit

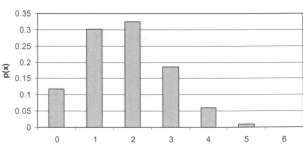

Geometric distribution:

$$p(x) = p(1-p)^x$$

  Number of failures before
  a success in a series of
  independent Bernoulli
  trials

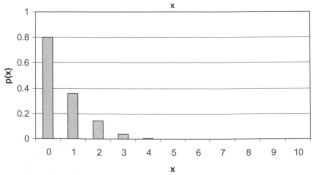

TABLE 3.1 *Continued*

Density Function	Graph
Uniform distribution: $f_U(x) = \dfrac{1}{b-a}, \quad a \le x \le b$ Random number generation	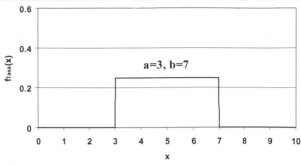
Normal distrbution: $f_N(x) = \dfrac{1}{\sqrt{2\pi\sigma^2}} \exp\left[-\dfrac{(x-\mu)^2}{2\sigma^2} \right]$ Natural phenomena of large population size	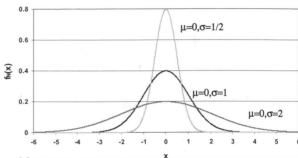

Exponential distribution:
 	
$f_{\exp}(x) = \lambda e^{-\lambda x}$
 	
Reliability models:
    Lifetime of a
    component
    Service time
    Time between arrivals
	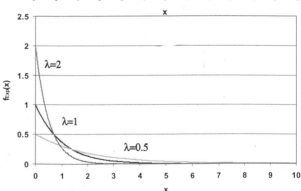

Triangular distribution: $f_{\text{tria}}(x) = \begin{cases} \dfrac{2(x-a)}{(b-a)(c-a)} \\ \quad \text{if } a \le x \le c \\ \dfrac{2(b-x)}{(b-a)(b-c)} \\ \quad \text{if } c < x \le b \end{cases}$	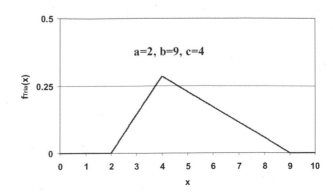

TABLE 3.1 *Continued*

Density Function	Graph

Gamma distribution:
 	
$$f_{\text{gamma}}(x) = \frac{\lambda}{\Gamma(\lambda)}\lambda x^{k-1}e^{-\lambda x}$$
 	
Failure due to repetitive
  disturbances
Duration of a multiphase
  task
	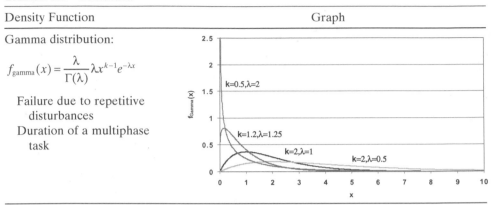

3.3 METHODS OF INPUT AND OUTPUT ANALYSIS

Statistical methods of input modeling, such as descriptive statistics, removing outliers, fitting data distributions, and others, play an important role in analyzing medical device historical data. The largest value added in modeling is achieved from analyzing outputs to draw statistical inferences and from optimizing the model parameters through experimental design and optimization. Models provide a flexible and cost-effective platform for running experimental design, what-if analysis, and optimization methods. Using the results obtained from the output analysis, design teams can draw better inferences about model behavior, compare multiple design alternatives, and optimize model performance.

Along with statistical and analytical methods, a practical sense of the underlying medical device and effective modeling techniques can greatly assist in the analysis of outputs of medical devices. Combined, such statistical and modeling techniques often lead to arriving at accurate analysis and clear conclusions. Several statistical methods and modeling skills are coupled at each main modeling activity to facilitate the analysis of output. Table 3.2 summarizes the statistical methods and modeling skills that are essential at each of the major modeling activities: input modeling and output analysis.

Output analysis in design focuses on measuring and analyzing certain model output variables. A variable, or in DFSS terminology a critical-to-quality characteristic (CTQ), is any measured characteristic or attribute that differs from one subject to another or from one time unit to another. For example, the biohuman material purity extracted from one device to another and the yield of a device vary over multiple collection times. A CTQ can be cascaded at lower device design levels (system, subsystem, or component), where measurement is possible and feasible to functional requirements (FRs). At the device level, the CTQs can be derived from all customer segment wants, needs,

TABLE 3.2   Modeling and Statistical Methods

Modeling Activity	Statistical Methods	Modeling Skills
Input modeling	Sampling techniques	Data collection
	Probability models	Random generation
	Histograms	Data classification
	Theoretical distributions	Fitting distributions
	Parameter estimation	Modeling variability
	Goodness of fit	Conformance test
	Empirical distributions	Using actual data
Output analysis	Graphical tools	Output representation
	Descriptive statistics	Results summary
	Inferential statistics	Drawing inferences
	Experimental design	Design alternatives
	Optimization search	Optimum design
	Transfer function	
	Scorecard	

and delights, which are then cascaded to functional requirements, the outputs at the various hierarchical levels.

Variables can be quantitative or qualitative. *Quantitative variables* are measured numerically in a discrete or continuous manner, whereas *qualitative variables* are measured in a descriptive manner. For example, device uniformity of medication mix is a quantitative variable, whereas device color options can be looked at as a qualitative variable. Variables are also dependent and independent. Design variables such as dimensions, spring constants, and material properties are *independent variables*; model outcomes such as medication flow rate and accuracy are *dependent variables*. Finally, variables are either continuous or discrete. A *continuous variable* is one for which any value is possible within the limits of the variable ranges. For example, the accuracy of a device is a continuous variable since it can take real values between an acceptable minimum and 100%. The variable cell count is a *discrete variable* since it can only take countable integer values such as 1, 2, 3, and 4. It is clear that statistics computed from continuous variables have many more possible values than do discrete variables.

The word *statistics* is used in several different senses. In its broadest sense, the word refers to a range of techniques and procedures for analyzing data, interpreting data, displaying data, and making decisions based on data. The term *statistic* refers to the numerical quantity calculated from a sample of size n. Such statistics are used for parameter estimation.

In analyzing outputs, it is also essential to distinguish between statistics and parameters. Whereas statistics are measured from data samples of limited size (n), a *parameter* is a numerical quantity that measures some aspect of the data population. A *population* consists of an entire set of objects, observations, or scores that have something in common. The distribution of a population can

TABLE 3.3   Examples of Parameters and Statistics

Measure	Parameter	Statistic
Mean	μ	$\bar{X}$
Standard deviation	σ	s
Proportion	π	p
Correlation	ρ	r

be described by several parameters, such as the mean and the standard deviation. Estimates of these parameters taken from a sample are called *statistics*. A sample is therefore a subset of a population. Since it is usually impractical to test every member of a population (e.g., 100% inspection of all design output variables), a sample from the population is typically the best approach available. For example, the average accuracy of five devices in 10 hours of run time is a statistics, and the accuracy mean over the device population history is a parameter. Population parameters are rarely known and are usually estimated by statistics computed using samples. Certain statistical requirements are, however, necessary in order to estimate the population parameters using computed statistics. Table 3.3 shows selected parameters and statistics.

3.4   DESCRIPTIVE STATISTICS

One important use of statistics is to summarize a collection of data in a clear and understandable way. Data can be summarized numerically and graphically. In a numerical approach a set of descriptive statistics are computed using a set of formulas. These statistics convey information about the data's central tendency measures (mean, median, and mode) and dispersion measures (range, interquartiles, variance, and standard deviation). Using the descriptive statistics, data central and dispersion tendencies are represented graphically (such as dot plots, histograms, probability density functions, stem and leaf, and box plot).

For example, a medical device yield in terms of nucleated cells produced every 2 hours for several patients is depicted in Table 3.4. The changing yield reflects the variability of design output that is typically caused by elements of randomness in device inputs and functional performance.

Graphical representations of yield as an output help us to understand the distribution and behavior of such functional requirements. For example, a histogram representation can be established by drawing the intervals of data points versus each interval's frequency of occurrence. The probability density function curve can be constructed and added to the graph by connecting the centers of data intervals. Histograms help in selecting the proper distribution that represents the data. Figure 3.1 shows the histogram and normal curve of the data in Table 3.4.

TABLE 3.4 Two-Hour Yield (× 109)

65	62	59	56	53	50	47	44	41	38
49	46	43	40	37	34	31	28	25	22
55	52	55	52	50	55	52	49	55	52
48	45	42	39	36	48	45	48	48	45
64	61	64	61	64	64	61	64	64	61
63	60	63	58	63	63	60	66	63	63
60	57	54	51	60	44	41	60	63	50
65	62	65	62	65	65	62	65	66	65
46	43	46	43	46	46	43	46	63	46
56	53	56	53	56	56	53	56	60	66

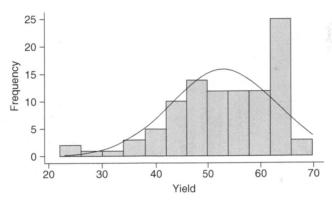

Figure 3.1 Histogram and normal curve of yield distribution in Table 3.4.

Several other types of graphical representation can be used to summarize and represent the distribution of a certain output. For example, Figures 3.2 and 3.3 show another two types of graphical representation of the yield requirement design output: the box plot and dot plot, respectively.

3.4.1 Measures of Central Tendency

Measures of central tendency are measures of the location of the middle or the center of a distribution of a functional requirement variable (y). The mean is the most commonly used measure of central tendency. The *arithmetic mean* is what is commonly called the *average*. The mean is the sum of all observations divided by the number of observations in a sample or in a population. The *mean of a population* is expressed mathematically as

$$\mu_y = \frac{\sum_{i=1}^{n} y_i}{N} \qquad \text{where } N \text{ is the number of population observations}$$

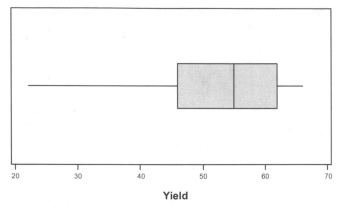

Figure 3.2   Box plot of yield data in Table 3.4.

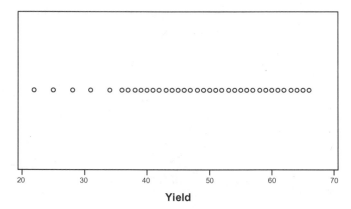

Figure 3.3   Dot plot of yield data in Table 3.4.

The *average of a sample* is expressed mathematically as

$$\bar{y} = \frac{\sum_{i=1}^{n} y_i}{n} \qquad \text{where } n \text{ is the sample size}$$

The mean is a good measure of central tendency for roughly symmetric distributions but can be misleading in skewed distributions since it can be influenced greatly by extreme observations. Therefore, other statistics, such as the median and mode, may be more informative for skewed distributions. The mean, median, and mode are equal in symmetric distributions. The mean is higher than the median in positively skewed distributions and lower than the median in negatively skewed distributions.

The *median* is the middle of a distribution: where half the scores are above the median and half are below. The median is less sensitive than the mean to

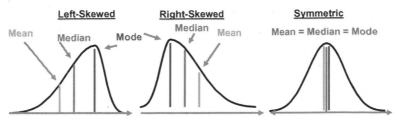

Figure 3.4 Symmetric and skewed distributions.

extreme scores, and this makes it a better measure than the mean for highly skewed distributions.

The *mode* is the most frequently occurring score in a distribution. The advantage of the mode as a measure of central tendency is that it has an obvious meaning. Further, it is the only measure of central tendency that can be used with nominal data (it is not computed). The mode is highly subject to sample fluctuation and is therefore not recommended to be used as the only measure of central tendency. A further disadvantage of the mode is that many distributions have more than one mode. These distributions are called *multi-modal*. Figure 3.4 illustrates the mean, median, and mode in symmetric and skewed distributions.

3.4.2 Measures of Dispersion

A functional requirement (FR) dispersion is the degree to which scores on the FR variable differ from each other. *Variability* and *spread* are synonyms for dispersion. There are many measures of spread. The *range* is the simplest measure of dispersion. It is equal to the difference between the largest and smallest values. The range can be a useful measure of spread because it is so easily understood. However, it is very sensitive to extreme scores since it is based on only two values. The range should almost never be used as the only measure of spread, but can be informative if used as a supplement to other measures of spread, such as the standard deviation and interquartile range. For example, the range is determined for a set of numbers as follows:

$$[10, 12, 4, 6, 13, 15, 19, 16] \qquad R = 19 - 4 = 15$$

The range is a useful statistic to know, but not as a stand-alone dispersion measure since it takes only two scores into account.

The *variance* is a measure of how spreadout a distribution is. It is computed as the average squared deviation of each number from its mean. Formulas for the variance are as follows: For a population,

$$\sigma_y^2 = \frac{\sum_{i=1}^{N}(y_i - \mu_y)^2}{N} \qquad \text{where } N \text{ is the number of population observations}$$

For a sample,

$$s_y = \frac{\sum_{i=1}^{n} (y_i - \overline{y})^2}{n-1}$$ where n is the sample size

The *standard deviation*, the square root of the variance, is the most commonly used measure of dispersion. An important attribute of the standard deviation is that if the mean and standard deviation of a normal distribution are known, it is possible to compute the percentile rank associated with any given observation. For example, the empirical rule states that in a normal distribution, about 68.27% of the data points are within 1 standard deviation of the mean, about 95.45% of the data points are within 2 standard deviations of the mean, and about 99.73% of the data points are within 3 standard deviations of the mean. Figure 3.5 illustrates the normal distribution curve percentage data points contained within a number of standard deviation from the mean.

The standard deviation is not often considered a good measure of spread in highly skewed distributions and should be supplemented in those cases by the interquartile range ($IQ_3 - IQ_1$). The interquartile range is rarely used as a measure of spread because it is not very mathematically tractable. However, it is less sensitive than the standard deviation to extreme data points, and is subsequently less subject to sampling fluctuations in highly skewed distributions.

For the data set shown in Table 3.4, a set of descriptive statistics, shown in Table 3.5, is computed using an Excel sheet to summarize the behavior of yield data in Table 3.4.

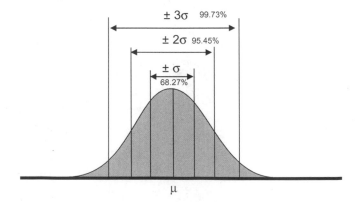

Figure 3.5 Normal distribution curve.

TABLE 3.5 Descriptive Statistics Summary for Data in Table 3.4 ($\times 10^9$)

Mean	53.06	Minimum	22
Standard error	1.01	Maximum	66
Median	55	First quartile (IQ_1)	46
Mode	63	Third quartile (IQ_3)	62
Standard deviation	10.11	Interquartile range	16
Sample variance	102.24	Count	100
Range	44	Sum	5306

3.5 INFERENTIAL STATISTICS

Inferential statistics are used to draw inferences about a population from a sample on n observations. Inferential statistics generally require that sampling be both random and representative. Observations are selected by random choice of the sample that resembles the population's functional requirement. This can be obtained through the following:

1. A sample is *random* if the method of obtaining the sample meets the criterion of randomness (each item or element of a population having an equal chance of being chosen). Hence, random numbers are typically generated from a uniform distribution $U[a,b]$.
2. Samples are drawn independently with no sequence, correlation, or autocorrelation between consecutive observations.
3. The sample size is large enough to be representative: usually, $n \geq 30$.

The two methods used most often in inferential statistics are parameter estimation and hypothesis testing.

3.5.1 Parameter Estimation

In parameter *estimation*, a sample is used to estimate a parameter and to construct a confidence interval around the parameter. Point estimates are used to estimate the parameter of interest. The mean (μ_y) and standard deviation (σ_y) are the most commonly used point estimates. As discussed earlier, the population mean (μ_y) and standard deviation (σ_y) are estimated using sample average ($\bar{y}$) and standard deviation (s_y), respectively.

A point estimate by itself does not provide enough information regarding variability encompassed into the response (output measure). This variability represents the differences between the point estimates and the population parameters. Hence, an interval estimate in terms of a *confidence interval* (CI) is constructed using the estimated average ($\bar{y}$) and standard deviation (s_y). A confidence interval is a range of values that has a high probability of containing the parameter being estimated. For example, the 95% confidence interval is constructed such that the probability that the estimated parameter is contained with the lower and upper limits of the interval is 95%. Similarly, 99% is the probability that the 99% confidence interval contains the parameter.

The confidence interval is symmetric about the sample mean $\bar{y}$. If the parameter being estimated is μ_y, for example, the 95% confidence interval constructed around an average of $\bar{y} = 28.0$ is expressed as follows:

$$25.5 \leq \mu_y \leq 30.5$$

This means that we can be 95% confident that the unknown performance mean (μ_y) falls within the interval [25.5, 30.5].

Three statistical assumptions must be met in a sample of data to be used in constructing the confidence interval. That is, the data points should normally be independent and identically distributed. The following formula is typically used to compute the confidence interval for a given significance level (α):

$$\bar{y} - t_{\alpha/2,n-1} \frac{s}{\sqrt{n}} \leq \mu \leq \bar{y} + t_{\alpha/2,n-1} \frac{s}{\sqrt{n}}$$

where $\bar{y}$ is the average of multiple data points, t_{n-1}, and $\alpha/2$ is a value from the Student's t distribution for an α level of significance. For example, using the data in Table 3.4, Figure 3.6 shows a summary of both graphical and descriptive statistics along with the 95% CI computed for the mean, median,

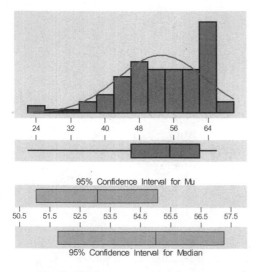

Anderson-Darling Normality Test
A-Squared: 1.852
P-Value: 0.000

Mean   53.0600
StDev   10.1113
Variance   102.239
Skewness   -7.4E-01
Kurtosis   4.19E-02
N   100

Minimum   22.0000
1st Quartile   46.0000
Median   55.0000
3rd Quartile   62.0000
Maximum   66.0000

95% Confidence Interval for Mu
51.0537   55.0663
95% Confidence Interval for Sigma
8.8778   11.7461
95% Confidence Interval for Median
51.7423   57.2577

Figure 3.6 Statistical and graphical summary for data in Table 3.4.

and standard deviation. The graph has been created with Minitab statistical software.

The normality assumption can be met by increasing the sample size (n) so that the central limit theorem (CLT) is applied. Each average performance, $\bar{y}$ (e.g., average yield) is determined by summing together individual performance values ($y_1, y_2, \ldots, y_n$) and dividing them by n. The CLT states that the variable representing the sum of several independent and identically distributed random values tends to be normally distributed. Since ($y_1, y_2, \ldots, y_n$) are not independent and identically distributed, the CLT for correlated data suggests that the average performance ($\bar{y}$) will be approximately normal if the sample size (n) used to compute $\bar{y}$ is large, $n \geq 30$. The $100\%(1 - \alpha)$ confidence interval on the true population mean is expressed as follows:

$$\bar{y} - Z_{\alpha/2} \frac{\sigma}{\sqrt{n}} \leq \mu \leq \bar{y} + Z_{\alpha/2} \frac{\sigma}{\sqrt{n}}$$

3.5.2 Hypothesis Testing

Hypothesis testing is a method of inferential statistics that is aimed at testing the feasibility of a *null hypothesis* about a certain population parameter based on some experimental data. It is common to put the null hypothesis forward and determine whether the available data are strong enough to reject it. The null hypothesis is rejected when the sample data are very different from what would be expected under a true null hypothesis assumption. It should be noted, however, that failure to reject the null hypothesis is not the same thing as accepting the null hypothesis.

In six sigma, hypothesis testing is used primarily for making comparisons. Two or more devices can be compared with the goal of identifying the superior design alternative relative to some functional requirement performance. In testing a hypothesis, the null hypothesis is often defined to be the reverse of what the team actually believes about the performance. Thus, the data collected are used to contradict the null hypothesis, which may result in its rejection. For example, if the design team has proposed a new device design alternative, he or she would be interested in testing experimentally whether the proposed design works better than the current baseline. To this end, the team would design an experiment comparing the two methods of production. The yield of the two devices could be collected and used as data for testing the feasibility of the null hypothesis. The null hypothesis would be, for example, that there is no difference between the two devices' yield (i.e., in the yield population the means of the two device populations μ_1 and μ_2 are identical). In such a case, the team would be hoping to reject the null hypothesis and conclude that the device proposed is the better one.

The symbol H_0 is used to indicate the null hypothesis, where *null* refers to the hypothesis of no difference. This is expressed as follows:

$$H_0: \mu_1 - \mu_2 = 0 \quad \text{or} \quad H_0: \mu_1 = \mu_2$$

The alternative hypothesis (H_1 or H_a) is simply set to state that the mean yield of the design proposed (μ_1) is higher than that of the current baseline (μ_2); that is,

$$H_a: \mu_1 - \mu_2 > 0 \quad \text{or} \quad H_a: \mu_1 > \mu_2$$

Although H_0 is called the null hypothesis, there are occasions when the parameter of interest is not hypothesized to be zero. For instance, it is possible for the null hypothesis to be that the difference (d) between population means is of a particular value ($H_0: \mu_1 - \mu_2 = d$). Or, the null hypothesis could be that the population mean is of a certain value ($H_0: \mu = \mu_0$).

The test statistics used in hypothesis testing depend on the hypothesized parameter and the data collected. In practical comparison studies, most tests involve comparisons of a mean performance with a certain value or with another device mean. When the variance (σ^2) is known, which is rarely the case in real-world applications, Z_0 is used as a test statistic for the null hypothesis $H_0: \mu = \mu_0$, assuming that the population observed is normal or the sample size is large enough so that the CLT applies. Z_0 is computed as follows:

$$Z_0 = \frac{\bar{y} - \mu_0}{\sigma/\sqrt{n}}$$

The null hypothesis $H_0: \mu = \mu_0$ would be rejected if $|Z_0| > Z_{\alpha/2}$ when $H_a: \mu \neq \mu_0$, $Z_0 < -Z_\alpha$ when $H_a: \mu < \mu_0$, and $Z_0 > Z_\alpha$ when $H_a: \mu > \mu_0$.

Depending on the test situation, several test statistics, distributions, and comparison methods can also be used in several hypothesis tests. Following are some examples. For the null hypothesis $H_0: \mu_1 = \mu_2$, Z_0 is computed as follows:

$$Z_0 = \frac{\bar{y}_1 - \bar{y}_2}{\sqrt{\sigma_1^2/n_1 + \sigma_2^2/n_2}}$$

The null hypothesis $H_0: \mu_1 = \mu_2$ would be rejected if $|Z_0| > Z_{\alpha/2}$ when $H_a: \mu_1 \neq \mu_2$, $Z_0 < -Z_\alpha$ when $H_a: \mu_1 < \mu_2$, and $Z_0 > Z_\alpha$ when $H_a: \mu_1 > \mu_2$.

When the process variance (σ^2) is unknown, which is typically the case in real-world applications, t_0 is used as a test statistic for the null hypothesis $H_0: \mu = \mu_0$; t_0 is computed as follows:

$$t_0 = \frac{\bar{y} - \mu_0}{s/\sqrt{n}}$$

The null hypothesis $H_0: \mu = \mu_0$ would be rejected if $|t_0| > t_{\alpha/2, n-1}$ when $H_a: \mu \neq \mu_0$, $t_0 < -t_{\alpha, n-1}$ when $H_a: \mu < \mu_0$, and $t_0 > t_{\alpha, n-1}$ when $H_a: \mu > \mu_0$.

For the null hypothesis H_0: $\mu_1 = \mu_2$, t_0 is computed as

$$t_0 = \frac{\bar{y}_1 - \bar{y}_2}{\sqrt{s_1^2/n_1 + s_2^2/n_2}}$$

Similarly, the null hypothesis H_0: $\mu_1 = \mu_2$ would be rejected if $|t_0| > t_{\alpha/2,v}$ when H_a: $\mu_1 \neq \mu_2$, $t_0 < -t_{\alpha,v}$ when H_a: $\mu_1 < \mu_2$, and $t_0 > t_{\alpha,v}$ when H_a: $\mu_1 > \mu_2$, where $v = n_1 + n_2 - 2$.

The examples of null hypotheses discussed involved the testing of hypotheses about one or more population means. Null hypotheses can also involve other parameters, such as an experiment investigating the variance (σ^2) of two populations, the proportion (π) and the correlation (ρ) between two variables. For example, the correlation between job satisfaction and performance on the job would test the null hypothesis that the population correlation (ρ) is zero. Symbolically, H_0: $\rho = 0$.

Sometimes it is necessary for the design team to compare more than two alternatives for a system design or an improvement plan with respect to a given performance measure. Most practical studies tackle this challenge by conducting multiple paired comparisons using several paired-t confidence intervals, as discussed above. *Bonferroni's approach* is another statistical approach for comparing more than two alternative medical devices. This approach is also based on computing confidence intervals to determine if the true mean performance of a functional requirement of one system (μ_i) is significantly different from the true mean performance of another system (μ_i') in the same FR. Analysis of variance (ANOVA; see Section 14.6) is another advanced statistical method that is often utilized for comparing multiple alternative medical devices. ANOVA's multiple comparison tests are widely used in experimental designs.

To draw the inference that the hypothesized value of the parameter is not the true value, a significance test is performed to determine if the value observed for a statistic is sufficiently different from a hypothesized value of a parameter (null hypothesis). The significance test consists of calculating the probability of obtaining a sample statistic that differs from the null hypothesis value (given that the null hypothesis is correct). This probability is referred to as the *p-value*. If this probability is sufficiently low, the difference between the parameter and the statistic is considered to be *statistically significant*. The probability of a type I error (α) is called the *significance level* and is set by the experimenter. The significance level (α) is commonly set to 0.05 and 0.01. The significance level used in hypothesis testing as follows:

1. Determine the difference between the results of the statistical experiment and the null hypothesis.
2. Assume that the null hypothesis is true.

3. Compute the probability (p-value) of the difference between the statistic of the experimental results and the null hypothesis.

4. Compare the p-value to the significance level (α). If the probability is less than or equal to the significance level, the null hypothesis is rejected and the outcome is said to be statistically significant.

5. The lower the significance level, therefore, the more the data must diverge from the null hypothesis to be significant. Therefore, the 0.01 significance level is more conservative since it requires a stronger evidence to reject the null hypothesis then that of the 0.05 level.

Two kinds of errors can be made in significance testing: *type I error* (α), when a true null hypothesis is rejected incorrectly, and *type II error* (β), when a false null hypothesis is accepted incorrectly. A type II error is an error only in the sense that an opportunity to reject the null hypothesis correctly was lost. It is not an error in the sense that an incorrect conclusion was drawn since no conclusion is drawn when the null hypothesis is accepted. Table 3.6 summarizes the two types of test errors.

Type I error is generally considered more serious than type II error since it results in drawing a conclusion that the null hypothesis is false when, in fact, it is true. The experimenter often makes a trade-off between type I and II errors. A design team protects itself against type I errors by choosing a stringent significance level, although this increases the chance of type II error. Requiring very strong evidence to reject the null hypothesis makes it very unlikely that a true null hypothesis will be rejected. However, it increases the chance that a false null hypothesis will be accepted, thus lowering the test power.

Test power is the probability of correctly rejecting a false null hypothesis. Power is therefore defined as $1 - \beta$, where β is the type II error probability. If the power of an experiment is low, there is a good chance that the experiment will be inconclusive. There are several methods for estimating the test power of an experiment. For example, to increase the test power, the team can be redesigned by changing one of the factors that determines the power, such as the sample size, the standard deviation (σ), or the size of difference between the means of the tested devices.

TABLE 3.6   The Two Types of Test Errors

Statistical Decision	True State of Null Hypothesis (H_0)	
	H_0 Is True	H_0 Is False
Reject H_0	Type I error (α)	Correct
Accept H_0	Correct	Type II error (β)

3.5.3   Experimental Design

In practical six sigma projects, experimental design is usually a main objective for building a transfer function model. Such models are built with an extensive effort spent on data collection, verification, and validation to provide a flexible platform for optimization and trade-offs. Experimentation can be done in hardware and software environments. Experimenting in a simulation environment is a typical practice for estimating performance under various running conditions, conducting "what-if" analysis, testing hypothesis, comparing alternatives, factorial design, and medical device optimization. The results of such experiments and methods of analysis provide the design team with insight, data, and necessary information for making decisions, allocating resources, and setting optimization strategies.

An *experimental design* is a plan based on a systematic and efficient application of certain treatments to an experimental unit or subject, a medical device. Being a flexible and efficient experimenting platform, the experimentation environment (hardware or software) represents the subject of experimentation at which various treatments (factorial combinations) are applied efficiently and systematically. The planned treatments may include both structural and parametric changes applied to the device. *Structural changes* include altering the type and configuration of hardware elements, the logic and flow of software entities, and the structure of the device configuration. Examples include adding a new component, changing the sequence of software operation, changing the concentration or the flow, and so on. *Parametric changes*, on the other hand, include making adjustments to device design parameters or variables, such as changes made to dimensions, or material.

Parameter design is, however, more common than that of structural design in medical device experimental design. In practical applications, design teams often adopt a certain concept structure and then use the experimentation to optimize its FR performance. Hence, in most experiments, design parameters are defined as decision variables and an experiment is set to receive and run at different levels of these decision variables to study their impact on a certain FR. Partial or full factorial design is used for two purposes:

1. To find those design parameters (variables) of greatest significance to system performance
2. To determine the levels of parameter settings at which the *best* performance level is obtained. Direction of goodness (i.e., best) performance can be maximizing, minimizing, or meeting a preset target of a functional requirement.

The success of experimental design techniques depends strongly on providing an efficient experiment setup. This includes appropriate selection of design parameters, functional requirements, experimentation levels of the parameters, and number of experimental runs required. To avoid conducting large numbers of experiments, especially when the number of parameters (i.e., factors in the design of experiment terminology) is large, certain experimental design techniques can be used. Examples of such handling include using screening runs to eliminate insignificant design parameter, and using Taguchi's fractional factorial designs instead of full factorial designs.

In experimental design, decision variables are referred to as *factors* and the output measures are referred to as *responses*. Factors are often classified into control and noise factors. *Control factors* are within the control of the design team, whereas *noise factors* are imposed by operating conditions and other internal or external uncontrollable factors. The objective of experiments is usually to determine settings to the device control factors so that device response (a functional requirement) is optimized and system random (noise) factors have the least impact on system response. You will read more about the setup and analysis of designed experiments in the following chapters.

3.6 NORMAL DISTRIBUTION AND THE NORMALITY ASSUMPTION

The *normal distribution* is used in various domains of knowledge and as such is standardized to avoid the taxing effort of generating specialized statistical tables. A standard normal has a mean of zero and a standard deviation of 1, and functional requirement (y) values are converted into Z-scores or sigma levels using $Z_i = (y_i - \mu)/\sigma$ transformation. A property of the normal distribution is that 68% of all its observations fall within a range of ± 1 standard deviation from the mean, and a range of ± 2 standard deviations includes 95% of the scores. In other words, in a normal distribution, observations that have a Z-score (or sigma value) of less than -2 or more than $+2$ have a relative frequency of 5% or less. A Z-score value means that a value is expressed in terms of its difference from the mean, divided by the standard deviation. If you have access to statistical software, you can explore the exact values of probability associated with different values in the normal distribution using the probability calculator tool; for example, if you enter a Z value (i.e., standardized value) of 4, the associated probability computed will be less than 0.0001, because in the normal distribution almost all observations (i.e., more than 99.99%) fall within the range ± 4 standard deviations. A population of measurements with normal or Gaussian distribution will have 68.3% of the population within $\pm 1\sigma$, 95.4% within $\pm 2\sigma$, 99.7% within $\pm 3\sigma$, and 99.9% within $\pm 4\sigma$ (Figure 3.7).

The normal distribution is used extensively in statistical reasoning (induction), called *inferential statistics*. If a sample size is large enough, the results of selecting sample candidates randomly and measuring an FR of interest is "normally distributed", thus, knowing the shape of a normal curve, we can calculate precisely the probability of obtaining "by chance" FR outcomes

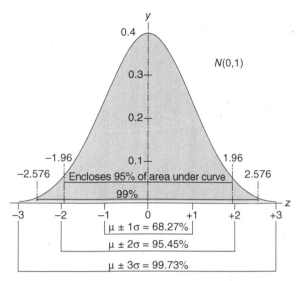

Figure 3.7   Standardized normal distribution $N(0,1)$ and its properties.

representing various levels of deviation from a hypothetical population mean of zero.

In hypothesis testing, if such a probability is so low that it meets the previously accepted criterion of statistical significance, we have only one choice: to conclude that our result gives a better approximation of what is going on in the population than does the null hypothesis. Note that this entire reasoning process is based on the assumption that the shape of the distribution of those data points (technically, the sampling distribution) is normal.

Are all test statistics normally distributed? Not all, but most of them are either based on the normal distribution directly or on distributions that are related to, and can be derived from the normal distribution, such as Student's *t*, Fisher's *F*, or chi-square. Typically, those tests require that the variables analyzed are themselves normally distributed in the population, that is, that they meet the *normality assumption*. Many variables observed are actually normally distributed, which is another reason why the normal distribution represents a general feature of empirical reality. A problem may occur when one tries to use a normal distribution–based test to analyze data from variables that are themselves not normally distributed. In such cases we have two general choices. First, we can use some alternative *nonparametric* (i.e., *distribution-free*) *test*, but this is often inconvenient because such tests are typically less powerful and less flexible in terms of types of conclusions that they can provide. Alternatively, in many cases we can still use a normal distribution–based test if we make sure that our sample size is large enough. The latter option is based on an extremely important principle which is largely responsible for the popularity of tests that are based on the normal function:

namely, that as the sample size increases, the shape of the sampling distribution (i.e., the distribution of a statistic from the sample, a term first used by Fisher in 1928) approaches the normal shape, even if the distribution of the variable in question is not normal. However, as the sample size (of samples used to create the sampling distribution of the mean) increases, the shape of the sampling distribution becomes normal. Note that for $n = 30$, the shape of that distribution is almost perfectly normal. This principle is the *central limit theorem* (a term first used by Pólya in 1920).

3.6.1   Violating the Normality Assumption

How do we know the consequences of violating the normality assumption? Although many of the statements made in preceding paragraphs can be proven mathematically, some of them do not have theoretical proofs and can be demonstrated only empirically using *Monte Carlo experiments*. In these experiments, large numbers of samples are generated by a computer following predesigned specifications, and the results are analyzed using a variety of tests. In this way we can evaluate empirically the type and magnitude of errors or biases to which we are exposed when certain theoretical assumptions of the tests we are using are not met by our data. Specifically, Monte Carlo studies have been used extensively with normal distribution–based tests to determine how sensitive they are to violations of the assumption of a normal distribution of the variables analyzed in the population. The general conclusion from these studies is that the consequences of such violations are less severe than thought previously. Although these conclusions should not entirely discourage anyone from being concerned about the normality assumption, they have increased the overall popularity of distribution-dependent statistical tests in many areas.

3.7   SUMMARY

In this chapter we provide a very basic review of appropriate statistical terms and methods that are described in this book. We review the collection, classification, summarization, organization, analysis, and interpretation of data. We use medical device examples to cover descriptive and inferential statistics. A practical view of common probability distributions, modeling, and statistical methods is presented throughout the chapter.

We express the criticality of understanding hypothesis testing and discuss examples of null hypotheses involving hypotheses testing involving one or more population means. Next, we move into an explanation of analysis of variance and types I and type II test errors. Experimental design and its objective in building the transfer function model are explained. Normal distribution and normality assumption are discussed and an answer is provided as to how we know the consequences of violating the normality assumption.

4

THE SIX SIGMA PROCESS

4.1 INTRODUCTION

In this chapter we overview six sigma and its development, as well as DMAIC, the traditional deployment for process/product improvement, and three components of the methodology. We also introduce the design application, which is detailed in Chapter 5 and beyond.

4.2 SIX SIGMA FUNDAMENTALS

Six sigma is a philosophy, a measure, and a methodology that provides businesses with perspective and tools to achieve new levels of performance in services, operations, processes, and products. The whole quality concept was discussed in Chapter 1. In six sigma, the focus is on process improvement to increase capability and reduce variation. A few vital inputs are chosen from the entire system of controllable and noise variables, and the focus of improvement is on controlling these inputs.

Six sigma as a philosophy helps companies achieve very low defect rates per million opportunities over long-term exposure. Six sigma as a measure gives us a statistical scale by which to measure our progress and benchmark other companies, processes, or products. The measurement scale of defects per million opportunities ranges from zero to 1 million, and the sigma scale

Medical Device Design for Six Sigma: A Road Map for Safety and Effectiveness,
By Basem S. El-Haik and Khalid S. Mekki
Copyright © 2008 John Wiley & Sons, Inc.

ranges from 0 to 6. The methodologies used in six sigma build on all of the tools that have evolved to date but put them into a data-driven framework. This framework of tools allows companies to achieve the fewest possible defects per million opportunities.

Six sigma evolved from early TQM efforts (see Chapter 1). Motorola initiated the movement, and it then spread to Asea Brown Boveri, the Texas Instruments Missile Division, and then Allied Signal. It was at this juncture that Jack Welch became aware of the power of six sigma, and in the nature of a fast follower, committed from Larry Bossidy General Electric to embracing the movement. It was GE that bridged the gap between a manufacturing process and product focus and what were first called *transactional processes* and later changed to *commercial processes*. One reason that Welch was so interested in this program was that a just-completed employee survey revealed that top-level managers at the company believed that GE had "invented" quality—after all, Armand Feigenbaum worked at GE, whereas the vast majority of employees didn't think that GE could spell "quality". Six sigma has turned out to be the methodology to accomplish Crosby's goal of zero defects. By recognizing the key process input variables and that variation and shift can occur, we could create controls that maintain six sigma performance on any product or service and in any process. Before we can clearly understand the process inputs and outputs, we need to understand process modeling.

4.3 PROCESS MODELING

Six sigma is a process-focused approach to achieving new levels of performance throughout any business or organization. We need to focus on a process as a system of inputs, activities, and output(s) in order to provide a holistic approach to all the factors and the way they interact to create value or waste. When used in a productive manner, many products and services are also processes. An ATM machine takes your account information, personal identification number, energy, and money and processes a transaction that dispenses funds or an account rebalance. A computer can take keystroke inputs, energy, and software to process bits into a word document. At the simplest level, the process model can be represented by a process diagram, often called an *input–process–output* (IPO) *diagram* (Figure 4.1).

If we take the IPO concept and extend it to include the suppliers of the inputs and the customers of the outputs, we have SIPOC (supplier–input–process–output–customer) (Figure 4.2). This is a very effective tool in gathering information and modeling any process. A SIPOC tool can take the form of a table with a column for each category in the name.

4.3.1 Process Mapping

Whereas SIPOC is a linear flow of steps, *process mapping* is a means of displaying the relationship between process steps and allows for the display of

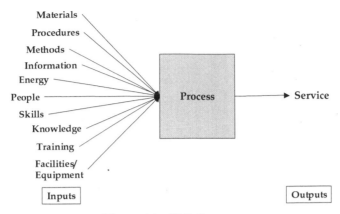

Figure 4.1 IPO diagram.

Suppliers	Inputs	Input Characteristics	Process	Outputs	Output Characteristics	Customers
			2a. What is the start of the process?			
7. Who are the suppliers of the inputs?	6. What are the inputs of the process?	8. What are the characteristics of the inputs?	1. What is the process?	3. What are the outputs of the process?	5. What are the characteristics of the outputs?	4. Who are the customers of the outputs?
			2b. What is the end of the process?			

Figure 4.2 SIPOC table.

various aspects of the process, including delays, decisions, measurements, and rework and decision loops. Process mapping builds on SIPOC information by using standard symbols to depict varying aspects of the processes flow linked together by lines, with arrows demonstrating the direction of flow.

4.3.2 Value Stream Mapping

Process mapping can be used to develop a *value stream map* to demonstrate how well a process is performing in terms of value and flow. Value stream maps can be created at two levels. In the first, each step of a process map is evaluated directly as being value added or non-value added (see Figures 4.3 and 4.4). This type of analysis has been in existence since at least the early

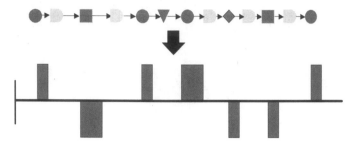

Figure 4.3 Process map transition to value stream map.

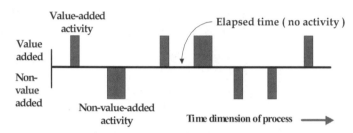

Figure 4.4 Value stream map definitions.

1980s, but a good reference is the book *The Hunters and the Hunted* (Swartz, 1995). This is effective if the design team is operating at a local level. However, if the design team is at more of an enterprise level and needs to be concerned about the flow of information as well as the flow of product or service, a higher-level value stream map is needed (see Figure 4.5). This methodology has best been described by Rother and Shook (2000).

4.4 BUSINESS PROCESS MANAGEMENT

Most processes are ad hoc or allow great flexibility to those who operate them. This, coupled with a lack of measurement of efficiency and effectiveness, results in the variation to which we have all become accustomed. In this case we use the term *efficiency* for the within-process-step performance (often called the *voice of the process*), whereas the *effectiveness* is how all the process steps interact to perform as a system (often called the *voice of the customer*). This variation is difficult to address, due to the lack of measures that allow traceability to root cause. Businesses that have embarked on six sigma programs have learned that they have to develop process management systems and implement them in order to establish baselines from which to improve. The deployment of a business process management system (BPMS) often results in a marked improvement in performance as viewed by the customer

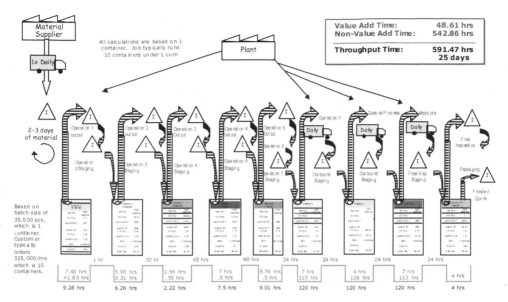

8% Value added Efficiency – most efficiency lost in Out Side Services

Figure 4.5 High-level value stream map example.

and by associates involved in the process. The benefits of implementing BPMS are magnified in cross-functional processes.

4.5 MEASUREMENT SYSTEMS ANALYSIS

Now that we have some form of documented process, with choices ranging from IPO, SIPOC, process map, and value stream map, to BPMS, we can begin our analysis of what to fix and what to enhance. Before we can focus on what to improve and how much to improve it, we must be certain of our measurement system. Measurements can start at benchmarking through to operationalization. We must determine how accurate the measurement system is versus a known standard, and how repeatable and reproducible the measurement is. Many measures are the results of manual calculations whose reproducibility and repeatability can astonish you if you take the time to perform a measurement system analysis.

In a supply chain, for example, we might be interested in promises kept, on-time delivery, order completeness, deflation, lead time, and acquisition cost. Many of these measures require an operational definition to provide repeatable and reproducible measures. Referring to Figure 4.6, is on-time delivery the same as on-time shipment? Many companies do not have knowledge of when a client takes delivery or processes a receipt transaction, so how do we measure these? Is it when the item arrives, when the paperwork has

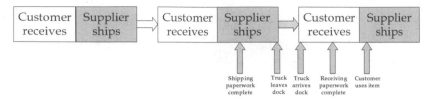

Figure 4.6   Supplier-to-customer cycle.

been completed or when a customer can actually use the item? We have seen a customer drop a supplier for a 0.5% lower cost component only to discover that the new multiyear contract that they signed did not include transportation and they ended up paying 3.5% more for three years.

The majority of measures in a process focus on:

- Speed
- Cost
- Quality
- Efficiency, as defined as first-pass yield of a process step
- Effectiveness, as defined as the rolled throughput yield of all process steps

All of these can be made robust by creating operational definitions, defining the start and stop times, and determining sound methodologies for assessing. The statement "If you can't measure it, you can't improve it" is worth remembering, as is ensuring that adequate measurement systems are available throughout a project's life cycle.

4.6   PROCESS CAPABILITY AND SIX SIGMA PROCESS PERFORMANCE

Process capability is determined by measuring a process's performance and comparing it to the customer's needs (specifications). *Process performance* may not be constant and, in fact, usually exhibits some form of variability. For example, we may have a molding process that has measures of injection speed and dwell time. For the first hour of a shift, the process has few defects, but when demand goes up, the molding process exhibits more defects.

If process performance is measurable in real numbers (continuous) rather than through pass or fail (discrete) categories, the process variability can be modeled using a normal distribution. A normal distribution is commonly used due to its robustness in modeling many real-world performance random variables. This distribution has two parameters quantifying the central tendency and variation. The center is the average performance and the degree of variation is expressed by the standard deviation. If the process cannot be measured in real numbers, we convert pass/fail or good/bad (discrete) into a yield and convert the yield into a sigma value. Several transformations from discrete distributions to continuous distributions can be borrowed from mathematical statistics.

If the process follows a normal probability distribution, 99.73% of the values will fall between the ±3σ limits (where σ is the standard deviation) and only 0.27% will be outside the ±3σ limits. Since the process limits extend from −3σ to +3σ, the total spread amounts to 6σ (six sigma) of total variation. This total spread is the process spread and is used to measure the range of process variability.

For any process performance metrics there are usually some performance specification limits. These limits may be single sided or two sided. For the molding process, the specification limit may be no less than 95% yield. For receipt of material into a plant, it may be 2 days early and 0 days late. For a call center, we may want a phone conversation to take between 2 and 4 minutes. For each of these two double-sided specifications, the limits can also be stated as a target and a tolerance. The material receipt could be 1 day early ±1 day, and for the phone conversation it could be 3 minutes ±1 minute.

If we compare the process spread with the specification spread, we can usually observe three conditions:

- *Condition 1: highly capable process* (see Figure 4.7). The process spread is well within the specification spread:

$$6\sigma < \text{USL–LSL}$$

The process is capable because it is extremely unlikely that it will yield an unacceptable performance.

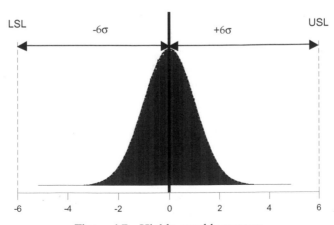

Figure 4.7 Highly capable process.

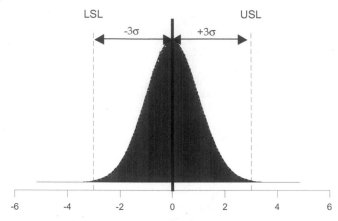

Figure 4.8   Marginally capable process.

- *Condition 2: marginally capable process* (see Figure 4.8). The process spread is approximately equal to the specification spread:

$$6\sigma = \text{USL–LSL}$$

When a process spread is nearly equal to the specification spread, the process is capable of meeting the specifications. If we remember that the process center is likely to shift from one side to the other, a significant amount of the output will fall outside the specification limit and will yield an unacceptable performance.

- *Condition 3: incapable process* (see Figure 4.9). The process spread is greater than the specification spread:

$$6\sigma > \text{USL–LSL}$$

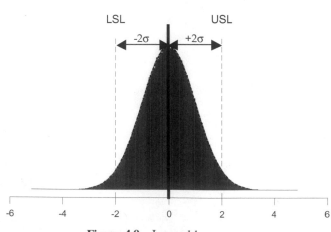

Figure 4.9   Incapable process.

When a process spread is greater than the specification spread, the process is incapable of meeting the specifications, and a significant amount of the output will fall outside the specification limit and yield an unacceptable performance.

As we have seen, the term *six sigma* comes from statistical terminology, where sigma (σ) represents standard deviation. For a normal distribution, the probability of falling within a $\pm 6\sigma$ range around the mean is 0.9999966 with a 1.5σ mean shift. In a production process, the *six sigma standard* means that the process will produce defectives at the rate of 3.4 defects per million units. Clearly, six sigma indicates a degree of extremely high consistency and extremely low variability. In statistical terms, the purpose of six sigma is to reduce variation to achieve very small process standard deviations of a functional requirement or a critical-to-quality requirement of interest, here denoted as y for ease of reference.

The six sigma strategy involves the use of statistical tools within a structured methodology for gaining the knowledge needed to achieve better, faster, and more cost-effective solutions. This involves repeated disciplined application of the master strategy on project after project, with the projects selected based on the need to resolve key business issues that directly affect the bottom line. The achievement of financial improvement results in increased profit margins and return on investment. Project leaders are called *black belts*. The six sigma initiative in a company is designed to change the culture through breakthrough improvement by focusing on out-of the-box thinking in order to achieve aggressive and stretched goals [see, e.g., Harry (1994, 1998) and Breyfogle (1999)].

A system is classified as *defective* if a desired requirement, denoted y, is outside the customer's upper specification limit (USL) or lower specification limit (LSL). The half-tolerance range of y, denoted t or Δy, equals half of the difference of the specification range (i.e., the design range). In addition to both limits, customers specify a target value, T, for y, which is typically the midpoint between the USL and the LSL. Let's say that the internal customer's specification of a shaft diameter is 50 ± 1 mm. In this example, $T = 50$ mm, LSL = 49 mm, USL = 51 mm, and the half-tolerance = 1 mm. There are many sources of variability in manufacturing processes, such as machine feed rate, speed, vibration, material properties, and setup variables, that will make the central limit theorem hold for a typical design parameter average. Therefore, the diameter can be treated as a normally distributed random variable. A sample is taken and the average, $\bar{y}$, and sample standard deviation, S, are used to estimate the process average, μ, and the process standard deviation, σ, respectively, from the sample. With this approximation, the terms *sigma* and *standard deviation* are used interchangeably (Tadikamalia, 1994).

The diameter, as a design parameter, is called *centered* (i.e., the average equals the target); otherwise, it is *off-center*. The sigma level is defined by a *z-score* (i.e., a sigma score), given by

TABLE 4.1   Sigma Levels (Normal Distribution)

Long-Term Yield (%)	Short-Term Sigma	Defects per 1,000,000	Defects per 10,000	Defects per 100
99.9996599	6	3.40	0.034	0.00034
99.9767327	5	232.67	2.327	0.02327
99.3790320	4	6,209.68	62.097	0.62097
93.3192771	3	66,807.23	668.072	6.68072
69.1462467	2	308,537.53	3,085.375	30.85375
30.8537533	1	691,462.47	6,914.625	69.14625
6.6807229	0	933,192.77	9,331.928	93.31928

$$z_{USL} = \frac{USL - \bar{y}}{\sigma}$$

$$z_{LSL} = \frac{\bar{y} - LSL}{\sigma} \tag{4.1}$$

When the process is centered in the design range and $\sigma = \Delta y/6, \Delta y/5, \Delta y/4, \Delta y/3, \ldots$, the z-scores are 6, 5, 4, 3, ..., respectively. As Table 4.1 shows, there are approximately 67,000 defects per million at the 3σ level and 6200 defects per million at the 4σ level, assuming a 1.5σ shift in the average over time. If $S = \Delta y/6$, and assuming that the diameter is off-center by as much as 1.5σ, the maximum number of defects is 3.4 defects (or, in this case, shafts) per million. Table 4.1 is derived from the normal distribution table.

When manufacturing companies embark on six sigma quality programs, what is their objective? Is it to reduce the process variance so that the half-tolerance of the product characteristic is equal to six times the standard deviation? From a technical viewpoint, it might make sense to talk in terms of the process variance. From a managerial or customer viewpoint, the quality standards can be described in terms of defects per million.

It is usually the case that an adjustment step to move the average closer to the target value is relatively easier than changing the system to reduce the variance. It is generally true that reducing process variance through programs such as six sigma involves extensive efforts, which may include use of statistical techniques and in some cases, capital investments in better technology. Alternatively, adjusting the process to the target value requires much less effort but may not result in significant improvement. Certainly, companies want to reduce process variance in the most cost-effective way. Both activities, variance reduction and adjustment of the mean to target, are steps usually taken to reduce design vulnerabilities or to solve a problem.

4.6.1   Motorola's Six Sigma Quality

In 1986, the Motorola Corporation won the Malcolm Baldrige National Quality Award. Motorola based its success in quality on its six sigma program.

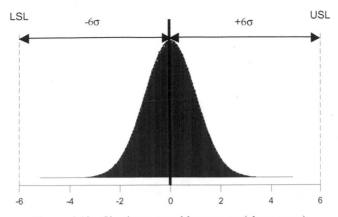

Figure 4.10 Six sigma capable process (short-term).

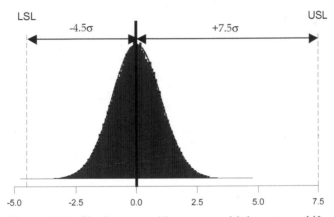

Figure 4.11 Six sigma capable process with long-term shift.

The goal of the program was to reduce the variation in every process such that a spread of 12σ (6σ on each side of the average) fits within the process specification limits (see Figure 4.10).

Motorola accounted for the process average shifting side to side over time. In this situation, one side shrinks to a 4.5σ gap and the other side grows to 7.5σ (see Figure 4.11). This shift accounts for 3.4 parts per million (ppm) on the small gap and a fraction of parts per billion on the large gap. So over the long term, a 6σ process will generate only 3.4 ppm defects.

To achieve six sigma capability, it is desirable to have the process average centered within the specification window and to have the process spread over approximately one-half of the specification window. There are two approaches to accomplishing six sigma levels of performance. When dealing with an existing process there is the process improvement method, also known as DMAIC, and if there is a need for a new process, it is DFSS. Both of these are discussed in the following sections.

4.7 OVERVIEW OF SIX SIGMA IMPROVEMENT

Applying six sigma methodology to improve an existing process or product follows a five-phase process:

1. *Define.* Define the opportunity and customer requirements.
2. *Measure.* Ensure adequate measures, process stability, and initial capability.
3. *Analyze.* Analyze the data and discover the critical inputs and other factors.
4. *Improve.* Improve the process based on the new knowledge.
5. *Control.* Implement adequate controls to sustain the gain.

This five-phase process, often referred to as DMAIC, is described in more detail below.

4.7.1 Phase 1: Define

First we create the project definition, which includes the problem/opportunity statement, the objective of the project, the benefits expected, which items are in scope and which are out of scope, the team structure, and the project time line. The scope includes details such as resources, boundaries, customer segments, and timing. The next step is to determine and define customer requirements. Customers can be both external consumers and internal stakeholders. At the end of this step you should have a clear operational definition of the project metrics (called *big Y*'s or *outputs*) and their link to critical business levers, as well as the goal for improving the metrics. Business levers can consist, for example, of return on capital invested, profit, customer satisfaction, and responsiveness. The last step in this phase is to define the process boundaries and high-level inputs and outputs using SIPOC as a framework and to define the data collection plan.

4.7.2 Phase 2: Measure

The first step is to make sure that we have good measures of the Y's through validation or measurement system analysis. Next, we verify that the metric is stable over time and then use the method discussed earlier to determine our baseline process capability. If the metric varies wildly over time, we must address the special causes creating the instability before attempting to improve the process. The result of stabilizing performance often provides all the improvement desired. Finally, we define all possible factors that affect the performance and use the qualitative methods of Pareto, cause-and-effect (fishbone) diagrams, cause-and-effect matrices, failure modes and their effects, and detailed process mapping to narrow down the potential influential (significant) factors (denoted as x's). See Appendix 4A for cause-and-effect tools.

4.7.3 Phase 3: Analyze

In the analyze phase, we first use graphical analysis to search out relationships between the input factors (x's) and the outputs (Y's). We follow this up with a suite of statistical analysis, including various forms of hypothesis testing, confidence intervals, or screening design of experiments to determine statistical and practical significance of the factors on the project Y's. A factor may prove to be statistically significant: that is, have a certain confidence that the effect is true and only a small chance that it could have occurred by mistake. The statistically significant factor is not always practical, in that it may account for only a small percentage of the effect on the Y's, in which case controlling the factor wouldn't provide much improvement. The transfer function $Y = f(x)$ for every Y measure usually represents the regression of several influential factors on the project outputs. There may be more that one project metric (output), hence the Y's.

4.7.4 Phase 4: Improve

In the improve phase, we first identify potential solutions through team meetings and brainstorming or the use of TRIZ (see Chapter 10). It is important at this point to have completed a measurement system analysis on the key factors (x's) and possibly to have performed some confirmation design of experiments. The next step is to validate the solution(s) identified through a pilot run or through optimization design of experiments. Following confirmation of the improvement, a detailed project plan and cost–benefit analysis should be completed. The last step in this phase is to implement the improvement. This is a point where change management tools can prove to be beneficial.

4.7.5 Phase 5: Control

The control phase consists of four steps. In the first we determine the control strategy based on the new process map, failure mode and effects, and a detailed control plan. The control plan should balance the output metric against the critical few input variables. The second step involves implementing the controls identified in the control plan. This is typically a blend of poka-yokes and control charts, clear roles and responsibilities, and operator instructions depicted in operational method sheets. Third, we determine the final capability of the process with all the improvements and controls in place. The final step is ongoing monitoring of the process based on the frequency defined in the control plan.

The DMAIC methodology has allowed businesses to achieve lasting break-through improvements which break the paradigm of reacting to causes rather than symptoms. This method allows design teams to make fact-based decisions using statistics as a compass and to implement lasting improvements that satisfy the external and internal customers.

4.8   SIX SIGMA GOES UPSTREAM: DESIGN FOR SIX SIGMA

The DMAIC methodology is excellent when dealing with an existing process in which reaching the entitled level of performance will provide all of the benefit required. *Entitlement* is the best the process or product is capable of performing with adequate control. Reviewing historical data, it is often evident as the best performance point. But what do we do if reaching entitlement is not enough or there is a need for an innovative solution never before deployed? We could continue with the typical build-it and fix-it process, or we can utilize the most powerful tools and methods available for developing an optimized, robust, "de-risked" design. These tools and methods can be aligned with an existing new product/process development process or used in a stand-alone manner. The rest of the book is devoted to explaining and demonstrating DFSS tools and methodology. Chapter 5 is the introductory chapter for DFSS, giving overviews of DFSS theory, the DFSS gated process, and DFSS applica-tion. In Chapter 6 we describe in detail how to deploy DFSS in a medical device firm, covering the training, organization support, financial manage-ment, and deployment strategy. Chapter 7 gives a very detailed road map of the entire DFSS project execution, which includes very detailed descriptions of the DFSS stages, task management, scorecards, and how to integrate all DFSS methods in developmental stages. Chapters 8 through 20 provide detailed descriptions, with examples, of all the major methods and tools used in DFSS.

4.9   SUMMARY

In this chapter we explain 6σ and how it has evolved over time. We describe it as a process-based methodology and introduce the reader to process model-ing with a high-level overview of IPO, process mapping, value stream mapping and value analysis, as well as the business process management system. The importance of understanding measurements used in a process or system and how this is accomplished with measurement systems analysis can not be stressed too much. Once we understand the goodness of our measures, we can evaluate the capability of the process to meet customer requirements and demonstrate six sigma (6σ) capability. Next, we describe DMAIC methodology and how it incorporates these concepts in a road map. Finally, we discussed how 6σ moves upstream to the design environment with the application of DFSS. In Chapter 5 we introduce the DFSS process.

APPENDIX 4A: CAUSE-AND-EFFECT TOOLS

A cause-and-effect diagram (i.e., the fishbone or Ishikawa diagram) and a cause-and-effect matrix are two tools commonly used to help an DFSS team to perform an FMEA exercise. The cause-and-effect diagram classifies the various causes thought to affect the operation of the design, using arrows to indicate the cause-and-effect relations among them. The diagram is formed from causes that can result in an undesirable failure mode. The causes are the independent variables, and the failure mode is the dependent variable. In the example depicted in Figure 4A.1, a company that manufactures consumer products suffers from warranty costs measured as a percentage of sales. The current performance is above the budgeted upper specification limit. Customers tend to have great sensitivity to warranty issues and equipment downtime, which results in dissatisfaction. Figure 4A.1 shows several causes for the warranty costs.

In a cause-and-effect matrix, a DFSS team lists the failure modes. The team then proceeds to rank each failure mode numerically using risk priority

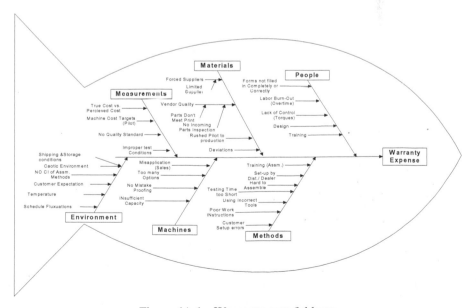

Figure 4A.1 Warranty cost fishbone.

numbers (RPNs). The team brainstorms to identify all potential causes that can affect the failure modes and lists these along the left-hand side of the matrix. It is useful to classify theses causes by type (e.g., variability, production environment) as design weaknesses or noise factor effects. The team then rates numerically the effect of each cause on each failure mode within the body of the matrix. This is based on the experience of the team and any information available. The team then cross-multiplies the rate of the effect by the FMEA (see Chapter 11) RPN, for example, to total each row (cause). The totals are then used to analyze and prioritize where to focus the effort when creating the FMEA. By grouping the causes according to classification (weakness, environment effect, production unit-to-unit effect, wear effect, etc.) the team will firm up several hypotheses about the strength of these types of causes to use to devise an attack strategy.

5

MEDICAL DEVICE DESIGN FOR SIX SIGMA

5.1 INTRODUCTION

The objective of this chapter is to introduce the theory on which the medical device design for six sigma (DFSS) process is based and to lay the foundation for the following chapters. DFSS combines design analysis (e.g., requirements cascading) with design synthesis (e.g., process engineering) within the framework of a medical device company's product development system. Emphasis is placed on CTS (critical-to-satisfaction requirements, or big Y's) identification, optimization, and verification using the transfer function and scorecard vehicles. In the lingo of medical devices, big Y's constitute the design input.

A transfer function in its simplest form is a mathematical relationship between CTSs and/or their cascaded functional requirements (FRs) and the critical or significant design parameters or process variables (i.e., the X's). Scorecards help predict risks to the achieving CTSs or FRs by monitoring and recording their mean shifts and variability performance.

In general, DFSS is a disciplined and rigorous approach to service, process, and product design by ensuring that new designs meet customer requirements at launch. It is a design approach that ensures complete understanding of deliverables, capabilities, and performance measurements by using scorecards, transfer functions, and tollgate reviews to ensure the accountability of all the

Medical Device Design for Six Sigma: A Road Map for Safety and Effectiveness,
By Basem S. El-Haik and Khalid S. Mekki
Copyright © 2008 John Wiley & Sons, Inc.

design team members, green and black belts, project champions, deployment champions,[1] and the remainder of the organizations.

The DFSS objective is to attack the design vulnerabilities at both the conceptual and operational levels by deriving and integrating tools and methods for their elimination and reduction. Unlike the DMAIC six sigma methodology discussed in Chapter 4, the phases or steps of DFSS are not defined universally, as evidenced by the many training curriculam available in the market place. Often, deployment companies will implement the version of DFSS used by their choice of vendor to assist in the deployment. A company may, on the other hand, implement DFSS to suit their business, industry, and culture, creating their own version. Nevertheless, all approaches share common themes, objectives, and tools.

In general, DFSS is used to design or redesign a product, process, or service, collectively called a *design entity*. The sigma level expected for a DFSS design entity in a given response (CTS, big Y or small y) is at least 4.5σ,[2] but can be 6σ or higher. The production of such a low defect level from launch means that customer expectations and needs must be understood completely before a design can be operationalized. That is, quality is defined by the customer as fitness for use. The material presented herein is intended to give the reader a high-level understanding of medical device DFSS and it uses and benefits. Following this chapter, readers should be able to assess how it could be used in relation to their jobs and to identify their needs for further learning.

As defined in this book, DFSS has two tracks, deployment and application. Deployment is the strategy adopted by the deploying company to launch six sigma and DFSS initiatives. It includes setting up the deployment infrastructure, strategy, and plan for initiative execution. Six sigma initiative deployment is covered in Chapter 6. In what follows we are assuming that the deployment strategy is in place as a prerequisite for application and project execution. The DFSS tools are laid on top of four phases, as outlined in Table 2.7, and are detailed in Chapter 7 in what we call the DFSS project road map.

There are two distinct tracks within the term *six sigma initiative* as discussed in earlier chapters. The retroactive six sigma DMAIC approach (see Section 4.7) takes existing process improvement as an objective. Proactive DFSS targets redesign and new product introductions in both the development and production (process) arenas.

The DFSS approach can be broken down into identify, characterize, optimize, and verify/validate (ICOV; see Figure 1.2).

- *Identify* customer wants and design inputs and map them to design outputs.
- *Characterize* the medical design entity and develop its conceptual .structure.

---

[1]We explore the roles and responsibilities of these six sigma operatives and others in Chapter 6.
[2]No more than approximately 1 defect per 1000 opportunities.

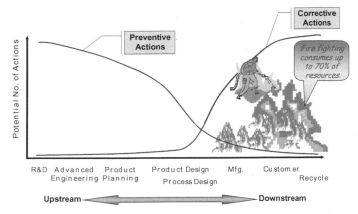

Figure 5.1 DFSS approach tackles problem prevention as a proactive strategy.

- *Optimize* the entity in its environment of use.
- *Verify/validate* that the entity delivers its functional outputs. This includes validation to customer wants.

In this book, the terms *ICOV* and *DFSS* are used interchangeably.

5.2 VALUE OF DESIGNING FOR SIX SIGMA

Generally, customer-oriented design is a developmental process of transforming customers' wants into design product solutions that are useful to a customer from a functionality standpoint. This process is carried over several development stages, starting at the idea generation stage. In the next, conceptual, stage, conceiving, evaluating, and selecting good design solutions are necessary tasks that have enormous consequences. It is usually the case that organizations operate in two modes: *proactive*, conceiving feasible and healthy conceptual entities, and *retroactive*, problem solving such that the design entity can live up to its potential. In the medical device industry, the latter mode expresses itself through a massive hidden factory commonly known as the *corrective action/preventive action*[3] (CAPA) *process*. Across other industries, unfortunately, the problem-solving mode consumes the largest portion of an organization's human and nonhuman resources. That is, DFSS has the potential to free resources by making a shift in the time at which issues can be prevented, before they manifest themselves as problems in the customers' hands (Figure 5.1), where they need to be solved.

---

[3]The acronym CAPA is a familiar one to those responsible for quality assurance in manufacturing facilities, particularly in the medical device and pharmaceutical industries. CAPA is the formal process of resolving existing problems and preventing potential problems.

DFSS is a premier approach to product development that is able to embrace and improve developed homegrown supportive processes (e.g., sales and marketing) as well within its development system (El-Haik and Roy, 2005). In the spirit of the whole quality concept discussed in Chapter 1, this advantage will enable the deploying company to build on current foundations while enabling them to reach unprecedented levels of achievement that exceed the targets set.

The link of the six sigma initiative and DFSS to the company vision and annual objectives should be direct, clear, and crisp. DFSS has to be the crucial mechanism to develop and improve product and business performance and to drive up customer satisfaction and quality metrics. Significant improvements in all health metrics are the fundamental source of DMAIC and DFSS projects, which will, in turn, transform the culture one project at a time. Achieving a six sigma culture is essential for the future well-being of medical device and health care–deploying companies and represents the biggest return on investment beyond the obvious financial benefits. Six sigma initiatives apply to all elements of company strategy in all areas of a business if a massive impact is really the objective.

Operational vulnerabilities takes variability reduction and mean adjustment of the critical-to-quality, critical-to-cost, and critical-to-delivery requirements, known collectively as the critical-to-satisfaction requirements, as an objective and have been the subject of many knowledge fields, such as parameter design, DMAIC six sigma, tolerance design, and tolerancing techniques. On the other hand, the conceptual vulnerabilities are usually overlooked, due to the lack of a compatible systemic approach to finding ideal solutions, the ignorance of the design team, the pressure of the deadlines, and budget limitations. This can be attributed, partly, to the fact that traditional quality methods can be characterized as after-the-fact disciplines since they use lagging information for developmental activities such as bench tests and field data. Unfortunately, this practice drives design toward endless cycles of design–test–fix–retest, creating what is broadly known as the "firefighting" mode of the design process (i.e., the creation of design-hidden factories; Figure 5.1). Companies that follow these practices usually suffer from high development costs, longer time to market, lower quality levels, and marginal competitive edge. In addition, corrective actions to improve the conceptual vulnerabilities via operational vulnerability improvement means (e.g., robustness DOEs) are marginally effective if at all useful. Typically, these corrections are costly and hard to implement as the medical device project progresses development process. Therefore, implementing DFSS as early as possible is a goal that can be achieved when systematic design methods are integrated with quality concepts and methods upfront. Specifically, on the technical side, we developed an approach to DFSS by borrowing from the following fundamental knowledge arenas: design engineering, quality engineering, TRIZ (Altshuller, 1988), axiomatic design (Suh, 1990), and applied probability and statistics concepts. At the same time, several venues in our DFSS approach enable transformation to a data-driven and customer-centric culture, such as concurrent design teams, deployment strategy, and planning.

In general, most current design methods are empirical in nature. They represent the best thinking of the design community, which, unfortunately, lacks a design scientific base and relies on subjective judgment. When a company suffers a detrimental decline in customer satisfaction, judgment and experience may not be sufficient to obtain an optimal solution, definitely not at the six sigma level—another motivation to devise a DFSS method to address such needs.

In the medical device industry, progress is very slow in shifting from improving performance during the later stages of the medical device design life cycle to the front-end stages, where design development takes place at higher levels of abstraction (i.e., prevention versus solving). This shift is also motivated by the fact that the design decisions made during the early stages of the medical device design life cycle have the largest impact on the total cost and quality of the system. It is often claimed that up to 80% of the total cost is committed in the concept development stage (Fredrikson, 1994). The research area of design is currently receiving increasing focus to address industry efforts to shorten lead times, cut development and manufacturing costs, lower total life-cycle cost, and improve the quality of the design entities in the form of products, services, and/or processes. It is the experience of the authors that at least 80% of the design quality is also committed in the early stages, as depicted conceptually in Figure 5.2 (see Yang and El-Haik, 2003). "Potential" in the figure is defined as the difference between the impact (influence) of the design activity at a certain design stage and the total development cost up to that stage. The potential is positive but decreasing as design progresses, implying reduced design freedom to make changes over time. As financial resources are committed (e.g., buying process equipment and facilities, hiring staff), the potential starts changing sign, going from positive to negative. In the consumers hands, the potential is negative and the cost outcomes the impact tremendously. At this stage, design changes for corrective actions can only be

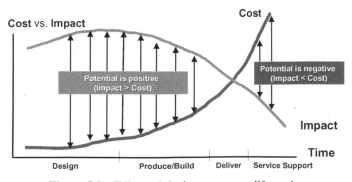

Figure 5.2　Effect of design stages on life cycle.

achieved at a high cost, including customer dissatisfaction, warranty, marketing promotions, and in many cases under the scrutiny of the government (e.g.,
recall costs), a CAPA process dilemma across the industry.

5.3 MEDICAL DEVICE DFSS FUNDAMENTALS

DFSS is a structured data-driven approach to design in all aspects of business
functions (e.g., human resources, marketing, sales, IT information technology)
where deployment is launched, used to eliminate the defects induced by the
design process and to improve customer satisfaction, sales, and revenue. To
deliver on these benefits, DFSS applies design methods such as axiomatic
design,[4] creativity methods such as TRIZ,[5] and statistical techniques such as
parameter design to all applicable levels of design decision making in every
corner of the business; identify and optimize the critical design factors (the
X's), and validate all design decisions in the use (or surrogate) environment
of the end user.

DFSS is not an add-on but represents a cultural change within various functions where deployment is launched. It provides the means to tackle weak or
new devices, driving customer and employee satisfaction. DFSS and six sigma
should be linked to the deploying company's annual objectives, medium- and
long-term plans, and vision and mission statements. It should not be viewed
as another short-lived initiative. It is a vital permanent component needed to
achieve leadership in design, customer satisfaction, and cultural transformation. From marketing and sales to development, operations, and finance, each
business function needs to be headed by a deployment leader or deployment
champion. This local deployment team will be responsible for delivering dramatic change, thereby removing customer issues and internal problems while
expediting growth. The deployment team can deliver on their objective
through six sigma operatives called black belts, master black belts, and green
belts, who will be executing scoped projects that are in alignment with the
objectives of the deployment plan. *Project champions* are responsible for
scoping projects from within their realm of control and handing project charters (contracts) over to the six sigma operatives. The project champion will
select projects consistent with corporate goals and remove any barriers to
execution. Six sigma operatives will complete successful projects using six
sigma methodology and will train and mentor the local organization personnel
on six sigma. The *deployment leader*, the highest initiative operative, sets
meaningful goals and objectives for deployment in his or her function and to
drive implementation of six sigma publicly.

---

[4]A perspective design method that employs two design axioms: the independence and information
axioms. See Chapter 9 for more details.
[5]TRIZ is the Russian acronym for the theory of inventive problem solving (TIPS). It is a systematic method of conceiving creative, innovative, and predictable design solutions. See Chapter 10
for more details.

Six sigma resources are full-time six sigma operatives, in contrast to *green belts*, who could be completing smaller projects of their own as well as assisting black belts. They play a key role in raising the core competency of a company, as they drive the initiative into day-to-day operations.

Black belts are the driving force of any DFSS deployment. They are project leaders who are removed from day-to-day assignments for a period of time (usually, two years) to focus exclusively on design and improvement projects with intensive training in six sigma tools, design techniques, problem solving, and team leadership. Black belts are trained by *master black belts*, who are initially hired, if not homegrown.

A black belt should possess process and organization knowledge, have some basic product development practices and statistical skills, and be eager to learn new tools. A black belt is a *change agent* to drive the initiative into his or her teams, staff function, and across the company. In doing so, their communication and leadership skills are vital. Black belts need effective intervention skills. They must understand why some team members may resist the six sigma cultural transformation. Some soft training on leadership should be embedded within their training curriculum. Soft-skills training may target deployment maturity analysis, team development, business acumen, and individual leadership. In training, it is wise to share several initiative maturity indicators that are being tracked in the deployment scorecard: for example, alignment of the project to company objectives in its own scorecard (the big Y's), readiness of the project's mentoring structure, preliminary budget, team member identification, and scoped project charter.

DFSS black belt training is intended to be delivered in tandem with a training project for hands-on application. The training project should be well scoped with ample opportunity for tool application and should have cleared tollgate 0 (kickoff) prior to class (i.e., project scoping). Usually, project presentations will be weaved into each training session. More details are given in Chapter 6.

While handling projects, the role of the black belts spans several functions, including learning, mentoring, teaching, and coaching. As a mentor, the black belt cultivates a network of experts in the project on hand, working with the process operators, design owners, and all levels of management. To become self-sustained, the deployment team may assign black belts to provide formal training to green belts and team members.

DFSS projects can be categorized as the design or redesign of an entity, whether a product, process, or service. *Creative design* is the term that we use to indicate a new design, or a design from scratch, and we use *incremental design* to indicate a redesign or design from a datum. In the latter case, some data can be used to provide a baseline for current performance. The degree of deviation of the redesign from a datum is the key factor in deciding on the usefulness of relative existing data. DFSS projects can come from historical sources (e.g., medical device redesign due to customer issues in a CAPA database) or from proactive sources such as growth and innovation (new medical device introduction). In either case, a medical device DFSS project requires greater emphasis on:

- A VOC collection scheme
- Addressing all (multiple) CTSs as cascaded by the customer
- Assessing and mitigating technical failure modes and project risks in the product's own environment as they are linked to tollgate process reviews
- Project management with some communication plan to all affected parties and budget management
- A detailed project change management process

5.4   THE ICOV PROCESS IN DESIGN

As discussed in Section 5.1, DFSS has four phases: identify, characterize, optimize, and verify/validate (ICOV), over seven development stages. The medical device life cycle is depicted in Figure 5.3. Notice the position of the ICOV phases of a design project.

Naturally, the process of medical device design begins when there is a need, an impetus. People create the need, whether it is a problem to be solved or a new invention. Design objective and scope are critical in the impetus stage.

A design project charter should describe simply and clearly what is to be designed. It cannot be vague. Writing a clearly stated design charter is just one step. In stage 2 the design team must write down all the information they may need and collect, in particular the voice of the customer, the voice of the regulation, and the voice of the business. With the help of quality function deployment methodology, such consideration will lead the definition of the medical device design product or functional requirements to be grouped later into modules such as systems, subsystems, and components. A product or functional requirement must contribute to an innovation or to a solution of the objective described in the design charter. Another question that should be on the minds of the team members relates to how the end result will look. The simplicity, comprehensiveness, and interfaces should make the medical device attractive. What options are available to the team? At what cost? Do they have the right physical properties, such as safety, quality, completeness, software language, and reliability? Will it be difficult to operate and maintain? Consider what methods you will need to process, store, and deliver the medical device.

In stage 3 the design team should produce a number of conceptual solutions. It is very important that they write or draw every concept on paper as it occurs to them. This will help them remember and describe them more clearly. It is also easier to discuss them with other people if drawings are avail-

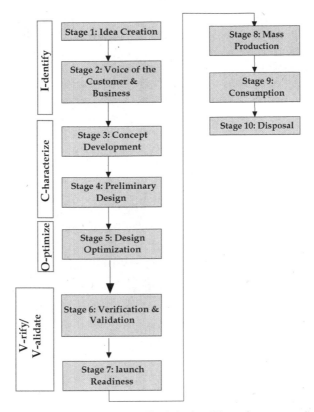

Figure 5.3 Medical device life cycle.

able. These first drawings do not have to be very detailed or accurate. Sketches will suffice and should be made quickly. The important thing is to record all ideas and develop solutions in the preliminary design stage (stage 4). The design team may find that they like several of the solutions. Eventually, the design team must choose one. Usually, careful comparison with the original design charter will help them to select the best, subject to the constraints of cost, technology, and skills available. Deciding among the several possible solutions is not always easy. It helps to summarize the design requirements and solutions and put the summary in a matrix called the *morphological matrix*, which is a way to show all functions and corresponding possible design parameters (solutions). An overall design alternative set is synthesized from this matrix, which is conceptually a highly potential feasible solution. Which solution would they choose? The Pugh matrix, a concept selection tool named after Stuart Pugh, can be used. The solution selected will be subjected to a thorough design optimization stage (stage 5). This optimization could be deterministic or statistical in nature. On the statistical front, the design solution will be made insensitive to uncontrollable factors (i.e., noise factors) that

may affect its performance. Factors such as customer usage profile, environment, and production device-to-device variation should be considered as
noise. To assist in this noise-insensitivity task, we rely on the transfer function
as an appropriate vehicle. In stage 5 the team needs to provide detailed documentation of the optimized solution. This documentation must include all of
the information needed to produce the medical device.

Consideration for design documentation, design and process mappings,
operational instructions, software code, communication, marketing, and so on,
should be put in place. In stage 6 the team can make a model assuming the
availability of the transfer functions and later a prototype, or they can go
directly to making a prototype or a pilot. A model is a full-sized or small-scale
simulation of a process or product. Architects, engineers, and most designers
use models. Models are expressive means to communicate the functionality
of the solution. For most people it is easier to understand when the project
end result is seen in three-dimensional form. A scale model is used when the
design scope is very large. A prototype is the first working version of the
design team's solution. It is generally full size and often using homegrown
expertise. Design verification and validation, stage 6, also includes testing and
evaluation, which is basically an effort to answer these very basic questions:
Does it work? Does it meet the design charter? Did we do the design right?
Did we do the right design? If failures are discovered, will modifications
improve the solution? These questions have to be answered. Upon having
satisfactory answers, the team can move to the next development and design
stage.

In stage 7 the team needs to prepare the production facilities where the
medical device will be produced for launch. Members from production/manu-
facturing engineering should be present at all times and at the start of the
project. At this stage they should assure that the medical device is marketable
and that no competitors beat them to the market. The team, together with the
project stakeholders, must decide how many to make. Similar to other products, a medical device may be mass-produced in low or high volume. The task
of making a medical device is divided into jobs. Each worker trains to do his
or her assigned job. As workers complete their special jobs, the medical device
takes shape. Post stage 7, the lean production saves time and other resources.
Since workers train to do a certain job, each becomes skilled in that job.

5.5   THE ICOV PROCESS IN PRODUCT DEVELOPMENT

In earlier sections we show how DFSS integrates with the medical device life-
cycle system. It is very apparent that it is an event-driven process: in particular,
the development (design) stages. In this stage, milestones occur when the
entrance criteria (inputs) are satisfied. At these milestones, the stakeholders,
including the project champion, process/design owner, and deployment cham-

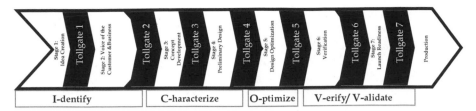

Figure 5.4   ICOV DFSS process.

pion (if necessary), conduct tollgate reviews. A development stage has some time *thickness*, that is, time needed to prepare the entrance and exit criteria for the bounding tollgates. The ICOV DFSS phases as well as the seven stages of the development process are depicted in Figure 5.4. In these reviews, a decision should be made as to whether to proceed to the next phase of development, recycle back for further clarification on certain decisions, or cancel the project altogether. Cancellation of problematic projects as early as possible is a good thing. It stops nonconforming projects from progressing further, consuming resources and frustrating people. In any case, the black belt should quantify the size of the benefits of the design project in language that will have an impact on upper management, identify major opportunities for improving customer dissatisfaction and associated threats to salability, and stimulate improvements through the DFSS approach.

In tollgate reviews, work proceeds when the exit criteria (required decisions) are developed. As a DFSS deployment bonus, a standard measure of development progress across the deploying company using a common development terminology is achieved. Consistent exit criteria from each tollgate comprise both the medical device DFSS's own deliverables, due to use of the approach itself, and business unit- or function-specific deliverables. The detailed entrance and exit criteria stage by stage are presented in Chapter 6.

The ICOV process offers a thread-through road map with overlaid tools that is based on nontraditional tools such as design mappings and design axioms, and creativity tools such as TRIZ, without ignoring the soft side of deployment, the cultural transformation. A major uniqueness of the ICOV DFSS approach adopted in this book is the employment of design principles. ICOV is principle-centered; that is, it demystifies not only *what* needs to be done and *how* it needs to be done, but also *why* it needs to be done as a prelude to regulatory requirements. As a green or black belt dives into his or her project execution, he or she may get mired in the complexity of the tools. A principle-based approach to training and project execution is best for handling many aspects of such complexity. Readers are encouraged to increase their acquaintance with ICOV principles by browsing Six Sigma Professionals, Inc.'s Web site, www.SixSigmaPI.com.

5.6 SUMMARY

Design for six sigma is a disciplined methodology that applies the transfer function $[CTSs = f(X)]$ to ensure that customer expectations are met, embeds customer expectations into the design, predicts design performance prior to the pilot study, builds performance measurement systems (scorecards) into the design to ensure effective ongoing process management, and leverages a common language for design within a design tollgate process.

DFSS offers a robust set of tools and processes that address many of today's complex medical device design problems. The DFSS approach helps design teams frame their project based on a process with financial, cultural, and strategic implications to the business. The DFSS comprehensive tools and methods described in this book for medical devices allow teams to assess medical device issues quickly and to identify financial and operational improvements that reduce costs, optimize investments, and maximize returns. Medical device DFSS leverages a flexible and nimble organization and maintains low development costs, allowing deploying companies to pass these benefits on to their customers. The ICOV DFSS approach employs a unique set of principles[6] and a gated process that allows teams to build tailormade approaches (i.e., not all the tools need to be used in each project). Therefore, it can be designed to accommodate the specific needs of the project charter. Project by project, the competency level of the design teams will be enhanced, leading to deeper knowledge and broader experience.

In this book we form and integrate several strategic and tactical and methodologies that produce synergies to enhance medical device DFSS capabilities to deliver a broad set of optimized solutions. The methods presented have widespread application to help design teams and the green and black belt population in different project portfolios (e.g., staffing and other human resources functions, finance, operations and supply chain functions, organizational development, financial services, training, technology, software tools and methods).

DFSS provides a unique commitment to medical device customers by guaranteeing agreed-upon financial and other results. Each design project must have measurable outcomes, and the design team is responsible for defining and achieving those outcomes. The medical device DFSS approach ensures these outcomes through risk identification and mitigation plans, variable (DFSS tools that are used over many stages)- and fixed (DFSS tool that is used once)-tool structures, and advanced conceptual tools. The DFSS principles and structure should motivate design teams to provide business and customers with a substantial return on their design investment.

---

[6]Browse Six Sigma Professionals, Inc.'s Web site: www.SixSigmaPI.com.

6

MEDICAL DEVICE DFSS DEPLOYMENT

6.1 INTRODUCTION

Medical device design for six sigma (DFSS) is a disciplined methodology that embeds customer expectations into the design, applies the transfer function approach to ensure that customer expectations are met, predicts design performance prior to pilot clinical studies, builds performance measurement systems (scorecards) into the design to ensure effective ongoing process management, leverages a common language for design, and uses tollgate reviews to ensure accountability.

In this chapter we take as an objective support of a medical device DFSS deployment team who will launch a six sigma program. A deployment team includes various levels of the deploying company's leadership, including initiative senior leaders, project champions and other deployment sponsors. As such, the material in this chapter should be used as deployment guidelines, with ample room for customization. It provides the considerations and general aspects required for a smooth and successful initial deployment experience.

The extent to which medical device DFSS produces the desired results is a function of the deployment plan adopted. Historically, we can observe that many sound initiatives became successful when commitment is secured from involved people at all levels. At the end, an initiative is successful when crowned as the new norm in the respective functions. Medical device six sigma and DFSS are no exception. A successful DFSS deployment is people depen-

Medical Device Design for Six Sigma: A Road Map for Safety and Effectiveness,
By Basem S. El-Haik and Khalid S. Mekki
Copyright © 2008 John Wiley & Sons, Inc.

dent, and as such almost every level, function, and division involved with the design process should participate, including the customer.

6.2 MEDICAL DEVICE DFSS DEPLOYMENT FUNDAMENTALS

The extent to which a medical device design for a six sigma program produces results affected directly by the plan with which it is deployed. In this section we present a high-level perspective of a sound plan by outlining the critical elements of successful deployment. We must point out up front that a successful DFSS initiative is the result of key contributions from people at all levels and functions of the company. In short, successful DFSS initiatives require buy-in, commitment, and support from officers, executives, and management staff before and while operational- and process-level employees execute improvement projects.

This top-down approach is critical to the success of any medical device DFSS program. While green and black belts are the focal point for executing projects and generating cash from process improvements, their success is linked inextricably to the way that leaders and managers establish the six sigma culture, create motivation, allocate goals, institute plans, set procedures, initialize systems, select projects, control resources, and maintain recognition and rewards.

Several scales of deployment may be used; however, maximum entitlement of benefits can only be achieved when all affected functions are engaged. A full-scale company-wide deployment program requires senior leadership to install the proper culture of change before they begin their support of the training, logistics, and other resources required. People empowerment is key, as well as leadership by example.

Benchmarking several DFSS deployment programs in several industries, we can conclude that a top-down deployment approach will work for medical device DFSS deployment as well. This conclusion reflects the critical importance of securing and cascading the buy-in from the top leadership level.

Black and green belts are the focused force of deployment under the guidance of master black belts and champions. Success can be measured by increases in revenue, customer satisfaction, and cash generated one project at a time. Belted projects should be scoped diligently and aligned to a company's objectives with some prioritization scheme. DFSS program benefits cannot be harvested without a sound strategy with the long-term vision of establishing the six sigma culture. In the short term, deployment success depends on motivation, management commitment, project selection and scoping, an institutionalized reward and recognition system, and optimized resources allocation. This chapter is organized into several sections, containing deployment models, roles, and responsibilities that can be employed readily by the deployment team. We categorize the deployment process, in terms of evolution time, into three phases:

1. A predeployment phase, to build infrastructure
2. A deployment phase, during which most activities will happen
3. A postdeployment phase, during which sustainment needs to be achieved

6.3 PREDEPLOYMENT PHASE

Predeployment is a phase representing the period of time when a leadership team lays the groundwork and prepares a company for medical device DFSS implementation, ensures the alignment of their individual deployment plans, and creates synergy and heightened performance.

The first step in an effective medical device DFSS deployment starts with the top leadership of the deploying company or organization. It is at this level that the team tasked with deployment works with senior executives in developing a strategy and plan for deployment that is designed for success. DFSS initiative marketing and selling should come from the top. Our observation is that senior leaders benchmark themselves across corporate America in terms of results, management style, and company aspirations. Six sigma, in particular DFSS, is no exception. The process usually starts with a senior leader or a pioneer who has researched six sigma and the benefits it brings to the culture, as well as its top- and bottom-line results. The pioneer starts the deployment one step at a time and begins challenging old paradigms. Guards of the old paradigm come to its defense and try to block deployment. Defense mechanisms fall one after another by the indisputable results in several benchmarked deploying companies (e.g., GE, 3M, Motorola, Textron, Allied Signal, Bank of America). Momentum builds up and a team is formed to be tasked with deployment. As a first step, it is advisable that select senior leadership meet off-site (for limited distractions) jointly as a team with the deployment team to consider a balanced mix of strategic thinking, six sigma high-level education, interaction, and hands-on planning. On the education side, overviews of six sigma concepts, presentation of successful deployment benchmarking, and demonstration of six sigma statistical methods, improvement measures, and management controls will be very useful. Specifically, the following should be a minimum set of objectives of this launch meeting:

- To understand the philosophy and techniques of medical device DFSS and six sigma, in general.
- To experience the application of some of the tools during the meeting.
- To brainstorm a deployment strategy and a corresponding deployment plan with high first-time through capability (benchmark other plans for comparison).
- To understand the organizational infrastructure requirements for deployment.

- To set financial and cultural goals, targets, and limits for the initiative.
- To discuss project pipeline and black belt resources in all phases of deployment.
- To put a mechanism in place to mitigate deployment risks and failure modes. See, for example, deployment failure mode and effect analysis (FMEA) of a typical medical device DFSS deployment. Failure modes such as the following are indicative of problematic strategy: training black belts before champions; deploying DFSS without multigenerational plans and, if possible, technology road maps; valid data and measurement systems; leadership development; a compensation plan; or a change management process.
- To design a mechanism for tracking the progress of the initiative. If desired, establish a robust financial management and reporting system for the initiative. The metrics to be used by stage would be different. A multidimensional deployment metric is suggested in Table 6.1.

TABLE 6.1 Suggested Deployment Metrics

Metric Category	Leading Metrics[a]	Lagging Metrics
Schedule	Number of simultaneous projects per resource Earned value analysis: money actually spent versus money that should have been spent based on schedule; deliverables complete versus deliverables that should have been complete based on the schedule	Development stage cycle time/ (complexity index: f(no. system functional requirements, no. new technologies, no. of disciplines)
Financial	Net present value (NPV) predicted (includes support costs)	NPV postlaunch (includes support costs)

Quality	Identify phase:
	  % of CTQs, FRs
	Characterize phase:
	  % of CTQs, FRs with transfer function
	  Capability growth index
	Optimize phase:
	  % of CTQs, FRs with transfer function defined
	  Capability growth index: optimize
	Verify/validate phase:
	  % of CTQs, FRs with transfer function validated
	  Capability growth index: validation
		Launch
		Capability growth index, postlaunch

Source: Suggested by Rob Gier of Baxter International.
[a]CTQ, critical to quality (Chapter 8); FRs, functional requirements (Chapter 9).

Once the initial joint meeting has been held, the deployment team could replicate to other tiers of leadership, whose buy-in is deemed necessary to *push* the initiative through the various functions of the company. A medical device six sigma *pull* system needs to be created and sustained in the deployment and postdeployment phases. Sustainment indicates the establishment of bottom-up pulling power. Medical device six sigma including DFSS has revolutionized many companies in the last 20 years. On the medical device side, companies in various markets can be found implementing medical device DFSS as a vehicle to improve profitability, plan growth, improve product/process quality and delivery performance, and to reduce cost. Parallel to many deploying companies, we find ourselves reaping the benefits of increased employee satisfaction through the true empowerment that six sigma provides. Factual study of several successful deployments indicates push and pull strategies that need to be adopted based on needs and differ strategically by objective and phase of deployment. A push strategy is needed in the predeployment and deployment phases (see below) to jump-start and operationalize deployment efforts. A pull system is needed in the postdeployment phase once sustainment is accomplished to improve deployment process performance on a continuous basis. In any case, top and middle management should be on board and leading the deployment proactively; otherwise, the DFSS initiative will fade away eventually.

6.3.1 Predeployment Considerations

The impact of a DFSS initiative depends on the effectiveness of deployment (i.e., how well the six sigma design principles and tools are practiced by the DFSS project teams). Intensity and constancy of purpose beyond the norm are required to improve deployment constantly. As an implicit requirement, a motivation system to maintain deployment should be institutionalized; otherwise, it will die. Rapid deployment of DFSS plus commitment, training, and practice characterize winning deploying companies.

In the predeployment phase, the deployment leadership should create a compelling business case for initiating, deploying, and sustaining DFSS as an effort. FDA design control violations, repetitive complaints over many device lines, and systematic CAPA are elements of a good predeployment business case. They need to raise general awareness about what DFSS is, why a company is pursuing it, what is expected of various people, and how it will benefit the company. Building commitment and alignment among executives and deployment champions to aggressively support and drive deployment throughout the designated functions of the company is a continuous activity. Empowerment of leaders and DFSS operatives to carry out their respective roles and responsibilities effectively is essential to success.

True empowerment is based on a belief, a belief that every employee, regardless of role, has the potential to be innovative, to solve problems, and to make a lasting contribution to overall DFSS deployment success. To describe empowerment at its most basic level, empowerment enables managers to manage and allows both employer and employee to contribute in the most effective and productive way possible. In an initiative such as DFSS, leaders need to understand their assumptions regarding empowerment and why they believe that empowerment will work in their organizations. Is it to improve the internal consultative process? Are they hoping to promote a more active approach to delegation? Or is their chief objective to extend responsibilities without expanding authority? Whatever the reason, having a clear understanding of leadership's own position will vastly improve the chances of DFSS deployment success.

A successful DFSS deployment requires the following prerequisites in addition to the senior leadership commitment just discussed.

Deployment Team Structure   The first step taken by a senior deployment leader is to establish a deployment team (usually, external master black belts with massive experience) to develop strategies and oversee deployment [see Yang and El-Haik (2003) for product DFSS perspectives]. With the help of the deployment team, the leader is responsible for designing, managing, and delivering successful deployment of the initiative throughout the company, locally and globally. He or she needs to work with human resources personnel to develop a policy to ensure that the initiative becomes integrated into the culture, which may include integration with internal leadership development programs, career planning for green and black belts and deployment champions, a reward and recognition program, and progress reporting to the senior leadership team. In addition, the deployment leader needs to provide training, communication (as a single point of contact to the initiative), and infrastructure support to ensure consistent deployment.

To ensure a smooth and efficient rollout, the critical importance of the team overseeing the deployment cannot be overemphasized. This team sets a DFSS deployment effort in the path to success in which the proper persons are positioned and support infrastructures are established. The deployment team is on the deployment forward edge, assuming responsibility for implementation. In this role, team members perform a company assessment of deployment maturity, conduct a detailed gap analysis, create an operational vision, and develop a cross-functional six sigma deployment plan that spans human resources, information technology (IT), finance, and other key functions. Conviction about the initiative must be expressed at all times, even though in the early stages there is no physical proof of a company's specifics. They also accept and embody the following deployment aspects:

- Visibility of the top-down leadership commitment to the initiative (indicating a push system).
- Development and qualification of a measurement system with defined metrics to track the deployment efficacy and progress. The objective here is to provide a tangible picture of deployment efforts. Later, in the matu-

rity stages (the end of the deployment phase), a new set of metrics that target effectiveness and sustainment needs to be developed.

- Stretching the goal-setting process in order to focus culture on changing the process by which work gets done rather than tweaking current products and processes, leading to quantum rates of improvement.
- Strict adherence to the devised strategy and deployment plan.
- Clear communication of success stories that demonstrate how DFSS methods, technologies, and tools have been applied to achieve dramatic operational and financial improvements.
- Providing a system that will recognize and reward those who achieve success.

A deployment structure should not be limited to the deployment team overseeing deployment both strategically and tactically, but should include project champions, functional area deployment champions, process and design owners where solutions will be implemented, and master black belts, who mentor and coach the green and black belts. All should have very crisp roles and responsibilities with defined objectives. A premier deployment objective can be that the black belts are used as a task force to improve customer satisfaction, company image, and other strategic long-term objectives of the deploying company. To achieve such objectives, the deploying division should establish a deployment structure formed from deployment directors, a centralized deployment team overseeing deployment, and master black belts with defined roles and responsibilities for long- and short-term planning. The structure can take the form of a committee or a council with a definite recurring schedule. *We suggest using DFSS to design the medical device DFSS deployment process and strategy.* The deployment team should:

- Develop a green belt structure of support to the black belts in every department.
- Cluster the green belts as a network around the black belts for synergy and to increase the velocity of deployment.
- Ensure that the scopes of the projects are within control and that the project selection criteria are focused on such company objectives as quality, cost, customer satisfiers, and delivery drivers.
- Hand off (match) the right scoped projects to the green and black belts.
- Support projects with key upfront documentation such as charters or contracts with financial analysis highlighting savings and other benefits, efficiency improvements, customer impact, and project rationale. Such documentation will be reviewed and agreed upon by primary stakeholders (deployment champions, design owners, black belts, and finance).
- Allocate the belt resources optimally across many divisions of the company, first targeting high-impact projects, and create a long-term

allocation mechanism to target a mix of DMAIC projects (on the corrective side of CAPA; see Section 5.2) versus the DFSS project (the preventive side of CAPA plus projects related to growth and innovation) that will be revisited periodically. In a healthy deployment, the number of DFSS projects should grow while the number of DMAIC projects should decay over time. However, this growth in the number of DFSS projects should be managed. A growth model, an S-curve, can be modeled over time to depict this deployment performance. The initiating condition of how many and where DFSS projects will be targeted is a significant growth control factor. This is a very critical aspect of deployment: in particular, when the deploying company chooses not to separate the training track of the black belts to DMAIC and DFSS and to train the black belts on both methodologies simultaneously.

- Use available external resources as leverage when advantageous, to obtain and provide the technical support required.
- Promote and foster work synergy through the various departments involved in the DFSS projects.
- Maximize utilization of a continually growing DFSS community by successfully closing most of the projects that are approaching the targeted completion dates.
- Keep leveraging significant projects that address the company's objectives: in particular, the customer satisfaction targets.
- Maximize belt certification turnover (set a target based on maturity).
- Achieve and maintain working relationships with all functions involved in DFSS projects that promote an atmosphere of cooperation, trust, and confidence among them. A proposed work breakdown structure is proposed in Table 6.2.

Deployment Operatives   A number of key people in a company are responsible for jump-starting engagement in the company for successful deployment. The same people are also responsible for creating momentum, establishing a culture, and driving DFSS through the company during the predeployment and deployment phases. In this section we describe these people in terms of their roles and responsibilities. The purpose is to establish clarity about what is expected of each deployment team member and to minimize the ambiguity that so often characterizes change initiatives, usually tagged as the "flavor of the month."

Deployment Champions   In the deployment structure, the deployment champion role is key. This position is usually an executive (e.g., vice president) handling various functions within the company (e.g., marketing, information technology, communication, sales). Their tasks as a part of the deployment team is to remove barriers within their functional area and to make things happen, review DFSS projects periodically to ensure that project champions

TABLE 6.2   Deployment Work Relationship High-Level Structure

Level 1	Level 2	Level 3
Commitment demonstration	Initiation event	
	Draft deployment plan	Deployment FMEA
Change management	Communication plan	
	Stakeholder analysis	
Organization definition process	Champion selection process	
	Belt selection process	
	Hiring/acquiring	Consultant
		Black belt
		Coop/intern
Project definition process	DMAIC project	
	DFSS project	
Training	Leadership training	
	DFSS ICOV/DMAIC process training	
	DFSS ICOV/DMAIC tool training	
Software support	Requirements management	
	Axiomatic design	
	Simulation	General
		Mechanical
		Electrical
		Software
		Simulation integration
Motivation systems	Project rewards	
	Performance management systems integration	
DFSS measurement systems	Deployment	See Table 6.1
	Product development up and running	See Table 6.1

Source: Suggested by Rob Gier of Baxter International.

are supporting their belts' progress toward goals, assist with project selection, and serve as change agents.

Deployment champions are full time into this assignment and should be at a level to execute the top-down approach, the push system, in the predeployment and deployment phases. They provide key employees with the managerial and technical knowledge required to create the focus and facilitate leadership, implementation, and deployment of DFSS in designated areas of their respective organizations. In medical device DFSS deployment, they are tasked with recruiting, coaching, and developing (i.e., mentoring, not training) green and black belts, identifying and prioritizing projects, leading product and process owners, removing barriers, providing the drum beat for results, and expanding project benefits across boundaries via the mechanism of replication. Champions should develop a big picture understanding of DFSS, deliverables, tools to the appropriate level, and how DFSS fits within the medical device life cycle.

The deployment champion will lead his or her function's total quality efforts toward improving growth opportunities, quality of operations, and operating margins among other people using medical device DFSS. This leader will have a blend of business acumen, management experience, and process improvement passion. The deployment champions need to develop and grow a master black belt training program for the purpose of certifying and deploying homegrown future master back belts throughout deployment. In summary, the deployment champions are responsible for broad-based deployment, common language, and culture transformation by weaving DFSS and six sigma into the company's DNA. They have a consistent, teachable point of view of their own.

Project Champions   The project champions are accountable for the performance of green and black belts and the results of projects and are responsible for selection, scoping, and successful completion of belt projects. Project champions remove roadblocks for belts within their span of control and ensure timely completion of projects. The following considerations should be the focus of the deployment team relative to project champions as they lay down their strategy relative to the champion role in deployment:

1. What does a DFSS champion need to know to be effective?
2. How should impact and progress projects be monitored?
3. What should be own expectations from senior leadership, the belt population, and others (expectations relative to the time line for full adoption of DFSS into their development process)?
4. What should be included in the playbook (reference guide) for champions ("must have" versus "nice to have" tools: lean DFSS project application)?
5. How do we use champions as change agents?
   a. Complete a deployment FMEA exercise in their area; identify deployment failure modes, ranking, and corrective actions. The FMEA will focus on potential failure modes in project execution.
   b. Plan for DFSS implementation; create a timely deployment plan within their span of control, project selection, project resources, and project pipeline.
   c. Develop guidelines, reference tools, and a checklist ("cheat sheet") for champions to help them understand (force) compliance with medical device DFSS project deliverables.

The roles and responsibilities of a champion in project execution is a vital dimension of successful deployment that needs to be iterated in the deployment communication plan. Champions should develop a teachable point of

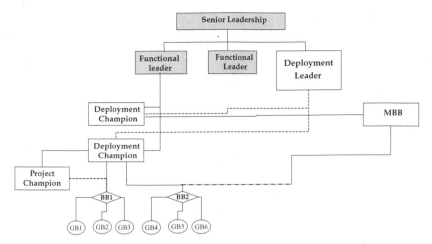

Figure 6.1   Suggested deployment structure.

view, "elevator speech," or resonant message. A suggested deployment structure is presented in Figure 6.1.

Design/Process Owners   This population of operatives comprises the owners of a process or design where DFSS project results and conclusions will be implemented. As the owners of a design entity and resources, their buy-in is critical, and they must be engaged early in the process. In predeployment, they are overwhelmed with the initiative and wonder why a belt was assigned to fix their design or process. They need to be educated, consulted on project selection, and be made responsible for the implementation of project findings. They are tasked with the sustainment of project gains by tracking project success metrics after full implementation. Typically, they should serve as team members on the project, participate in reviews, and push the team to find permanent innovative solutions. In the deployment and postdeployment phases, process owners should be the first in line to staff their projects with green and black belts.

Master Black Belts   A medical device master black belt (MBB) should possess expert knowledge of the full six sigma tool kit, including proven experience with DFSS. As a full-time assignment, he or she will also have experience in training, mentoring, and coaching black belts, green belts, champions, and leaders. MBBs are ambassadors for the business and the DFSS initiative, people who will be able to go to work in a variety of business environments and with varying scales of six sigma penetration. An MBB is a leader with good command of statistics as well as the practical ability to apply six sigma in an optimal manner for a company. An MBB should be adaptable to deployment phase requirements. Some businesses trust MBBs with the management of large projects relative to deployment and objective achievements. They also need to get involved with project champions relative to project scoping, and coach the senior teams at each key function.

Black Belts   Black belts[1] are a critical deployment resource, as they initiate projects, apply medical device DFSS tools and principles, and close them with tremendous benefits. Selected for technical proficiency, interpersonal skills, and leadership ability, a black belt is a person who solves difficult business issues for the last time. Typically, black belts have a life of a couple of years in the deployment phase. Nevertheless, their effect as disciples of medical device DFSS when they finish their DFSS life (postdeployment for them) and move on as the next generation of leaders cannot be trivialized. It is recommended that a fixed population of green and black belts (usually computed as a percentage of the functions affected when medical device DFSS is deployed) be kept in the pool during the deployment life designated. This population is not static, however; it is kept replenished every year by new blood. Repatriated black belts, in turn, replenish the disciple population, and the cycle continues until sustainment is achieved: that is, until medical device DFSS becomes the way of doing design business.

Black belts will learn and understand DFSS methodologies and principles and find application opportunities within a project, cultivate a network of experts, train and assist others (e.g., green belts) in new strategies and tools, leverage surface business opportunities through partnerships, and drive concepts and methodology into the way that work is done.

The deployment of black belts is a subprocess within the deployment process itself, with the following steps: (1) black belt identification, (2) black belt project scoping, (3) black belt training, (4) black belt deployment during the medical device life, and (5) black belt repatriation into the mainstream.

The deployment team prepares designated training waves or classes of medical device black belts to apply DFSS and associated technologies, methods, and tools on scoped projects. Black belts are developed by project execution, training in statistics and design principles with on-the-project application, and mentored reviews. Typically, with a targeted quick cycle time, a black belt should be able to close at least three projects a year. Our observations indicate that black belt productivity, on average, increases after their training, following which black belt projects can get more complex and evolve into cross-function, supply chain, and customer projects.

The black belts are the leaders of the future. Their visibility should be apparent to the rest of the organization, and they should be chosen to join the DFSS program with "leader of the future" stature. Armed with the right tools, processes, and DFSS principles, black belts are the change-agent network that

---

[1]Although black belts are deployment supportive persons who could have been included in the preceding section, we chose to separate them in a separate section, due to the significance of their role.

the deploying company should utilize to achieve its vision and mission statements. They need to be motivated and recognized for their good efforts while being mentored at both the technical and leadership fronts by the master black belt (MBB) and the project champions. Oral and written presentation skills are crucial to their success. To increase the effectiveness of the black belts, we suggest building a black belt collaboration mechanism for the purpose of maintaining structures and environments to foster individual and collective learning of the initiative and DFSS knowledge, including direction, vision, and prior history. In addition, the collaboration mechanism, whether virtual or physical, could serve as a focus for black belt activities to foster team building, growth, and inter- and intrafunction communication and collaboration. Another important reason for establishing such a mechanism is to ensure that the deployment team gets accurate and timely information, to prevent and mitigate failure modes downstream from the deployment and postdeployment phases. Historical knowledge might include lessons learned, best practices sharing, and deployment benchmarking data.

Green Belts   A green belt is an employee of a deploying company who has been trained on six sigma and will participate on project teams as part of his or her full-time job. Green belt penetration of knowledge and six sigma skills is less than that of a black belt. A green belt's knowledge of the company must be thorough to ensure success of his or her process improvement task. Green belt employees play important roles in executing the six sigma process through day-to-day operations by completing smaller scope projects. Black belts should be networked around green belts to support and coach green belts. Green belt training is not for awareness; the deployment plan should enforce certification while tracking their project status as control mechanisms over deployment. Like black belts, green belts should be closing projects as well.

Green belts are thus employees trained in six sigma methodologies who are conducting or contributing to a project that requires six sigma application. Following successful completion of training, green belts will be able to participate in larger projects being conducted by a black belt, lead small projects, and apply six sigma tools and concepts to their daily work.

Deployment Operative Roles Summary   The roles and responsibilities of the deployment operatives presented in this section may be summarized as follows:

- Project champions
  - Manage projects across the company.
  - Approve the resources.
  - Remove the barriers.
  - Create vision.

- Master black belts
  - Review the project status.
  - Teach tools and methodology.
  - Assist the champion.
  - Develop local deployment plans.
- Black belts
  - Train their teams.
  - Apply the methodology and lead projects.
  - Drive projects to completion.
- Green belts
  - Same responsibilities as those of black belts (but done in conjunction with other full-time job responsibilities).
- Project teams
  - Implement process improvements.
  - Gather data.

Figure 6.2 depicts the growth curve of six sigma deployment operatives. It is the responsibility of the deployment team to shape the duration and slopes of growth curves subject to the deployment plan. The pool of black belts is replenished periodically. The 1% rule (i.e., one black belts per 100 employees) has been adopted by several successful deployments. The number of MBBs is a fixed percentage of the black belt population. Current practice ranges from 10 to 20 black belts per MBB.

Communication Plan   To ensure the success of medical device DFSS, the deployment team should develop a communication plan that highlights the key steps as DFSS is being deployed. In doing so, they should target

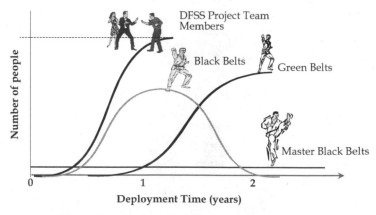

Figure 6.2   Deployment operatives growth curves.

the audiences that will receive necessary communication at various points in the deployment process through the media of communication deemed most effective by the company. The deployment team should outline the overriding communication objectives at each major phase of DFSS deployment and provide a high-level communications plan for each of the communicators identified during company DFSS initialization.

As DFSS is deployed in a medical device company, we recommend that various people communicate certain messages at certain relative times. For example, at the outset of deployment, the CEO should send a strong message to all executives that the corporation is adopting DFSS, why it is necessary, who will be leading the effort at the leadership and deployment team levels, why their commitment and involvement are absolutely required, and other important items. Among other communiqués sent to other audiences, the CEO sends a message to the deployment champions explaining why they have been chosen, what is expected of them, and how they are empowered to enact their respective roles and responsibilities.

As DFSS is initialized, deployed, and sustained, several key people will need to communicate key messages to key audiences: for example, the training and development leader, finance leader, human resources leader, IT leader, project champions, deployment champions (functional leaders), mangers and supervisors, and black belts and green belts, to name a few. To avoid derailment, every leader involved in the DFSS process must believe in the cause. As the principal communicators, leaders must believe completely if they are to enable the cultural evolution driven by DFSS. Every leader must seek out information from the deployment team to validate their conviction as to the value of the process.

To assist further in achieving effective communications, everyone responsible for communicating DFSS deployment should delineate who delivers messages to whom during the predeployment period. It is obvious that certain people have primary communication responsibility during the initial stages of six sigma deployment, including the CEO, the DFSS deployment leader, and the deployment champions. The company communications leader plays a role in supporting the CEO, deployment leader, and other leaders as they formulate and deliver their communiqués in support of predeployment. The communication plan should include the following minimum communiqués:

- Why the company is deploying DFSS, along with several key points about how six sigma supports and is integrated with the company's vision, including other business initiatives

- A set of financial targets, operational goals, and metrics that will provide structure and guidance to DFSS deployment effort; to be done with the discretion of the targeted audience

- A breakdown of where DFSS will be focused within the company; a rollout sequence by function, geography, product, or other scheme; a general time frame for how quickly and aggressively DFSS will be deployed

- A firmly established and supported long-term commitment to the DFSS philosophy, methodology, and anticipated results
- Specific managerial guidelines to control the scope and depth of deployment for the corporation or function
- Reviews and interrogates key performance metrics to ensure the progressive utilization and deployment of DFSS
- Commitment of part- and full-time deployment champions, a project champion, and full-time black belt resources

Medical Device DFSS Project Sources   Successful deployment of the DFSS initiative within a company is tied to projects derived from the company's break-through objectives, multigeneration planning, growth and innovation strategy, and chronic pressing redesign issues exposed through the corrective action/preventive action (CAPA) process. Such DFSS project sources can be categorized as retroactive and proactive sources. In either case, an active measurement system should be in place for both internal and external critical-to-satisfaction (CTS) metrics, sometimes called "big Y's." The measurement system should pass a gauge R&R study in all big Y metrics. How to define big Y's? This question underscores why we need to determine, as early as possible, the primary customer (internal and external) of our potential DFSS project. What is the big Y (CTS) in customer terms? It does us no good, for example, to develop a delivery system to shorten delivery processes if the customer is upset primarily with quality and reliability. Similarly, it does us little good to develop a project to reduce tool breakage if the customer is actually upset about inventory cycle losses. It pays dividends, later, to project success to know the big Y's. No big Y (CTS) means simply no project! Potential projects with hazy big Y definitions are setups for belt failure. Again, it is unacceptable not to know the big Y's of top problems (retroactive project sources such as the corrective side of CAPA) or those of proactive project sources (the preventive side of CAPA plus projects launched for innovation and growth) aligned with the annual objectives, growth and innovation strategy, benchmarking, and multigeneration product planning and technology road maps.

On the proactive side, black belts will be claiming projects from a multigenerational medical device/process plan or from the big Y replenished prioritized project pipeline. Green belts should be clustered around these key projects for the deploying function or business operations and tasked with assisting the black belts, as suggested by Figure 6.3.

We need some useful measure of the big Y's, in *variable terms*,[2] to establish the transfer function, $Y = f(y)$. The transfer function is a means for dialing

---

[2]The transfer function will be weak and questionable without it.

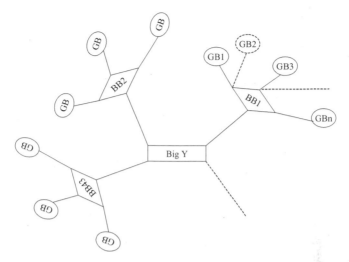

Figure 6.3 Green belt (GB) and black belt (BB) clustering scheme.

customer satisfaction, or other big Y's, and can be identified by a combination of design mapping and design of experiment (if transfer functions are unavailable or cannot be derived). A transfer function is a mathematical relationship in the design mapping that links controllable and uncontrollable factors. Transfer functions can be derived, obtained empirically from a design of experiments, or regressed using historical data. In some cases, no closed mathematical formula can be obtained and the DFSS team can resort to modeling. In our DFSS project road map, there is a transfer function for every functional requirement, for every design parameter, for every process variable, and ultimately for every big Y.

Sometimes we find that measurement of the big Y's opens windows to the mind with insights powerful enough to solve a problem immediately. It is not rare to find customer complaints that are very subjective or unmeasured. The black belt needs to find the best measure available to his or her project big Y to help describe the variation faced and to support $Y = f(x)$ analysis. The black belt may have to develop a measuring system for the project to be true to the customer and the big Y definition!

We need measurements of the big Y that we trust. Studying problems with false measurements leads to frustration and defeat. With variable measurements, the issue is handled as a straightforward gauge R&R question. With attribute or other subjective measures, it is an attribute measurement system analysis (MSA) issue. It is tempting to ignore MSA of the big Y, but that is not a safe practice. More that 50% of the black belts that we coached encountered MSA problems in their projects. This issue in big Y measurement is probably worse because little thought is conventionally given to MSA at the customer level. Black belts should make every effort to assure themselves that their big Y's measurement is error-minimized. We need to be able to establish a distribution of Y from which to model or draw samples for $Y = f(x)$ study. The better the measurement of the Big Y, the better the black belt can see the distribution contrasts needed to yield or confirm the $Y = f(x)$ study.

What is the value to the customer? This should be a mute point if the project is a top issue, as the value decisions have already been made. *Value* is a relative term with numerous meanings. It may be cost, or appearance, or status, but the currency of value must be decided. It is a common practice in six sigma to ask that each project generate benefits (on average) greater than $250,000. This is seldom a problem in top projects that are aligned with business issues and opportunities.

The black belt, together with the financial personnel assigned to the project, should decide in a value standard and do a final check for potential project value greater than the minimum. High-value projects are not necessarily more difficult than low-value projects to carry out. Projects usually hide their level of complexity until solved. Many low-value projects are just as difficult as high-value projects to complete, so the deployment champions should leverage their effort by value. Deployment management, including the local master black belt, has the lead in identifying redesign problems and opportunities as good potential projects. However, the task of going from a potential to an assigned six sigma project belongs to the project champion. A deployment champion selects a project champion, who then carries out the next phases. The champion is responsible for the project scope, black belt assignment, ongoing project review, and ultimately, the success of the project and the black belt assigned. This is an important and responsible position and must be taken very seriously. A suggested project initiation process is depicted in Figure 6.4.

It is a significant piece of work to develop a good project, but black belts, particularly those already certified, have a unique perspective that can be of great assistance to the project champions. Green belts, as well, should be taught fundamental skills useful in developing a project scope. Black and green belt engagement is key to help champions fill the project pipeline, investigate potential projects, prioritize them, and develop achievable project scopes (albeit with stretched targets). It is the observation of many skilled problem solvers that defining the problem adequately and setting up a solution strategy consumes the most time on the path to a successful project. The better we define and scope a project, the faster the deploying company and its customer base benefit from a solution! That is the primary six sigma objective.

It is the responsibility of management, deployment champions, and project champions, with the help of the design/process owner, to identify both retroactive and proactive sources of DFSS projects that are important enough to assign the company's limited valuable resources to find a six sigma solution. Managers are the caretakers of the business objectives and goals. They set policy, allocate funds and resources, and provide the personnel necessary to carry out the business of the company. Individual black belts may contribute to building a project pipeline, but it is entirely management's responsibility.

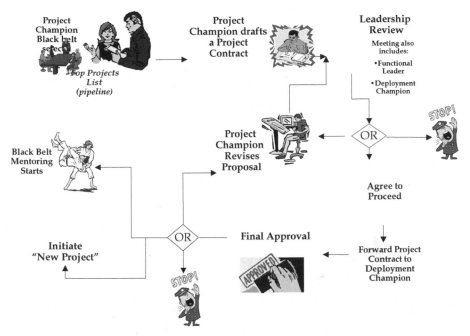

Figure 6.4 Project initiation process.

It is expected that an actual list of projects will always exist and be replenished frequently as new information or policy directions emerge. Sources of information from which to populate the list include all retroactive sources, support systems such as a field corrective action system, a CAPA system, as internal manufacturing and production systems related to problematic metrics such as scrap and rejects, customer repairs/complaints database, and many others. In short, the information comes from the strategic vision and annual objectives, multigeneration medical device plans, from voice-of-the-customer surveys or other engagement methods, and from the daily business of deployment champions, and it is their responsibility to approve what gets into the project pipeline and what does not. In general, medical device DFSS projects usually come from processes that have reached their ultimate capability (entitlement) and are still problematic, or from those targeting new products presently nonexistent.

In the case of retroactive sources, projects derive from problems that champions agree need solution. Project levels can be reached by applying the "five why" technique (see Figure 6.5) to dig into root causes prior to assignment of a black belt.

A scoped project will always give the black belt a good starting ground and reduce the identify phase cycle time within the ICOV DFSS approach (Yang and El-Haik, 2003). They must prioritize because the process of going from a potential project to a properly scoped black belt project requires significant

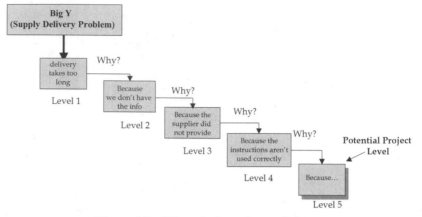

Figure 6.5   "Five why" scoping technique.

work and commitment. There is no business advantage in spending valuable time and resources on something with a low priority. A typical company scorecard may include metrics relative to safety, quality, delivery, cost, and environment. We accept these as big sources (buckets), yet each category has a myriad of its own problems and opportunities to drain resources quickly if champions do not prioritize. Fortunately, the Pareto principle applies, so we can find leverage in the significant few. It is important to assess each of the buckets to the 80–20 principles of Pareto. In this way, the many are reduced to a significant few that still control over 80% of the problems in question. These need review and renewal by management routinely as the business year unfolds. The top project list emerges from this as a living document.

From the individual bucket Pareto lists, champions must again give us their business insight to plan an effective attack on the top issues. Given key business objectives, they must look across the several Pareto diagrams, using the 80–20 principle, and again sift through until we have a few top issues that have the biggest impact on the business. If the champions identify their biggest problem elements well, based on management business objectives and the Pareto principle, how could any manager or supervisor refuse to commit resources to achieving a solution? Solving any problems but these gives only marginal improvement.

Resource planning for black belts, green belts, and other personnel is visible and simplified when they are assigned to top projects on the list. Opportunities to assign other personnel, such as project team members, are clear in this context. Your local deployment champion and/or master black belt needs to manage the list. Always remember: A project focused on the top problems is worth a lot to a business. All possible effort must be exerted to scope problems and opportunities into projects that black belts can drive to a six sigma solution. The process steps shown in Figure 6.6 help us turn a problem into a scoped project.

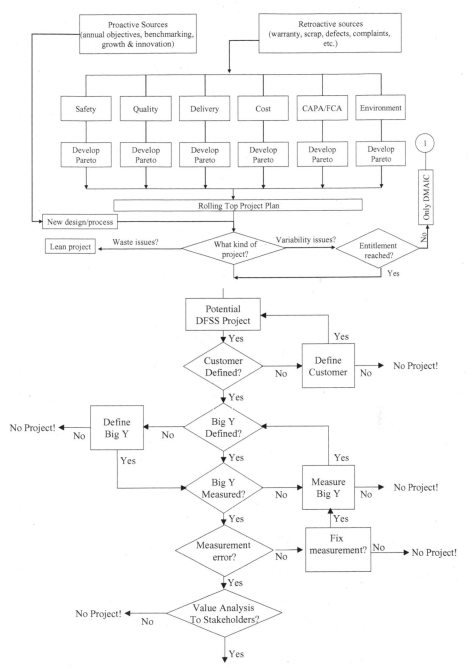

Figure 6.6 Six sigma project identification and scoping process.

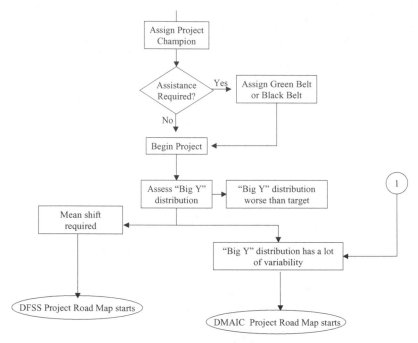

Figure 6.6 *Continued*

A critical step in the process is to define the customer. This is not a matter that can be taken lightly! How can we satisfy customers, either internal or external to the business, if the MBB is not sure who they are? The MBB and his team must know the customers so as to understand their needs, delights, and satisfiers. Never guess or assume what your customers need—ask them. Several customer interaction methods are described in the next chapters. For example, the customer of a medical device project on improving company image is the buyer of the device, the consumer. On the other hand, if the potential project is to reduce tool breakage in a manufacturing process, the buyer is too far removed to be the primary customer. Here the customer is more likely to be the process owner or other business unit manager. Certainly, if we reduce tool breakage, we gain efficiency that may translate to cost or availability satisfaction, but this is of little help in planning a good project to reduce tool breakage.

No customer, no project! Know your customer. It is unacceptable, however, not to know your customer in the top project pipeline. These projects are too important to allow this type of lapse.

Proactive DFSS Project Sources: Multigenerational Planning   A multigenerational plan is concerned with developing timely design evolution of a medical device and for finding optimal resource allocation. An acceptable plan must be capable of dealing with uncertainty about the future market and the availability of medical devices when demanded by the customer. Product generational planning is the responsibility of people handling R&D or core technology development. The incorporation of uncertainty into a resource-planning model of a medical device multigenerational plan is essential. For example, on the personal financial side, it was not that long ago that a family was only three generations deep: grandparent, parent, and child. But as life expectancies have increased, four generations are now common, and five generations are no longer unheard of. The financial impact of this demographic change has been dramatic. Instead of a family focused only on its own finances, it may have to deal with financial issues that cross generations. Where once people lived only a few years into retirement, now they live 30 years or more. If the parents can not take care of themselves, or can not afford to pay for high-cost, long-term care either at home or in a facility, their children may need to step forward. A host of financial issues are involved, such as passing on the estate, business succession, college versus retirement, life insurance, and loaning money. These are only a smattering of the many multigenerational financial issues that may arise. Now you can extend this thinking to medical device multigenerational planning.

Medical device design requires multigenerational planning that takes into consideration demand growth and the level of coordination in planning and resource allocation among functions within a company. The plan should take into consideration uncertainties in demand and technology and other factors by means of defining strategic design generations, which reflect gradual and realistic possible evolutions of the medical device of interest. Decision analysis framework needs to be incorporated in order to quantify and minimize risks for all design generations. Advantages associated with generational design in mitigating risks, financial support, economies of scale, and reductions of operating costs are key incentives for growth and innovation.

The main step is to produce generational plans for medical device design CTSs and functional requirements or other metrics with an assessment of uncertainties around achieving them. One key aspect for defining the generation is to split the plan into periods where flexible generations can be decided. The beginning of generational periods may coincide with milestones or relevant events. For each period, a generational plan provides an assessment of how each generation should perform against an adopted set of metrics. Figure 6.7 depicts a multigenerational plan that lays out the key metrics and the enabling technologies by a time horizon for a generic device.

Training To jump-start the deployment process, DFSS training is usually outsourced in the first years of deployment. The deployment team needs to devise a qualifying scheme for training vendors once their strategy is finalized and approved by the senior leadership of the company. Specific training

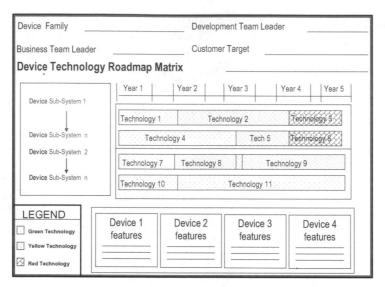

Figure 6.7 Generic multigenerational product plan.

session content for executive leadership, champions, and green and black belts should be planned with heavy participation by the vendor selected. This facilitates a coordinated effort, allowing better management of the training schedule and a more prompt medical device. In this section, simple guidelines for training deployment champions, project champions, and any others whose scope of responsibility intersects with the training function need to be discussed. Attendance is required all day of each day of training. To get the full benefit of the training course, each attendee needs to be present for all of the material that is conveyed. Each training course should be developed carefully and condensed into the shortest possible period by the vendor. Missing any part of a course will result in diminished understanding of the topics covered, and as a result, may severely delay the progression of projects.

Medical Device Program Development Management System Our experience is that a project road map is required for successful DFSS deployment. The road map works as a compass leading green and black belts to closure by laying out the full picture of DFSS project. We would like to think of the road map as a recipe that can be further tailored to a customized application within the company's management system that spans the design life cycle (see Chapter 1). Usually, the DFSS deployment team encounters two venues at this point. The first is to develop a new product development process[3] (PDP) to include

---

[3]For example, advanced product quality planning in the automotive industry, integrated product and process design in the aerospace industry, project management institute process, and James Martin in the software industry.

the DFSS road map proposed. It is the experience of the authors that many companies lack such universal discipline in a practical sense. This venue is suitable for such companies and those practicing a variety of PDPs hoping that alignment will evolve. The PDP should span the medical device life cycle presented in Chapter 1. The second venue is to integrate with the current PDP by laying this road map over and to synchronize when and where needed.

In either case, the DFSS project will be paced at the speed of the leading program from which the project was derived in the PDP. Initially, high-leverage projects should target subsystems to which the business and the customer are sensitive. A sort of requirement flow-down, a cascading method, should be adopted to identify the subsystems. Later, when DFSS becomes the way of doing business, system-level DFSS deployment becomes the norm, and the issue of synchronization with the PDP will eventually diminish. Actually, the PDP will be crafted to reflect the DFSS learning experience that the company has gained over years of experience.

6.4 DEPLOYMENT PHASE

This phase is the period of time when champions are trained and initial belt projects selected, as well as when the initial wave of black belts are trained and projects are completed that yield a significant operational benefit from both soft and hard types. The training encompasses most of the deployment activities in this phase, and it is discussed in the following section. Additionally, this phase includes the following assignment of the deployment team:

- Reiterate to key personnel their responsibilities at critical points in the deployment process.
- Reinforce the commitment among project champions and black belts to execute selected improvement projects aggressively. Mobilize and empower both populations to carry out their respective roles and responsibilities effectively.
- Recognize exemplary performance in execution and in culture at the project champion and black belt levels.
- Inform the general employee population about the tenets of six sigma and the deployment process.
- Build information packets for project champions and black belts that contain administrative, logistical, and other information that they need to execute their responsibilities at given points in time.
- Document and publicize successful projects and the positive consequences for the company and its employees.
- Document and distribute project savings data by business unit, product, or other appropriate area of focus.

- Hold six sigma events or meetings with all employees at given locations where leadership is present and involved and where such topics are covered.

6.4.1 Training

The critical steps in DFSS training are (1) determining the content and outline, (2) developing the materials, and (3) deploying training classes. In doing so, the deployment team and their training vendor of choice should be very cautious about cultural aspects and careful to weave into the soft side of the culture change into training. Training is the significant mechanism within deployment that in addition to equipping trainees with the right tools, concepts, and methods will expedite deployment and help shape a data-driven culture. In this section we present a high-level perspective of the training recipients and the type of training they should receive. They are arranged below by level of complexity.

Senior Leadership   Training for senior leadership should include an overview, business and financial benefits of implementation, benchmarking of successful deployments, motivation systems, and specific training on tools to ensure successful implementation.

Deployment Champions   Training for deployment champions is more detailed than that provided to senior leadership. Topics include the DFSS concept, methodology, and "must-have" tools and processes to ensure successful deployment within their functions. A class focused on how to be an effective champion as well as on their roles and responsibilities is often beneficial.

Master Black Belts   Initially, experienced master black belts (MBBs) are hired from the outside to jump-start the system. Additional homegrown MBBs may need to go to additional training beyond their black belt training. Training for MBBs must be rigorous about the concept, methodology and tools, as well as detailed statistics training, computer analysis, and other tool application. Their training should include soft and hard skills to get them to a level of proficiency compatible with their roles. On the soft side, topics such as strategy, deployment lesson learned, their roles and responsibilities, presentation and writing skills, leadership and resource management, and critical success factors benchmarking history and outside deployment. On the hard side, typical training may go into the theory of topics such as DOE and ANOVA, axiomatic design, theory of inventive problem solving (TIPS or TRIZ), hypothesis testing of discrete random variables, and lean tools.

Black Belts   The black belts as project leaders will implement the DFSS methodology and tools within a function on projects aligned with the business objectives. They lead projects, institutionalize a timely project plan, determine appropriate tool use, perform analyses, and act as the central point of contact for their projects. Training for black belts includes detailed information about the concept, methodology, and tools. Depending on the curriculum, the duration is usually between three and six weeks on a monthly schedule. Black belts will come with a training-focused scoped project that has an ample opportunity for tool application to foster learning while delivering to deployment objectives. The weeks between the training sessions will be spent on gathering data, forming and training their teams, and applying concepts and tools where necessary. DFSS concepts and tools in conjunction with some soft skills from the core of the curriculum. Of course, DFSS training and deployment will be synchronous with the medical device development process adopted by the deploying company. In Chapter 7 we provide a suggested medical device DFSS project road map serving as a design algorithm for a six sigma team. The road map will work as a compass, leading black belts to closure by laying out the full picture of a typical DFSS project.

Green Belts   Where there needs to be more focus, green belts may take training courses developed specifically for black belts. Short-circuiting theory and complex tools to meet the allocated short training time (usually less than 50% of the black belt training period) may dilute many subjects. Green belts can resort to the black belt network for help on complex subjects and for coaching and mentoring.

6.4.2   Project Financials

In general, DFSS project financials can be categorized as hard or soft savings and are mutually calculated or assessed by the black belt and the financial analyst assigned to the project. Generally, DFSS projects need to be assessed on an NPV basis, and the NPV has to include after-launch support costs. The emphasis on hard savings results in a portfolio of smaller-return six sigma projects as opposed to higher-return DFSS projects. The finance analyst assigned to a DFSS team should act as the lead in quantifying the financials related to project "actions" at the initiation and closure phases, assist in identification of "hidden factory" savings, support the black belt on an ongoing basis, and if financial information is required from areas outside his or her area of expertise, he or she needs to direct the black belt to the appropriate contacts, to followup, and to ensure that the black belt receives the appropriate data. At project closure, the analyst should ensure that the appropriate stakeholders concur with the savings. This affects primarily processing costs, design expense, and nonrevenue items for rejects not led directly by black belts from those organizations. In essence, the analyst needs to provide more than an audit function.

Hard savings are defined as measurable savings associated with improvements in repairs, rework, absorptions, write-offs, concessions, inspection, material cost, warranty, labor savings (will be achieved and collectable through work rebalances), revenue associated with reductions in customer dissatisfaction, cash flow savings (i.e., inventory), and other values of lost customer satisfaction. Hard savings are calculated against present operating levels, not against a budget or a plan. They represent the bottom-line savings that directly affects the company's income statement and cash flow, and are the results of measurable medical device and process improvements. The effect on company financial statements will be determined off-line by the appropriate company office. *Soft savings* are less direct in nature, and include projects that open floor space (as a side benefit) to allow for the location of future operations and projects that reduce vehicle weight to enable other design actions to delete expensive lightweight materials and cost avoidance. Cost avoidance is usually confused with cost savings. For example, employing software instead of an operator to collect real-time data to reduce operating cost is avoidance rather than saving.

The financial analyst should work with the black belt to assess the projected annual financial savings based on the information available at that time (e.g., scope, expected outcome). This is not a detailed review but a rough order-of-magnitude approval. These estimates are expected to be revised as the project progresses and more accurate data become available. The project should have the potential to achieve the annual target. The analyst confirms the business rationale for the project where necessary.

Yang and El-Haik (2003) developed a scenario of black belt target cascading that can be customized to different applications. It is based on project cycle time, the number of projects handled simultaneously by the black belt, and their importance to the organization.

6.5   POSTDEPLOYMENT PHASE

This phase spans the period of time when subsequent waves of black belts are trained, when the synergy and scale of six sigma builds to a critical mass, and when additional elements of DFSS deployment are implemented and integrated. In what follows we present some of the thoughts and observations that have been gained through our deployment experience with six sigma and, in particular, DFSS. The purpose is to determine factors that will sustain keeping and expanding the momentum of DFSS deployment.

In this book we present the medical device DFSS methodology, which exhibits the merging of many tools at both the conceptual and analytical levels and penetrates dimensions such as conceptualization, optimization, and validation by integrating tools, principles, and concepts. This vision of DFSS is a core competency in a company's overall technology strategy to accomplish its goals. An evolutionary strategy that moves the deployment of DFSS method toward the ideal culture is discussed. In the strategy we have identified the critical elements, needed decisions, and deployment concerns.

The literature suggests that more innovative methods fail immediately after initial deployment than at any other stage. Useful innovation attempts that are challenged by cultural change are not terminated directly but allowed to fade slowly and silently. A major reason for the failure of technically feasible innovations is the inability of leadership to commit to an integrated, effective, and cost-justified evolutionary program for sustainability, which is consistent with the company's mission. In many aspects, the DFSS deployment parallels the technical innovation challenges from a cultural perspective. The DFSS initiatives are particularly vulnerable if they are too narrowly conceived, built on only one major success mechanism, or lack fit with the larger organizational objectives. The tentative top-down deployment approach has been working where the top leadership support should be the significant driver. However, this approach can be strengthened when built around much mechanisms as the superiority of DFSS as a design approach and the attractiveness of the methodologies to designers who want to become more proficient in their jobs.

Although there are needs to customize a deployment strategy, it should not be rigid. The strategy should be flexible enough to meet expected improvements. The deployment strategy itself should be DFSS driven and robust to anticipated changes. It should be insensitive to expected swings in the financial health of the company and should be attuned to the company's objectives on a continuous basis.

The strategy should consistently build coherent linkages between DFSS and daily design business. For example, engineers and architects need to see how all the principles and tools fit together, complement one another, and build toward a coherent, complete process. DFSS needs to be seen, initially, as an important part, if not the central core, of an overall effort to increase technical flexibility.

6.6 DFSS SUSTAINABILITY FACTORS

In our view, DFSS possesses many inherent sustaining characteristics that are not offered by current design practices. Many design methods, some called *best practices*, are effective if the design is at a low level of complexity and need to satisfy a minimum number of functional requirements (e.g., a component). As the number of requirements increases (i.e., the design becomes more complex), the efficiency of these methods decreases. In addition, these methods are hinged on heuristics and developed algorithms (e.g., design for manufacturability/assembly, design for packaging, design for reliability), limiting their application across the various development phases.

The process of design can be improved by constant deployment of DFSS, which begins from a different premise: namely, the principle of design. The design axioms and principles are central to the conception part of DFSS. As will be defined in Chapter 9, axioms are general principles or truths that cannot be derived except that there are no counterexamples or exceptions. Axioms are fundamental to many engineering disciplines, such as the laws of thermodynamics, Newton's laws, and the concepts of force and energy. Axiomatic design provides the principles to develop a good design systematically and can overcome the need for customized approaches.

In a sustainability strategy, the following attributes would be persistent and pervasive features:

- Developing a deployment measurement system to tracks the critical-to-deployment requirements and failure modes, and to implement corrective actions, with a parallel measurement system for the overall profitability or effectiveness of new product development
- Continued improvement in the effectiveness of DFSS deployment by benchmarking successful deployment elsewhere
- Enhanced control (over time) over the company's objectives via selected DFSS projects that really "move the needle"
- Extending involvement of all levels and functions
- Embedding DFSS into the everyday operations of the company

The prospectus for sustaining success will improve if the strategy yields a consistent day-to-day emphasis of recognizing that DFSS represents a cultural change and a paradigm shift and allow the time necessary for the project's success. In several deployment efforts it was found very useful to extend the DFSS initiative to key suppliers, and then beyond the component level to the subsystem and system levels. Some call these projects *interprojects* when they span different areas, functions, and business domains. Ultimately, this will lead to integrating the DFSS philosophy as a superior design approach within the product development process and aligning the issues of funding, timing, and reviews with the embedded philosophy. As an added bonus of the deployment, conformance to narrow design protocols will start fading away. In all cases, sustaining leadership and managerial commitment to adopting an appropriate, consistent, relevant, and continuing reward and recognition mechanism for black belts and green belts is critical to the overall sustainment of the initiative.

The vision is that DFSS as a consistent, complete, fully justified, and usable process should be expanded to other new areas. The deployment team should keep an eye on the changes that are needed to accommodate altering belt tasks from individualized projects to broader-scope intrateam assignments. A prioritizing mechanism for such future projects, which targets the location, size, complexity, involvement of other units, type of knowledge to be gained, and potential for fit within the strategic plan, should be developed.

Another sustaining factor lies in providing relevant on-time training and opportunities for competency enhancement of black and green belts. The capacity to continue learning and the alignment of rewards with competency and experience must be fostered. Instituting an accompanying accounting and financial evaluation that enlarges the scope of consideration of the impact of the project on both fronts' hard and soft savings is a lesson learned. To accommodate DFSS methodology, finance and other resources should be moving upfront toward the beginning of the design cycle.

If the DFSS approach is to become pervasive as a central culture underlying a development strategy, it must be linked to larger company objectives. In general, the DFSS methodology should be linked to:

1. The societal contribution of the company in terms of developing more reliable, efficient, environmentally friendly products, processes, and medical devices
2. The goals of the company, including profitability and sustainability in local and global markets
3. The explicit goals of management embodied in the company's mission statement, including such characteristics as greater design effectiveness, efficiency, cycle time reduction, responsiveness to customers, and the like
4. A greater capacity for the deploying company to adjust and respond to customers and competitive conditions
5. The satisfaction of mangers, supervisors, and designers

A deployment strategy is needed to sustain the momentum achieved in the deployment phase. The strategy should show how DFSS allows green and black belts and their teams to respond to a wide variety of externally induced challenges and that complete deployment of DFSS will fundamentally increase the yield of company operations and its ability to provide a wide variety of design responses. DFSS deployment should be a core competence of a company. DFSS will enhance the variety of quality-of-design entity and design processes. These two themes should be stressed continuously in strategy presentations to more senior leaders. As deployment proceeds, the structures and processes used to support deployment will also need to evolve. Several factors need to be considered to build the overall sustainability strategy. For example, the future strategy and plan for sustaining DFSS needs to incorporates more modern learning theory on the usefulness of the technique for green belts and other members at the time they need the information. On sustaining DFSS deployment, we suggest that the DFSS community (i.e., black belts, green belts, master black belts, champions, and deployment directors) commit to the following:

- Supporting their company image and mission as a highly motivated producer of choice of world-class, innovative, complete product, process, or medical device solutions that lead in quality and technology and that exceed customer expectations in satisfaction and value
- Taking pride in their work and in the contribution they make internally and externally
- Constantly pursuing the policy of doing it right the first time as a means of reducing the cost to their customers and the company
- Striving to be recognized as a resource that is vital to both current and future development programs and management of operations
- Establishing and fostering a partnership with subject matter experts, the technical community in their company
- Treating DFSS lessons learned as a corporate source of returns and savings through replicating solutions and processes in other relevant entities
- Promoting the use of DFSS principles, tools, and concepts where possible in both project and day-to-day operations and promote a data-driven decision culture, the crest of six sigma culture

6.7   BLACK BELTS AND THE DFSS TEAM: CULTURAL CHANGE

This first step is to create an environment of teamwork. One thing that the black belt will eventually learn is that team members have very different abilities, motivations, and personalities. For example, some team members will be pioneers and others will want to vanish. If black belts allow the latter behavior, they become dead weight and a source of frustration. The black belt must not allow this to happen. When team members vanish, it is not entirely their fault. For example, people who are introverted find it stressful to talk in a group. They like to think things through before they start talking. They consider others' feelings and do not find a way to participate. It is the extroverts' specific responsibility to include introverts, not talk over them, and not take the floor away from them. If the black belt wants the team to succeed, he or she has to accept that you must manage others actively. One of the first things the black belt should do is to make sure that every member knows every other member, beyond name recognition. It is important to have an idea as to what each person is good at and what resources he or she can bring to the project.

One thing to realize is that when teams are new, each person wonders about his or her identity within the team. Identity is a combination of personality, competencies, behavior, and position on the organization chart. The black belt needs to push for another dimension of identity: that is, belonging to the same team, with the DFSS project as the task on hand. Vision is, of course, a key. Besides the explicit DFSS project activities, what are the real project goals? A useful exercise, a deliverable, is to create a project charter, with a vision statement, to use among themselves and with the project stakeholders. The charter is basically a contract that says what the team is about, what their objectives are, what they are ultimately trying to accomplish, where to get resources, and what types of benefits will be gained as a return upon their investment upon closing the project. The best charters are usually those that synthesize from each member's input. A vision statement may also be useful. Each member should figure out what they think the team should accomplish, then together see if there are any common elements out of which they can build a single, coherent vision to which each person can commit. The reason that it is helpful to use common elements of member input is to capitalize on the common direction and to motivate the team going forward.

It is a critical step in a DFSS project endeavor to establish and maintain a DFSS project team that has a shared vision. Teamwork fosters the six sigma transformation and instills the culture of execution and pride. It is difficult for teams to succeed without a leader, the black belt, who should be equipped with several leadership qualities acquired by experience and training. It is a fact that there will be team functions to be performed and that he or she can do all of them or split up the job among pioneer thinkers within the team. One key function is that of facilitator. The black belt will call meetings, keep members on track, and pay attention to team dynamics. As a facilitator, the black belt makes sure that the team focuses on the project, ensures participation from all members, prevents personal attacks, suggests alternative procedures when the team is stalled, and summarizes and clarifies the team's decisions. In doing so, the black belt should stay neutral until the data start speaking, and stop any meeting from running too long, even if it's going well, or people may avoid coming next time. Another key function is that of liaison. The black belt will serve as liaison between the team and the project stakeholders for most of the work in progress. Finally, there is the project management function. As manger of a DFSS project, the black belt organizes the project plan and sees that it is implemented. He or she needs to be able to take a whole project task and break it down into scoped and bounded activities with crisp deliverables to be handed out to team members as assignments. The black belt has to be able to budget time and resources and get members to execute their assignments at the right time.

Team meetings can be very useful if done right. One simple thing that helps a lot is having an updated agenda. Having a written agenda, the black belt will make it useful for the team to steer things back to the project activities and assignments, the compass.

There will be many situations in which the black belt needs to give feedback to other team members. It is extremely important to avoid any negative comment that would seem to be about the member rather than about the work or the behavior. It is very important that teams assess their performance from time to time. Most teams have good starts and then drift away from their original goals and eventually collapse. This is much less likely to happen if from time to time the black belt asks everyone how they are feeling about the team, and takes a "performance pulse" of the team against the project charter. It is just as important to the black belt to *maintain* the team to improve its performance continuously. This function is therefore an ongoing effort throughout the project's full cycle.

The DFSS teams emerge and grow through systematic efforts to foster continuous learning, shared direction, interrelationships, and a balance between intrinsic motivators (a desire that comes from within) and extrinsic motivators (a desire stimulated by external actions). Winning is usually contagious. Successful DFSS teams foster other teams. Growing synergy arises from ever-increasing numbers of motivated teams and accelerates improvement throughout the deploying company. The payback for small up-front investment in team performance can be enormous.

DFSS deployment will shake many guarded and old paradigms. People's reaction to change varies from denial to pioneering, passing through many stages. In this venue the objective of the black belt is to develop alliances for his or her efforts as he or she progresses.

What about six sigma culture? What we are finding powerful in cultural transformation is the premise that the company results wanted represents the culture wanted. Leadership must first identify objectives that the company must achieve. These objectives must be defined carefully so that other elements, such as employee beliefs, behaviors, and actions, support them. A company has certain initiatives and actions that must be maintained in order to achieve the new results. But to achieve six sigma results, certain things must be stopped while others must be started (e.g., deployment). These changes will cause a behavioral shift that people must make for the six sigma cultural transition to evolve. True behavior change will not occur, let alone last, unless there is an accompanying change in leadership and deployment team belief. Beliefs are powerful in that they dictate action plans that produce desired results. Successful deployment benchmarking (initially) and experiences (later) determine the beliefs, and beliefs motivate actions, so ultimately, leaders must create experiences that foster beliefs in people. The bottom line is that for a six sigma data-driven culture to be achieved, the company cannot operate with the old set of actions, beliefs, and experiences; otherwise, the results it gets are the results that it is currently having. Experiences, beliefs, and actions—these have to change.

The biggest significant element in the culture of a company is the initiative of the founders themselves, starting from the top. The new culture is then maintained by the employees once the transition is complete—they keep it alive. Leaders set up structures (deployment team) and processes (deployment plan) that consciously perpetuate the culture. A new culture includes both a new identity and a new direction, the DFSS way.

In implementing large-scale change through six sigma deployment, a company identifies and understands the key characteristics of the current culture. Together with the deployment team, leaders then develop the six sigma culture characteristics and a deployment plan for how to get there. Companies with great internal conflicts or with accelerated changes in business strategy are advised to move with more caution in deployment.

Several topics that are vital to deployment success should be considered from a cultural standpoint, such as:

- Elements of cultural change in the deployment plan
- The amount of resistance
- Ways to handle change resistance relative to the culture
- The types of leaders and leadership needed at different points in the deployment effort
- How to communicate effectively when very little is certain initially
- The readiness to change and maturity measurement or assessment

A common agreement between senior leadership and the deployment team should be achieved on major deployment priorities and timing relative to cultural transformation and those areas where further work is needed to reach consensus.

At the team level, there are several strategies that a black belt could use to his or her advantage in order to deal with team change. To help reconcile much change, the black belt needs to listen with empathy, acknowledge difficulties, and define what is out of scope and what is not. To help stop the old paradigm and reorient the team to the DFSS paradigm, the belt should encourage redefinition, utilize management to provide structure and strength, rebuild a sense of identity, gain a sense of control and influence, and encourage opportunities for creativity. To help recommit the team in the new paradigm, the black belt should reinforce the new beginning, provide a clear purpose, develop a detailed plan, be consistent in the spirit of six sigma, and celebrate success.

6.8 SUMMARY

In this chapter we cover the medical device design for six sigma process as a disciplined methodology supported by the deployment team who will launch the design for six sigma program as an objective. Along with that we present a high-level perspective of a sound plan by outlining the critical elements of a successful deployment. The deployment process is categorized, in terms of evolution time, into three phases: a predeployment phase to build the infra-structure; a deployment phase, where most of activities will happen; and a postdeployment phase, where sustainment needs to be made a reality. Finally, the deployment process phases structure is discussed in detail together with roles and responsibilities.

7

MEDICAL DEVICE DFSS PROJECT ROAD MAP

7.1 INTRODUCTION

This chapter is written primarily to present the DFSS project road map to support the black belt and his or her team and the functional champion in the project execution mode of deployment. The design project is the core of DFSS deployment and has to be executed consistently using a road map that lays out the DFSS principles, tools, and methods within a chosen gated design process (see Section 5.4). From a high-level perspective, this road map provides the immediate details required for a smooth and successful DFSS deployment experience.

Figure 7.1 depicts the road map proposed. The road map objective is to develop six sigma–level medical devices with unprecedented level of fulfillment of customer wants, needs, and delights for its total life cycle (see Section 1.3).

The DFSS road map has four phases: identify, characterize, optimize, and verify/validate (ICOV) in seven developmental stages (see Chapter 5). In addition, Chapter 2 presents those stages in the context of regulations and design controls. While FDA regulations could have been included in this chapter together with the DFSS methodology technical project deliverables, we elected to present it in a stand-alone chapter to highlight its importance. An ICOV phase may contain more that one stage of the development life cycle depicted in Figure 2.3. Stages are separated by milestones called *tollgates* (see the glossary).

Medical Device Design for Six Sigma: A Road Map for Safety and Effectiveness,
By Basem S. El-Haik and Khalid S. Mekki
Copyright © 2008 John Wiley & Sons, Inc.

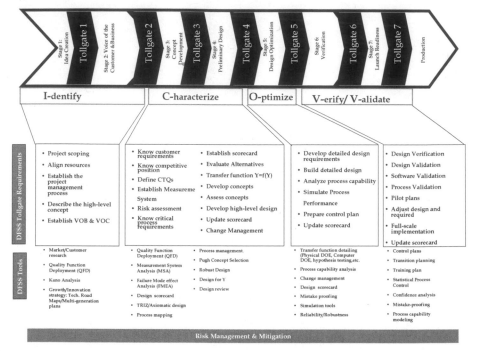

Figure 7.1   DFSS project road map.

The verify/validate phase of the DFSS ICOV process has a dual meaning in the context of the medical device industry. It encompasses design verification, software validation and design, and process validation activities. As noted in Chapter 1, FDA regulations differentiate between activities that *verify and validate* a design versus activities that *validate* the manufacturing process (Chapter 17).

As the device design matures, design transfer becomes more prominent. In DFSS it is a common practice for sections and modules of a design to be transferred before the entire device is completed, with the caveats that transfer is to be performed only for completed elements of the design device, and multiple transfers may not be used to bypass design, labeling, or other requirements. The DFSS design transfer procedure needed to cover the generation of device master record documents based on information in the design output documents is given in Chapter 18.

Coupled with design principles and tools, the objective of this chapter is to mold all DFSS elements in a comprehensive implementable sequence in a manner that enables deployment companies to systematically achieve desired benefits from executing projects. In Figure 7.1 a *design stage* constitutes a collection of design activities and can be bounded by entrance and exit tollgates. A tollgate represents a milestone in the product development cycle and has some formal meaning defined by the company's own development process coupled with management decision-making events for budget and resources, team recognition, and support function involvement. The ICOV process depicted in this chapter design need not be adopted blindly, but customized to reflect synchronization with company's own medical device development process and its DFSS deployment objective.

Generally, the life cycle of a medical device starts with some form of idea generation, whether in a free invention format or using a more disciplined format, such as multigenerational medical device planning and growth strategy.

Prior to starting on the DFSS road map, the black belt team needs to understand the rationale of the project. We advise that they assure the feasibility of advancing the project by validating the project scope, the project charter, and the project resource plan. A session with the champion is advised to take place once the black belt and the project charter have been matched. The objective is to make sure that every one is aligned with the objectives and to discuss the next steps. The DFSS team needs to understand the assignment from the system perspective, device, manufacturing processes, documentation (design master record, design history file), and software development as depicted in Figure 7.2. The relation of software to DFSS is presented in Section 7.4.

In medical device DFSS deployment, we emphasize the synergistic DFSS cross-functional team. A well-developed team has the potential to design winning six sigma–level solutions. The growing synergy, which arises from ever-increasing numbers of successful teams, accelerates deployment throughout a company. The payback for upfront investments in team performance can be enormous. Continuous vigilance on the part of the black belt toward improving and measuring team performance throughout a project life cycle will be rewarded with ever-increasing capability and commitment to deliver winning device solutions. Given time, there will be a transition from resistance to embracing the methodology, and the company culture will be transformed.

7.2 MEDICAL DEVICE DFSS TEAM

It is plausible that medical devices intended to serve the same purpose and the same market may be designed and produced in radically different variations, depending on the design team's approach, creativity, experience, and understanding of customer wants. Look at any product that is produced by two different companies and you will start to notice differences. From the perspective of the design process, it is obvious that the device developed from a series of decisions, and that different decisions made at the tollgates resulted in such differentiation. This is simply common sense; however, it has significant consequences. It suggests that a design can be understood not only in

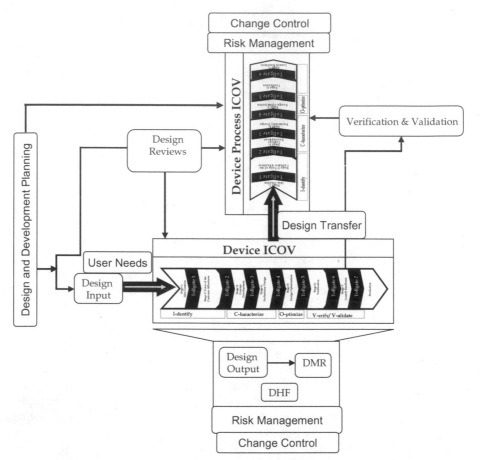

Figure 7.2 DFSS encompasses device and manufacturing processes.

terms of the design process adopted, but also in terms of the decision-making process used to arrive at it. Measures to address both sources of design variation need to be institutionalized in a DFSS deployment. We believe that the adoption of the customized ICOV DFSS process presented in this chapter will address one issue: the consistency of development activities. For medical device design teams, this means that the company functions used to facilitate coordination during the project execution have an effect on the core of the development process. In addition to coordination, the primary intent of an organizing design function (e.g., project/program management) is to control the decision-making process. It is thus logical to conclude that we must consider the design implications of the types of organizing structures that we deploy in the ICOV process to manage design practice. When flat organizing structures are adopted with design teams, members must negotiate design decisions among themselves, because a top-down approach to decision making may not be available. Members of a medical device design team negotiating decisions with one another during design projects is an obvious practice. A common assumption seems to be that these decision-making negotiations proceed in a reasonable manner, this being a basic premise of concurrent design. Patterns and outcomes of decision making are best explained as a dynamic behavior of the teams. Even if two teams develop similar devices using the same process, members of the otherwise comparable design teams may have varying levels of influence as decisions are made. The rank differences among members of a design team can play a substantial role in team dynamics from the perspective of day-to-day decisions. It is the responsibility of the black belt to balance such dynamics in his or her team. As team leaders, black belts and master black belts need to understand that design teams must make decisions, and that invariably, some set of principles and values must drive these decisions.

Decision making and team structure in companies that use hierarchical structures follow known patterns. Although day-to-day decision making is subject to team dynamics, the milestone decisions are not. In the latter, decisions are made based on formal rank. That is, decisions made by higher-ranking persons override those made by lower-ranking ones. Such an authoritatively decision-making pattern makes sense as long as the rank copes with expertise and appreciation of company goals. This pattern will also assure that those higher in rank can coordinate and align the actions of others with the goals of the company. In Chapter 6 we adopted this model for DFSS deployment. Despite these clear benefits, a number of factors make this traditional form of hierarchical structure less attractive, particularly in the context of the design team. For example, risk caused by increased technological complexity of the medical device being designed, market volatility, and others make it difficult to create a decision-making structure for day-to-day design activities. To address this problem, we suggest a flatter, looser structure that empowers team members, black belts, and master black belts to assert their own expertise, when needed, in day-to-day activities. In our view, an ideal design team should consist of team members who represent every phase of a medical device's life cycle. This concurrent structure combined with the road map will assure a company of consistent (i.e., minimal design process variation) and successful DFSS deployment. This approach allows information to flow freely across the bounds of time and distance: in particular, for geographically challenged companies. It also ensures that in making design decisions, representatives of later stages of the life cycle have an influence similar to that of representatives of earlier stages (e.g., customer service, maintenance, vendors, aftermarket). Although obvious benefits such as these can result from a flattened structure, it need not to be taken to the extreme. It is apparent that having no structure means the absence of a sound decision-making process. Current practice indicates that a design project is far from a rational process of simply identifying day-to-day activities and then assigning the expertise required to handle them. Rather, the truly important design decisions are more likely to be subjective decisions made based on judgments, incomplete information, or personally biased values, even though we strive to minimize these gaps in voice-of-the-customer and technology road mapping. In milestones, the final say over decisions in a flat design team remains with the champions or tollgate approvers. It must not happen at random, but rather, in a mapped way.

Our recommendation is twofold. First, a deployment company should adopt a common design process that is customized with its design needs and flexibility to adapt the DFSS process to obtain design consistency and to assure success. Second, choose flatter, looser design team structures that empower team members to assert their own expertise when needed. This practice is optimum in companies servicing advanced device development work in high-technology domains.

A cross-functional synergistic design team is one of the ultimate objectives of any deployment effort. The black belt needs to be aware of the fact that full participation in design is not guaranteed simply because members are assigned into a team. The structural barriers and interests of others on the team are likely to be far too formidable as the team travels through the ICOV DFSS process.

The success of development activities depends on the performance of this team, which is fully integrated, with representation from internal and external (suppliers and customers) members. Special efforts may be necessary to create a multifunctional DFSS team that collaborates to achieve a shared project vision. Roles, responsibilities, membership, and resources are best defined up front, collaboratively, by the teams. Once the team is established, however, it is just as important to maintain the team to improve its performance continuously. This first step is therefore an ongoing effort throughout the device's DFSS ICOV cycle of planning, formulation, and production.

The primary challenge for a design organization is to learn and improve faster than the competitor. Lagging competitors must go faster to catch up. Leading competitors must go faster to stay in front. A medical device DFSS team should learn rapidly, not only about what needs to be done, but about how to do it—how to implement a DFSS process pervasively.

Learning without application is really just gathering information, not learning. No company becomes first class simply by knowing what is required, but rather, by practicing, by training day in and day out, and by using the best contemporary DFSS methods. The team needs to monitor competitive performance using benchmarking of devices and processes to help guide directions of change and employ lessons learned to help identify areas for their improvement. In addition, they will benefit from deploying program and risk management best practices throughout the project life cycle (Figure 7.1). This activity is key to achieving a winning rate of improvement by avoiding or eliminating risks. The team is advised to practice design principles and systems thinking continuously (i.e., thinking in terms of the total profound knowledge).

7.3 · MEDICAL DEVICE DFSS ROAD MAP

In Chapter 5 we learned about the ICOV process and the seven developmental stages spaced by bounding tollgates indicating a formal transition between the entrance and exit. As depicted in Figure 7.3, tollgates or design milestones events include reviews to assess what has been accomplished in the current developmental stage and preparation for the next stage. The medical device design stakeholders, including the project champion, design owner, and deployment champion, conduct tollgate reviews. In a tollgate review, three decision options are available to the champion or his or her delegate or tollgate approver: (1) proceed to the next stage of development, (2) recycle back for further clarification on certain decisions, or (3) cancel the project.

In tollgate reviews, work proceeds when the exit criteria (required decisions) are made. Consistent exit criteria from each tollgate blend medical device DFSS deliverables due to application of the approach itself with the company's or it's business unit's deliverables.

In this section we first expand on the ICOV DFSS process activities by stage, with comments on the applicable key DFSS tools and methods over what was outlined in Chapter 5. A subsection per phase is presented in Figure 7.4.

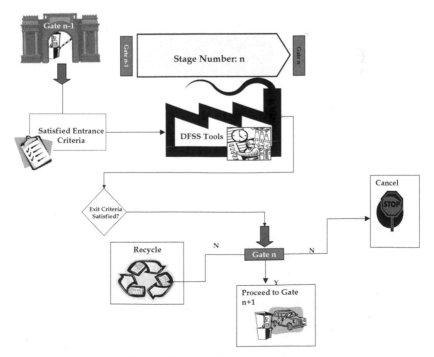

Figure 7.3 DFSS tollgate process.

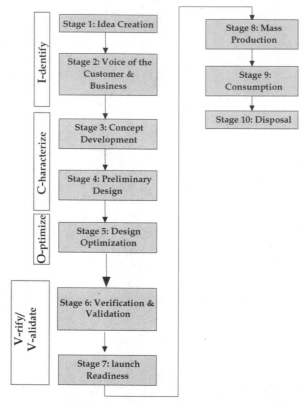

Figure 7.4   Medical device life cycle.

7.3.1   Phase 1: Identify Requirements

This phase includes two stages: idea creation (stage 1) and voice of the customer and business (stage 2).

Stage 1: Idea Creation

Stage 1 Entrance Criteria   Entrance criteria may be tailored by the deploying company for the particular program/project provided that in the opinion of the company, the modified entrance criteria are adequate to support the exit criteria for this stage. They may include a business case with:

- A target customer or market
- A market vision with an assessment of marketplace advantages
- An estimate of development cost
- A project risk assessment

Tollgate 1: Stage 1 Exit Criteria

- Decision to collect the voice of the customer to define customer needs, wants, and delights
- Verification that adequate funding is available to define customer needs
- Identification of the tollgate keepers'[1] leader and the appropriate staff

Stage 2: Customer and Business Requirements Study

Stage 2 Entrance Criteria

- Closure of tollgate 1: approval of the gate keeper obtained
- A medical device DFSS project charter that includes the project's objective, medical device design statement, big Y's, and other business levers, metrics, resources, and team members. These are almost the same criteria as those required for DMAIC-type projects. However, project duration is usually longer and the initial cost is probably higher. Relative to DMAIC, the DFSS team typically experiences a longer project cycle time. The goal here is either designing or redesigning a different entity, not just patching up the holes in an existing one. Higher initial cost is due to the fact that the value chain is being energized from the venue of medical device development and not from the manufacturing or production arenas. There may be new customer requirements to be satisfied, adding cost to the developmental effort. For DMAIC projects, we may work only on improving a very limited subset of the critical-to-satisfaction characteristics (the CTSs or big Y's).
- Completion of a market survey to determine customer needs critical to satisfaction (CTS): the voice of the customer. In this step, customers are fully identified and their needs collected and analyzed, with the help of quality function deployment (QFD) and Kano analysis (Chapter 8). Then the most appropriate set of CTS or big Ys metrics is determined in order to measure and evaluate the design. Again, with the help of QFD and Kano analysis, the numerical limits and targets for each CTS are established. In summary, here is a list of tasks in this step. A detailed explanation is provided in later chapters.
  - Determine methods of obtaining customer needs and wants.
  - Obtain customer needs and wants and transform them into a list of the voice of the customer.
  - Finalize requirements.
  - Establish minimum requirement definitions.

---

[1]A tollgate keeper is a person or a group who will assess the quality of work done by the design team and initiate a decision to approve, reject or cancel, or recycle the project to an earlier gate. Usually, a project champion is assigned this task.

- Identify and fill gaps in customer-provided requirements.
- Validate application and usage environments.
- Translate the VOC to CTSs as critical-to-quality, critical-to-delivery, critical-to-cost, and so on.
- Quantify CTSs or big Y's.
- Establish metrics for CTSs.
- Establish acceptable performance levels and operating windows.
- Start flow-down of CTSs.
- An assessment of required technologies
- A project development plan (through TG2)
- A risk assessment
- Alignment with business objectives: voice of the business relative to growth and innovation strategy
- Alignment with FDA safety requirements

Tollgate 2: Stage 2 Exit Criteria

- Assessment of market opportunity
- Commanding a reasonable price or being affordable
- Commitment to development of the conceptual designs
- Verification that adequate funding is available to develop the conceptual design
- Identification of the gatekeeper's leader (gate approver) and the appropriate staff
- Continue flow-down of CTSs to functional requirements

DFSS Tools Used in This Phase

- Market/customer research
- Quality function deployment (QFD) phase I
- Kano analysis
- Growth/innovation strategy

Medical Device Company Growth and Innovation Strategy: Multigenerational Planning[2]   Even within best-in-class companies, there is need and opportunity to strengthen and accelerate progress. The first step is to establish a set of clear and unambiguous guiding growth principles as a means to characterize company position and focus. For example, growth in emerging markets might be the focus abroad, while effectiveness and efficiency of resource us

[2]Adapted from http://216.239.57.104/search?q=cache:WTPP0iD4WTAJ:cipm.ncsu.edu/symposium/docs/Hutchins_text.doc+product+multi-generation+plan&hl=en by Scott H. Hutchins.

within the context of enterprise productivity and sustainability may be the local position. Growth principles and vision at a high level are adequate to find agreement and focus debate within the zone of interest and to exclude or diminish nonrealistic targets. The second key step is to assess the current know-how and solutions of a medical device portfolio in the context of these growth principles: an inventory of what the senior leadership team knows they have, and how it integrates into the set of guiding growth principles. Third, establish a vision of the ultimate state for the company. Finally, develop a *multigenerational plan* to focus the research, product development, and integration efforts in planned steps to move toward that vision. The multigenerational plan is key because it helps the deploying company stage progress in realistic developmental stages, one DFSS project at a time, but always with an eye on the ultimate vision.

In today's business climate, successful companies must be efficient and market-sensitive to supersede their competitors. By focusing on new medical devices, companies can create custom solutions to meet customer needs, enabling customers to keep in step with new medical device industry trends and changes that affect them. As the design team engages customers (through surveys, interviews, focus groups, etc.) and processes the QFD, they gather competitive intelligence. This information helps increase design team awareness of competing medical devices and of how they stack up competitively with a particular key customer. By doing this homework, the team identifies potential gaps in their development maturity. Several in-house tools to manage the life cycle of each medical device needs to be developed to include the multigenerational plan coupled with a customized version of the ICOV DFSS process, if required. The multigenerational plan evaluates the market size and trends, medical device positioning, competition, and technology requirements. This tool provides a means to easily identify any gaps in the portfolio while directing the DFSS project road map. The multigenerational plan needs to be supplemented with a decision-analysis tool to determine the financial and strategic value of potential new applications over a medium time horizon. If the project passes this decision-making step, it can be lined up with others in the six sigma project portfolio to develop a start schedule.

Researching Customer Activities   This is usually done by the medical device planning departments or market research experts, who should be on the DFSS team. The black belt and his or her team start by brainstorming all possible customer groups of the product. Use the affinity diagram method to group the brainstormed potential customer groups. Categories of markets, user types, or medical device and process applications types will emerge. From these categories, the DFSS team should work toward a list of clearly defined customer groups from which individuals can be selected.

External customers might be drawn from customer centers, independent sales organizations, regulatory agencies, societies, and patient advocate groups. Clinics, hospitals, and most important, the patient, should be included. The selection of external customers should include both existing and loyal customers, recently lost customers, and new conquest customers within the market segments. Internal customers might be drawn from production, functional groups, facilities, finance, employee relations, design groups, distribution organizations, and so on. Internal research might assist in selecting internal customer groups that would be most instrumental in identifying wants and needs in operations and medical device operations.

The ideal medical device definition, in the eye of the patient, may be extracted from several engagement activities. This will help turn the knowledge gained from continuous monitoring of patient trends, competitive benchmarking, and user likes and dislikes into a preliminary definition of an ideal medical device. In addition, it will help identify areas for further research and dedicated efforts. The design should be described from a customer's viewpoint (external and internal) and should provide the first insight into what a good medical device should look like. Concept models and design studies using innovation (Chapter 10) and axiomatic design (Chapter 9) are good sources for developing areas of likes or dislikes.

The array of customer attributes should include all customer and regulatory requirements and social and environmental expectations. It is necessary to understand requirement and prioritization similarities and differences in order to understand what can be standardized and what needs to be tailored.

7.3.2 Phase 2: Characterize Design

This phase spans the following two stages: concept development (stage 3) and preliminary design (stage 4).

Stage 3: Concept Development

Stage 3 Entrance Criteria

- Closure of tollgate 2: approval of the gatekeeper obtained
- Defined system technical and operational requirements: Translate customer requirements (CTSs or big Y's) to the medical device and its manufacturing process functional requirements: Customer requirements (CTSs) give us ideas about what will make the customer satisfied, but they usually cannot be used directly as the requirements for product or process design. We need to translate customer requirements to medical device and process functional requirements. Another phase of QFD can be used to develop this transformation. Axiomatic design principles will also be very helpful in this step.
- Medical device conceptual design
- Trade-off of alternative conceptual designs with the following steps:
  - *Generate design alternatives.* After determination of the functional requirements for the new design entity (medical device), we need to

conceptualize (develop) design entities, which are able to deliver those functional requirements. In general, there are two possibilities. The first is that the existing technology or known design concept is able to deliver all the requirements satisfactorily; then this step becomes almost a trivial exercise. The second possibility is that the existing technology or known design is not able to deliver all requirements satisfactorily; then a new design concept has to be developed. This new design could be *creative* or *incremental*, reflecting the degree of deviation from the baseline design, if any. TRIZ method (Chapter 10) and axiomatic design (Chapter 9) will be helpful to generate many innovative design concepts in this step.

- *Evaluate design alternatives.* Several design alternatives might be generated in the last step. We need to evaluate them and make a final determination as to which concept will be used. Many methods can be used to design evaluation, which include Pugh concept selection technique, design reviews, and FMEA. After design evaluation, a winning concept will be selected. During the evaluation, many weaknesses of the initial set of design concepts will be exposed, and the concepts will be revised and improved. If we are designing a medical device manufacturing processes, process management techniques will also be used as an evaluation tool.

- Functional, performance, and operating requirements allocated to medical device design components (subsystems)
- Development cost estimate (tollgates 2 through 5)
- Target medical device unit production cost assessment
- Software development deliverables
- Market:
  - Profitability and growth rate
  - Supply chain assessment
  - Time-to-market assessment
  - Share assessment
- Overall risk assessment
- Project management plan (tollgates 2 through 5) with schedule and test plan
- Team member staffing plan

Tollgate 3: Stage 3 Exit Criteria

- Assessment that the conceptual development plan and cost will satisfy the customer base
- Decision that the medical device design represents an economic opportunity (if appropriate)

- Verification that adequate funding will be available to perform preliminary design
- Identification of the tollgate keeper and the appropriate staff
- Action plan to continue flow-down of the design functional requirements
- Software development deliverables

Stage 4: Preliminary Design

Stage 4 Entrance Criteria

- Closure of tollgate 3: approval of the gatekeeper obtained
- Flow-down of system functional, performance, and operating requirements to subprocesses and steps (components)
- Documented design data package with configuration management, a systematic approach to defining design configurations and managing the change process, at the lowest level of control
- Development-to-production operations transfer plan published and in effect
- Subsystems functionality, performance, and operating requirements verified
- Development of testing objectives complete under nominal operating conditions
- Software development deliverables
- Testing with design parametric variations under critical operating conditions
    - Tests might not utilize the intended operational production processes
- Design, performance, and operating transfer functions
- Reports documenting the design analyses as appropriate
- Procurement strategy (if applicable)
- Make-or-buy decision
- Sourcing (if applicable)
- Risk assessment

Tollgate 4: Stage 4 Exit Criteria

- Acceptance of the medical device solution/design selected
- Agreement that the design is likely to satisfy all design requirements
- Agreement to proceed with the next stage of the medical device solution/design selected
- Software development deliverables

- Action plan to finish flow-down of the design functional requirements to design parameters and process variables

DFSS Tools Used in This Phase

- QFD
- TRIZ/axiomatic design
- Measurement system analysis
- Failure mode effect analysis
- Design scorecard
- Process mapping
- Process management
- Pugh concept selection
- Robust design
- Design for X
- Design reviews

7.3.3 Phase 3: Optimize Requirements

This phase spans stage 5 only, the design optimization stage.

Stage 5: Design Optimization

Stage 5 Entrance Criteria

- Closure of tollgate 4: approval of the gatekeeper obtained
- Design documentation defined; the design includes complete information specific to the operations processes (in the opinion of the operating functions)
- Design documents under the highest level of control
- Formal change configuration in effect
- Operations validated by the operating function to preliminary documentations
- Software development deliverables
- Demonstration test plan put together that must demonstrate functionality and performance under operational environments; full-scale testing, load testing
- Risk assessment

Tollgate 5: Stage 5 Exit Criteria

- Agreement that functionality and performance meet the customers and business requirements under the intended operating conditions

- Decision to proceed with a verification test of a pilot built to preliminary operational process documentation
- Software development deliverables
- Analyses to document the design optimization to meet or exceed functional, performance, and operating requirements
  - Optimized transfer functions: Design of experiments (DOE) is the backbone of process design and redesign improvement. It represents the most common approach to quantify the transfer functions between the set of CTSs and/or requirements and the set of critical factors, the X's, at different levels of design hierarchy. DOE can be conducted by hardware or software (e.g., simulation). From the subset of the few, vital X's, experiments are designed to actively manipulate the inputs to determine their effect on the outputs (big Y's or small y's). This phase is characterized by a sequence of experiments, each based on the results of the preceding study. Critical variables are identified during this process. Usually, a small number of X's account for most of the variation in the outputs.

The result of this phase is an optimized medical device entity with all functional requirements released at the six sigma performance level. As the concept design is finalized, there are still a lot of design parameters that can be adjusted and changed. With the help of computer simulation and/or hardware testing, DOE modeling, Taguchi's robust design methods, and response surface methodology, the optimal parameter settings will be determined. It is very probable that this parameter optimization stage may be followed by a tolerance optimization step. The objective is to provide a logical and objective basis for setting requirements and process tolerances. If the design parameters are not controllable, we may need to repeat stages 1 to 3 of medical device DFSS.

DFSS Tools Used in This Phase

- Transfer function detailing (physical DOE, computer DOE, hypothesis testing, etc.)
- Process capability analysis
- Design scorecard
- Simulation tools
- Mistake-proofing plan
- Robustness assessment (Taguchi methods: parameter and tolerance design)

7.3.4   Phase 4: Verify/Validate the Design

This phase spans the following two stages: verification (stage 6) and launch readiness (stage 7).

Stage 6: Verification and Validation

Stage 6 Entrance Criteria

- Closure of tollgate 5: approval of the gatekeeper obtained
- Software development deliverables
- Risk assessment

Tollgate 6: Stage 6 Exit Criteria   After the parameter and tolerance design is finished, we move to the final verification and validation activities, including testing. The key actions are:

- Auditing of pilot tests for conformance with design and operational process documentation
- Software development deliverables
- Pilot test and refining: no medical device may go directly to market without first piloting and refining and mostly with clinical trials; here we can use design failure mode effect analysis (DFMEA; see Chapter 11) as well as pilot and small-scale implementations to test and evaluate real-life performance
- Design verification
- Design validation
- Software validation
- Process validation and control: verifying devise design and validating the manufacturing processes to make sure that the medical device, as designed, meets the requirements and establishes process controls in operations to ensure that critical characteristics are always produced to the specifications of the optimize phase

Stage 7: Launch Readiness

Stage 7 Entrance Criteria

- Closure of tollgate 6: approval of the gatekeeper obtained
- Operational processes demonstrated
- Software development deliverables
- Risk assessment
- Control plans in place
- Final design and operational process documentation published
- Process achieves or exceeds all operating metrics
- Operations demonstrated continuous operations without the support of design development personnel
- Planned sustaining development personnel transferred to operations

- Optimize, eliminate, automate, and/or control a vital few inputs deemed so in the preceding phase.
- Document and implement the control plan.
- Sustain the gains identified.
- Reestablish and monitor long-term delivered capability.
- Transfer plan in place for the design development personnel
- Risk assessment

Tollgate 7: Stage 7 Exit Criteria

- Decision made to reassign the DFSS black belt team
- Software development deliverables
- Full commercial rollout and handover to new process owner: As the medical device is validated and process control is established, we launch full-scale commercial rollout, and the new designed medical device, together with the supporting operations processes, can be handed over to design and process owners, complete with requirements settings, and control and monitoring systems.
- Closure of tollgate 7: approval of the gatekeeper obtained

DFSS Tools Used in This Phase

- Process control plan
- Control plans
- Design transfer planning
- Training plan
- Statistical process control
- Confidence analysis
- Mistake-proofing
- Process capability modeling

7.4 SOFTWARE DFSS ICOV PROCESS

As the device and its manufacturing processes are being designed, there is a mirrored path for the information and control of an intelligent device. That is the software DFSS ICOV process as depicted in Figure 7.5.

There are many ongoing iterative interfaces with the device DFSS ICOV process that are not depicted in the figure. Software development deliverables are embedded in device deliverables to strengthen the linkage between the two processes.

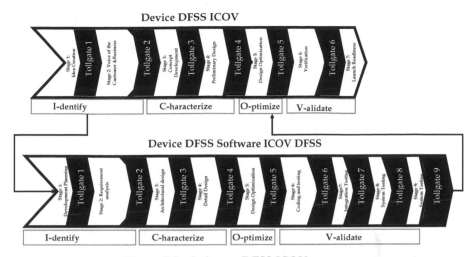

Figure 7.5 Software DFSS ICOV process.

A decades-long goal has been to find repeatable, predictable processes or methodologies that improve software productivity and quality. Some try to systematize or formalize the seemingly unruly task of writing software. Others apply project management techniques to writing software. Without project management, software projects can easily be delivered late or over budget. With large numbers of software projects not meeting their expectations in terms of functionality, cost, or delivery schedule, effective project management is proving difficult. The best-known and oldest process is the *waterfall model*, where developers (roughly) follow contain steps in order: State requirements, analyze requirements, design a solution approach, architect a software framework for that solution, develop code, test (perhaps unit tests, then system tests), deploy, and carry out postimplementation. The DFSS ICOV process goes beyond the waterfall process, applying tools, design principles, and best practices from product domain to software domain.

A growing number of medical devices implement process methodologies. The international standard for describing the method of selecting, implementing, and monitoring the life cycle for a software is ISO 12207. The IEC 62304 standard specifies software life-cycle processes, including software development, software maintenance, software risk management, software configuration management, and software problem resolution requirements for medical device software. It requires manufacturers to assign one of three defined safety classes to the software system, makes normative reference to ISO 14971, the application of risk management to medical devices, partitioning and safety classification of software items, and selection of software processes.

Device-critical software needs to have high integrity. Software integrity depends on software development processes. Software safety is part of device safety, and device safety depends on a risk management process (Chapter 11). The IEC 60601-1 standard, 3rd edition, Medical Electrical Equipment, Part 1: General requirements for safety and essential performance, Clause 14, covers programmable electrical medical systems. In addition, ANSI/AAMI SW 68, Medical Device Software: Software Life Cycles, satisfies FDA requirements but not for all levels of concern. Other standards include IEC 61508, Functional Safety Electrical/Electronic/Programmable Electronic Safety-Related Systems, claims to be a "standard for standards" covering all software safety. ISO 14971, Application of Risk Management to Medical Devices, is well established.

The *capability maturity model* (CMM) is another of the leading models. Independent assessments grade organizations on how well they follow their defined processes, not on the quality of those processes or the software produced. CMM is gradually being replaced by CMMI. ISO 9000 describes standards for formally organizing processes with documentation. ISO 15504, also known as *software process improvement capability determination* (SPICE), is a "framework for the assessment of software processes." This standard is aimed at setting out a clear model for process comparison. SPICE is used much like CMM and CMMI. It models processes to manage, control, guide, and monitor software development. This model is then used to measure what a development organization or project team actually does during software development. This information is analyzed to identify weaknesses and drive improvement. It also identifies strengths that can be continued or integrated into common practice for that organization or team.

Often, the first step in attempting to design a new piece of device software, whether it be an addition to existing software, a new application, a new subsystem, or an entirely new device, is what is generally referred to as the software identify phase. Assuming that the DFSS team (including the analysts) are not sufficiently knowledgeable in the subject area of the new software, the first task is to investigate the *domain* of the software. The more knowledgeable they already are about the domain, the less the work that is required. Another objective of this work is to make the analysts who will later try to elicit and gather the requirements from area experts or professionals, speak with these experts in the domain's own terminology better understand what is being said by these people. Otherwise, they will not be taken seriously.

In the software identify DFSS phase, the most important task in creating a device software is extracting the requirements. Customers typically know what they want but not what software should do, whereas incomplete, ambiguous, or contradictory requirements are recognized by skilled and experienced software engineers. Demonstrating live code may help reduce the risk that the requirements are incorrect.

Specification is the task of precisely describing the software to be written, possibly in a rigorous way. In practice, most successful specifications are written to understand and fine-tune applications that were already well developed, although safety-critical software systems are often specified carefully prior to application development. Specifications are most important for external interfaces that must remain stable.

In the software characterize phase, the architecture of a software system refers to an abstract representation of that system. Architecture is concerned with making sure that the software system will meet the requirements of the product as well as ensuring that future requirements can be addressed. This phase also addresses interfaces between the software system and other software products, the underlying hardware, or the host operating system.

In the optimize phase, reducing a design to code may be the most obvious part of the software engineering job, but it is not necessarily the largest portion.

In the validate phase, testing of parts of software, especially where code by two different engineers must work together, falls to the software engineer. An important (and often overlooked) task is documenting the internal design of software for the purpose of future maintenance and enhancement. Documentation is most important for external interfaces.

A large percentage of software projects fail because the developers fail to realize that it doesn't matter how much time and planning a development team puts into creating software if nobody in an organization uses it. People are occasionally resistant to change and avoid venturing into an unfamiliar area, so as part of this deployment phase, it is very important to have training classes for the most enthusiastic software users (build excitement and confidence), shifting the training toward neutral users intermixed with avid supporters, and finally, incorporate the rest of the organization into adopting the new software. Users will have lots of questions and software problems, which lead to the next version of software.

Maintaining and enhancing software to cope with newly discovered problems or new requirements can take far more time than the initial development of the software. Not only may it be necessary to add code that does not fit the original design, but just determining how software works at some point after it is completed may require significant effort by a software engineer. About two-thirds of all software engineering work is maintenance, but this statistic can be misleading. A small part of that is fixing bugs. Most maintenance is extending systems to do new things, which in many ways can be considered new work.[3]

7.5 SUMMARY

In this chapter we present the medical device DFSS road map. The map is depicted in Figure 7.1, which highlights at a high level the identify, characterize, optimize and verify/validate phases, the seven medical device development stages (idea creation, voice of the customer and business, concept

---

[3]See http://en.wikipedia.org/wiki/Software_development_process and Pressman (2000).

development, preliminary design, design optimization, verification/validation, and launch readiness). The road map also recognizes the tollgate design milestones where DFSS teams update stockholders on development and ask for decisions to be made, whether to approve going into the next stage, to recycle back to an earlier stage, or to cancel the project altogether. The road map also highlights most appropriate DFSS tools by the ICOV phase. It indicates when it is mot appropriate to start tool use. These tools are presented in Chapters 8 to 10.

8

QUALITY FUNCTION DEPLOYMENT

8.1 INTRODUCTION

In this chapter we cover the history of quality function deployment (QFD; see El-Haik, 2007), describe the methodology of applying the QFD within the DFSS project road map (Chapter 7), and apply QFD to a medical device example. QFD is a planning tool that allows the flow-down of high-level customer needs and wants, a major component of design inputs, through to design parameters and then to process variables critical to fulfilling the high-level needs. By following the QFD methodology, relationships are explored between quality characteristics expressed by customers and substitute quality requirements expressed in engineering terms (Cohen, 1988, 1995). In the context of medical device DFSS, we call these requirements *critical-to characteristics*. These characteristics can be expanded along the dimensions of safety (*critical to safety*), quality (*critical to quality*) and cost (*critical to cost*), as well as the other dimensions. In the QFD methodology, customers define their wants and needs using their own expressions, which rarely carry any actionable engineering technical terminology. The voice of the customer can be affinitized into a list of needs and wants that can be used as input to a relationship matrix, which is called QFD's *house of quality*.

Knowledge of customer needs and wants is paramount in designing effective products and services with innovative and rapid means. Utilizing the QFD methodology allows the developer to attain the shortest

Medical Device Design for Six Sigma: A Road Map for Safety and Effectiveness,
By Basem S. El-Haik and Khalid S. Mekki
Copyright © 2008 John Wiley & Sons, Inc.

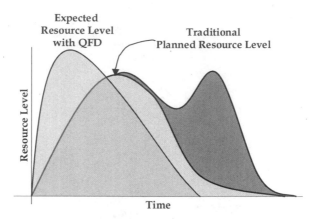

Figure 8.1   Time-phased effort for DFSS versus traditional design.

development cycle while ensuring the fulfillment of customer needs and wants.

Figure 8.1 shows that teams which use QFD place more emphasis on responding to problems early in the design cycle. Intuitively, it incurs more effort, time, resources, and energy to implement a design change at production launch than at the concept phase because more resources are required to resolve problems than to prevent their occurrence in the first place.

With QFD, quality is defined by the customer. Customers want products and services that throughout their lives meet customer needs and expectations at a value that exceeds cost. QFD methodology links these needs through design and into process control. At the same time, QFD's ability to link and prioritize provides a sharp focus to guide the design team as to where to focus energy and resources. In this chapter we provide the detailed methodology to create the four QFD houses and evaluate them for completeness and goodness, to introduce the Kano model for the voice of the customer, and to relate the QFD with the DFSS road map introduced in Chapter 7.

8.2   HISTORY OF QFD

As we mentioned in Chapter 1, QFD was developed in Japan by Yoji Akao and Shigeru Mizuno in 1966 but not Westernized until the 1980s. Their purpose was to develop a quality assurance method that would design customer satisfaction into a product before it was manufactured. For six years the methodology was developed from the initial concept of Kiyotaka Oshiumi of the Bridgestone Tire Corporation. Following the publication in 1972 of *Hinshitsu Tenkai* (Quality Deployment) by Akao, the pivotal development work was conducted at the Kobe shipyards for Mitsubishi Heavy Industry. The stringent government regulations for military vessels coupled with the large capital outlay forced management at the shipyard to seek a method of ensuring upstream quality which cascaded down throughout all activities. The team developed a matrix that related all the government regulations, critical design requirements, and customer requirements to company technical controlled characteristics of how the company would achieve them. Within the matrix the team depicted the importance of each requirement, which allowed for prioritization. Following successful deployment within the shipyard, Japanese automotive companies adopted the methodology to resolve the problem of rust on cars. Next, it was applied to car features—and the rest, as they say, is history. In 1978 the detailed methodology was published in Japanese and was translated into English in 1994 (Mizuno and Akao, 1978, 1994).

8.3 QFD FUNDAMENTALS

The benefits of utilizing the QFD methodology are primarily to ensure that high-level customer needs are met, that the development cycle is efficient in terms of time and effort, and that the control of specific process variables is linked to customer wants and needs for continuing satisfaction.

To complete a QFD, three key conditions are required to ensure success. Condition 1 is that a multidisciplinary DFSS team is required to provide a broad perspective. Condition 2 is that more time is expended upfront in the collecting and processing of customer needs and expectations. Condition 3 is that the functional requirements defined in house of quality 2 will be solution-free.

All of the theory sounds logical and achievable, but three realities must be overcome to achieve success. Reality 1 is that the interdisciplinary DFSS team will not work together well in the beginning. Reality 2 is the prevalent culture of heroic problem solving in lieu of drab problem prevention. People get visibly rewarded and recognized for firefighting and no recognition for problem prevention that drives a culture focused on correction rather than prevention. The final reality is that the team members and even customers will jump right to solution all too early and frequently instead of following the details of the methodology and remaining solution-free until design requirements are specified.

8.4 QFD METHODOLOGY

Quality function deployment is accomplished by multidisciplinary DFSS teams using a series of matrixes, called *houses of quality* (HOQs), to deploy critical customer needs throughout phases of design development. The QFD methodology is deployed through the four-phase sequence shown in Figure 8.2: phase 1, critical-to-satisfaction planning: HOQ 1; phase 2, functional requirements planning: HOQ 2; phase 3, design parameters planning: HOQ 3; phase

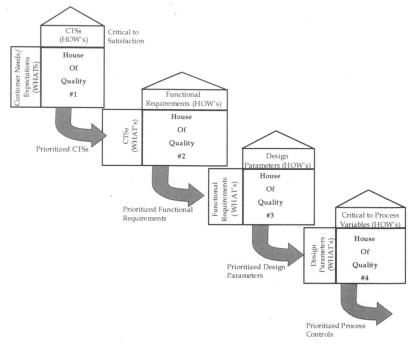

Figure 8.2   The four phases of QFD.

4, process variable planning: HOQ 4. Each of these phases is covered in detail in this chapter.

It is interesting to note that the QFD is linked to the voice of the customer (VOC) tools at the front end and then to design scorecards and customer satisfaction measures throughout the design effort. These linkages, along with adequate analysis, provide feed-forward (requirements flow-down) and feed-backward (capability flow-up) signals that allow for the synthesis of design concepts (Suh, 1990).

Each of the four phases deploys the HOQ, with the only content variation occurring in rooms 1 and 3. Figure 8.3 depicts the generic HOQ. Going room by room, we see that the input is into room 1, in which we answer the question "what?". The "whats" are either the results of VOC synthesis, the design inputs for HOQ 1, or a rotation of the hows from room 3 into the following HOQs. The "whats" are rated in terms of their overall importance and placed in the importance column. The analytical hierarchical process (AHP) can be used to prioritize the "whats."

AHP helps capture both subjective and objective evaluation measures in the "whats," providing a useful mechanism for checking the consistency of the evaluation suggested by the team, thus reducing bias in decision making. AHP can minimize common pitfalls of the team decision-making process, such as lack of focus, planning, participation, or ownership, which ultimately

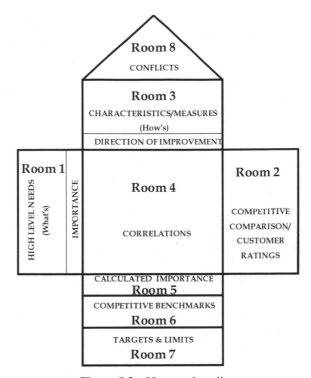

Figure 8.3 House of quality.

are costly distractions that can prevent DFSS teams from making the right choices.

Another technique that can be used in room 1 is the *affinity diagram*, which comprises a group decision-making technique designed to sort a large number of ideas, process variables, concepts, and opinions into naturally related groups. These groups are connected by a simple concept, in our case, for example, a high-level "what" and its siblings. The purpose of the affinity diagram is to sort a list of "whats" into groups.

Next, we move to room 2 and compare our performance and the competition's performance against these "whats" in the eyes of the customer. This is usually a subjective measure and is generally scaled from 1 to 5. A different symbol is assigned to the various providers, so that a graphical representation is depicted in room 2. Next, we must populate room 3 with the "hows." For each "what" in room 1, we ask "How can we fulfill this?" The answer are the design outputs, the high-level critical-to-satisfaction/quality characteristics. We also indicate in which direction improvement is required to satisfy the "what": maximize, minimize, or target. This classification is in alignment with robustness methodology (Chapter 15) and indicates an optimization direction. In HOQ 1 these become "How does the customer measure the 'what'?" In HOQ 1 we call these critical-to-satisfaction/quality (CTS/CTQ) measures. In

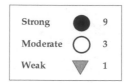

Figure 8.4   Rating values for affinities.

HOQ 2 the "hows" are measurable, solution-free functions that are required to fulfill the "whats" of CTSs. In HOQ 3 the "hows" become design parameters, and in HOQ 4 the "hows" become process variables. A word of caution: Teams involved in designing new devices often jump right to specific solutions in HOQ 1. It is a challenge to stay solution-free until HOQ 3. There are some rare circumstances where the VOC is a specific function that flows straight through each house unchanged.

Within room 4 we assign the weight of the relationship between each "what" and each "how" using 9 for strong, 3 for moderate, and 1 for weak. In an actual HOQ, these weightings will be depicted with graphical symbols, the most common being the solid circle for strong, an open circle for moderate, and a triangle for weak (Figure 8.4).

Once the relationship assignment has been completed, by evaluating the relationship of every "what" to every "how," the importance can be derived by multiplying the weight of the relationship and the importance of the "what" and summing for each "how." This is the number in room 5. For each of the "hows" we can also derive quantifiable benchmark measures of the competition and us; in the eyes of industry experts; this is what goes in room 6. In room 7 we can state the targets and limits of each of the "hows." Finally, in room 8, often called the *roof*, we assess the interrelationship of the "hows" to each other. If we were to maximize one of the "hows," what happens to the other "hows"? If it were also to improve in measure, we classify it as a *synergy*, whereas if it were to move away from the direction of improvement, it would be classified as a *compromise*. Wherever a relationship does not exist, it is just left blank. For example, if we wanted to improve a device stem cells yield, accuracy may degrade. This is clearly a compromise. Although it would be ideal to have correlation and regression values for these relationships, they are often just based on common sense or business laws. This completes each of the eight rooms in the HOQ. The next step is to sort based on the importance in rooms 1 and 5 and then evaluate the HOQ for completeness and balance.

8.5   HOQ EVALUATION

Completing the HOQ is the first important step; however, the design team should take the time to review their efforts toward quality, checks and balances, and design resource priorities. The following diagnostics can be utilized on the sorted HOQ.

1. Is there a diagonal pattern of strong correlations in room 4? This will indicate good alignment of the "hows" (room 3) with the "whats" (room 1)?
2. Do all "hows" (room 3) have at least one correlation with "whats" (room 1)?
3. Are there empty or weak rows in room 4? This indicates unaddressed "whats" and this could be a major issue. In HOQ 1 this would be unaddressed customer wants or needs.
4. Evaluate the highest score in room 2. What should our design target be?
5. Evaluate the customer rankings in room 2 versus the technical benchmarks in room 6. If room 2 values are lower than room 6 values, the design team may need to work on changing the customer's perception, or the correlation between the want or need and the CTS will not be correct.
6. Review room 8 trade-offs for conflicting correlations. For strong conflicts or synergies, changes in one characteristic (room 3) could affect other characteristics.

8.6   HOQ 1: THE CUSTOMER'S HOUSE

Quality function deployment begins with the voice of the customer (VOC), the voice of the business (VOB), and the voice of regulation (VOR). This is the first step required for HOQ 1. VOC can be collected by many methods and from many sources. Some common methods are historical research methods, focus groups, interviews, councils, clinical trials, surveys, and observations. Sources range from passive historical records of complaints, testimonials, warranty records, customer records, and call centers through to active customers, lost customers, or target customers. Stick with the language of the customer (e.g., a clinic, hospital, or patient) and think about how they speak when angered or satisfied; this is generally their natural language. These voices need to be prioritized and synthesized into a rank order of importance. The two most common methods are the affinity diagram (see Figure 8.5) and Kano analysis. We will cover the Kano model (see Figure 8.6) before taking the prioritized CTSs into room 1 of HOQ 2.

Affinity diagramming is a very simple but powerful technique for grouping and understanding information. It provides a good way to identify and analyze cutomer voices. There are several variations of the technique. Use affinity diagramming in a DFSS team workshop environment when you want participants to work together identifying, grouping, and discussing issues. Affinity

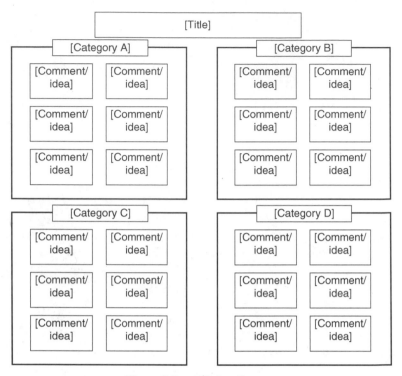

Figure 8.5 Affinity diagram.

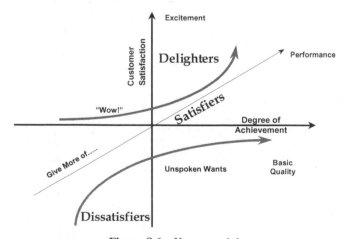

Figure 8.6 Kano model.

diagramming consists simply of placing related items together. Although this can be done electronically for very small sets of data (using a word processor or spreadsheet program), it is better to work with paper (Post-It notes or 3 × 5 cards are ideal). If you have a preexisting set of information, you can print these on labels or cards or print on paper and trim to a convenient size. Here are some tips:

- Inquire whether ideas are clarified adequately.
- Use only three to five words in the phrase on the header card to describe the group.
- If possible, have groupings reviewed by nonteam personnel.
- While sorting, get up and gather around the area where the cards are placed.
- Team members will ultimately reach agreement on placement, if for no other reason than exhaustion.
- Sorting should not start until all team members are ready.
- If an idea fits in more than one category or group, and consensus about placement cannot be reached, make a second card and place it in both groups.

When collecting the VOC, make sure that it isn't the voice of the engineer, the voice of the employee, or the voice of the boss. Although the QFD is a robust methodology, if you start with a poor foundation, it will be exacerbated throughout the process.

8.6.1 Kano Model

In the context of DFSS, customer attributes are potential benefits that the customer could receive from the design and are characterized by qualitative and quantitative data. Each attribute is ranked according to its relative importance to the customer. This ranking is based on the customer's satisfaction with similar design entities featuring that attribute.

The understanding of customer expectations (wants, needs) and delights ("wow" factors) by the design team is a prerequisite to further development and is therefore the most important action prior to starting the other functional mappings (Chapter 9). The fulfillment of these expectations and the provision of differentiating delighters (unspoken wants) will lead to satisfaction. This satisfaction will ultimately determine what medical devices the customer is going to endorse and consume or buy. In doing so, the design team needs to identify constraints that limit the delivery of such satisfaction. Constraints present opportunities to exceed expectations and create delighters.

The Kano model, a theory of product development developed in the 1980s by Noriaki Kano, classifies customer preferences into five categories: attractive, one-dimensional, must-be, indifferent, and reverse. These categories have been translated into English using various names (delighters/exciters, satisfiers, dissatisfiers, etc.), but all refer to the original articles written by Kano. For example, Cadotte and Turgeon (1988) used *dissatisfier, satisfier, critical,* and *neutral.* Brandt (1988) had the following categorization: *minimum requirement, value enhancing, hybrid,* and *unimportant* as determinants. Venkitaraman and Jaworski (1993) used *flat, value-added, key,* and *low.* Brandt and Scharioth (1998) use *basic, attractive, one-dimensional,* and *low impact.*

The Kano model offers some insight into the device attributes that are perceived to be important to customers. The purpose of the tool is to support product specification and discussion through better development team understanding. Kano's model focuses on differentiating medical device features rather than focusing initially on customer needs. Kano also produced a methodology for mapping consumer responses to questionnaires into his model.

QFD makes use of the Kano model in terms of the structuring of QFD matrices. Mixing Kano types in QFD matrices can lead to distortions in the customer weighting of product characteristics. For instance, mixing must-be product characteristics such as cost, reliability, workmanship, safety, and technologies used in the medical device initial house of quality will usually result is completely filled rows and columns with high correlation values. Other QFD techniques using additional matrices are employed to avoid such issues. Kano's model provides insights into the dynamics of customer (e.g., the patient, clinician, doctor, clinic, hospital) preferences to understand these methodology dynamics.

The identification of customer expectations is a vital step in the development of six sigma devices the customer will buy in preference to those of competitors. Kano's model relating design characteristics to customer satisfaction (Cohen, 1995) (see Figure 8.6) divides the characteristics into categories, each of which affects customers differently: dissatifiers, satisfiers, and delighters. We use a mix here of the category names suggested by Brandt, Cadotte, and Turgeon.

Dissatisfiers are also known as basic, "must-be," or expected attributes and can be defined as a characteristic that a customer takes for granted and which, when missing, causes dissatisfaction, such as an operational manual shipped with a device. *Satisfiers* are known as performance, one-dimensional, or straight-line characteristics and are defined as being something the customer wants and expects; the more, the better, such as better quality or higher reliability. *Delighters* are features that exceed competitive offerings in creating pleasant, unexpected surprises, such as charting and statistical functionality recording and reporting readings of critical CTQs. Not all customer satisfaction attributes are equal from an importance standpoint. Some are more important to customers than others, in subtly different ways. For example, dissatisfiers may not matter when they are met but subtract from overall medical device satisfaction when they are not delivered.

When customers interact with the design team, delighters are often surfaced that would not have been conceived independently. Another source of delighters may emerge from design team creativity, as some features have the unintended result of becoming delighters in the eyes of customers. Any design feature that fills a latent or hidden need is a delighter, and with time, becomes a want. A good example of this is the remote controls introduced with television sets. Early on, these were "differentiating delighters", today they are common features of television sets, radios, and even automobile ignitions and door locks. Today, if you received a television set without a remote control, it would be a dissatisfier. Delighters can be sought in the areas of weakness, competitor benchmarking, technical, customer leadership, social, and strategic innovation. Social aspects are becoming more important as educated customers want to preserve the environment and human rights, and cycling of medical devices and disposable attachments is gaining more attention.

The design team should conduct a customer evaluation study, although this is difficult to do in creative design situations. Customer evaluation is conducted to assess how well the current or proposed design delivers on the needs and desires of patients. The method used most frequently for this evaluation is to ask the customer (e.g., interview, focus group, survey) how well the design project is meeting each customer's expectations. In order to leap ahead of the competition, the team must also study the evaluation and performance of their toughest competitors. In HOQ 1, the team has the opportunity to grasp and compare how well current, proposed, or competitive devices are delivering on customer needs.

The objective of the HOQ 1 room 2 evaluation is to broaden a team's strategic choices for setting targets for customer performance goals. For example, armed with meaningful customer desires, the team could aim their efforts at either the strengths or weaknesses of best-in-class competitors (if any). In another choice, the team might explore other innovative avenues to gain competitive advantages.

The list of customer wants and needs should include all customer input as well as regulatory requirements and social and environmental expectations. It is necessary to understand requirements and prioritization similarities and differences in order to understand what can be standardized and what needs to be tailored.

Customer wants and needs in HOQ 1, social, environmental, and other company wants can be refined in a matrix format for each market segment identified. The customer importance rating in room 1 is the main driver for assigning priorities from both the customer and corporate perspectives, as obtained through direct or indirect engagement with the customer.

The traditional method of using the Kano model is to ask functional and dysfunctional questions around known wants and needs or CTQs. Functional questions take the form "How would you feel if the CTQs were present in the medical device?" Dysfunctional questions take the form of "How would you feel if the CTQs were not present in the medical device?"

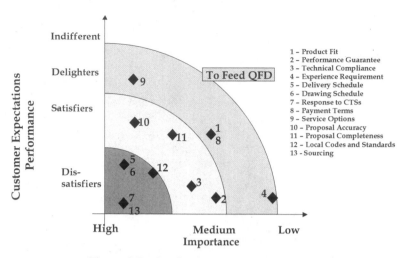

Figure 8.7   Qualitative Kano analysis plot.

Collection of this information is the first step. Detailed analysis is then required but is beyond the scope of this book. For a good reference on processing the voice of the customer, see Burchill et al. (1997).

In addition to the traditional method, it is possible to use qualitative assessment to put things into a Kano analysis plot and then have it validated by the end user. Figure 8.7 shows an example of this method. In a Kano analysis plot, the y-axis consists of the Kano model dimensions of dissatisfiers, satisfiers, delighters, and indifferent. The top item, indifferent, is where they customer chooses opposite items in the functional and dysfunctional questions. The x-axis is based on the importance of the CTQs to the customer. The type of plot can be completed from the Kano model or can be arranged qualitatively by the design team, but it must be validated by the customer or we will fall again into the trap of the voice of the engineer.

8.7   HOQ 2: TRANSLATION HOUSE

The critical-to (CTs) characteristics (critical to quality, critical to safety, critical to delivery, etc.) list is a set of metrics derived by the design team from the customer attributes list. The CT list rotates into HOQ 2 room 1 in this QFD phase. The objective is to determine a set of functional requirements (FRs) by which the CT requirements can be made to materialize. The answering activity translates customer expectations into such requirements as yield, purity, and uniformity. For each CT there should be one or more FRs that describe means of attaining customer satisfaction.

At this stage, only overall CTs that can be measured and controlled need to be used. We call these CTs, technical CTs. As explained in section 8.1, CTSs are traditionally known as substitute quality characteristics. Relationships between technical CTs and FRs are often used to prioritize CTs filling the relationship matrix of HOQ 2 rooms. For each CT, the design team has to assign a value that reflects the extent to which the defined FRs contribute to meeting it. This value, along with the calculated importance index of the CT, establishes the contribution of the FRs to overall satisfaction and can be used for prioritization.

An analysis of the relationships of FRs and CTs allows a comparison to other indirect information which needs to be understood before prioritization can be finalized. The new information from room 2 in the QFD HOQ needs to be contrasted with the device information available (if any) to ensure that reasons for modification are understood.

The purpose of QFD HOQ 2 activity is to define the design functions in terms of customer expectations, benchmark projections, institutional knowledge, and interface management with other systems, and to translate this information into technical functional requirement targets and specifications. This will facilitate the design mappings (Chapter 9). Since the FRs are solution-free, their targets and the specifications for them are flowed down from the CTs. For example if a CT is for *yield*, the measure is the number of cells counted.

A major reason for customer dissatisfaction is that the design specifications do not adequately link to customer use of the medical device. Often, the specification is written after the design has been completed (e.g., design history file remediation). It may also be a copy of outdated specifications. This reality may be attributed to current planned design practices that do not allocate activities and resources in areas of importance to customers and waste resources by spending too much time in activities that provide marginal value, a gap that is nicely filled by the QFD activities. The targets and tolerance setting activity in QFD phase 2 should also be stressed.

8.8 HOQ 3: DESIGN HOUSE

The FRs are a list of solution-free requirements derived by the design team to answer the CT array. The FR list is rotated into HOQ 3 room 1 in this QFD phase. The objective is to determine a set of design parameters that will fulfill the FRs. Again, the FRs are the "whats," and we decompose them into the "hows." This is the phase that most design teams want to jump right into, so hopefully, they have completed the HOQ 1 and HOQ 2 phases before arriving here. The design parameters must be tangible physical solutions.

8.9 HOQ 4: PROCESS HOUSE[1]

The DPs are a list of tangible entities derived by the design team to answer the FR array. The DP list is rotated into HOQ 4 room 1 in this QFD phase.

[1]See Chapter 20 for the complete case study.

The objective is to determine a set of process variables which, when controlled, ensure DP delivery. Again the DPs are the "whats," and we decompose them into the "hows," the process variables (PVs).

8.10   APPLICATION: AUTO 3D

The *automatic dissolving and dosing device* (Auto 3D) is a device that comprises a system of hardware, disposable materials, and software that is used by a nurse, pharmacist, and/or caregiver at home to automatically reconstitute a prescribed dose of medication to be administered in one or multiple doses. The system goal is to consistently, safely, and effectively dissolve and dose the required pharmaceutical. Auto 3D is depicted in Figure 20.1.

Early on, the design team realized that the actual customer base would include the corporate parent, looking for results; a local management team that wanted no increased cost; and the operational caregiver, who needed the device to service patients. The latter is closest to the end user, the patient. In this segment, the customer needs for the Auto 3D device were defined based on marketing research (through interviews laced with common sense), and the following list of needs was obtained:

- Safety and effectiveness
- Medication security
- Device ease of use
- Device reliability and availability
- Device value cost
- Device visual appearance

The high-level wants were prioritized as shown in Table 8.1 using the analytical hierarchy process (AHP). Developed by Thomas Saaty, AHP provides a proven, effective means to deal with complex decision making and can assist with identifying and weighting selection criteria, analyzing the data collected for the criteria, and expediting the decision-making process. The first step is for the team to decompose the customer wants, the "whats," into their constituent elements, progressing from the general to the specific. In its simplest form, this structure comprises a goal, criteria, and alternative levels. Each set of alternatives would then be further divided into an appropriate level of detail, recognizing that the more "whats" criteria are included, the less important each individual criterion may become.

Next, assign a relative weight to each "what," all of which have a local (immediate) and a global priority. Its global priority shows its relative importance within the overall model. Finally, after the criteria are weighted and the information is collected, the DFSS team puts the information into the model. Scoring is on a relative, not an absolute basis, comparing one choice to another.

			A3D Needs							
			1	2	3	4	5	6		
Analytical Hierarchy Process			Safety and effectiveness	Medication security	Ease of use	Reliability and availability	Value cost	Visual appearance	Total	Importance
A3D Needs	1	Safety and effectiveness	1.0	5.0	10.0	10.0	10.0	10.0	46.0	5.0
	2	Medication security	0.2	1.0	10.0	5.0	10.0	10.0	36.2	4.0
	3	Device ease of use	0.1	0.1	1.0	5.0	10.0	10.0	26.2	1.0
	4	Device reliability and availability	0.1	0.2	0.2	1.0	1.0	5.0	7.5	1.0
	5	Device value cost	0.1	0.1	0.1	1	1.0	5.0	6.3	1.0
	6	Device visual appearance	0.1	0.1	0.1	0.2	0.2	1.0	1.7	0.0
		Total	1.6	6.5	21.4	22.2	32.2	41.0		
		Importance	5.0	4.0	3.0	1.0	1.0	0.0		

Figure 8.8   Auto 3D prioritized need using AHP.

Relative scores for each choice are computed within each leaf of the hierarchy. Scores are then synthesized through the model, yielding a composite score for each choice at every tier, as well as an overall score. This process is depicted in Figure 8.8. The importance column will be used in Auto 3D QFD for all customer segments.

The list of "whats" is not directly actionable and needs further detailing using affinity diagramming. Figure 8.9 shows the affinity diagram that was used to determine these high-level needs. The DFSS development team then used the affinity diagram in a brainstorming session and defined the set of "whats" shown in Figure 8.9. In applying the affinity process, the team collected a list of Auto 3D "whats," clarified the list, recorded them on small Post-It notes, and then randomly laid the notes out on a table. The team, without speaking, sorted the notes into "similar" groups based on their gut reactions. If a team member didn't like the placement of a particular note, he or she moved it until consensus was reached. Later, header notes consisting of concise three- to five-word descriptions were created as the unifying concept for each group and placed at the top of each group. The team discussed the groupings to understood how the groups related to each other. The output of the affinity diagramming is depicted in Figure 8.9.

We take these affinity elements and begin to build our HOQ 1 (HOQ 2 was omitted in this study). Figure 8.10 shows the completed HOQ 1.

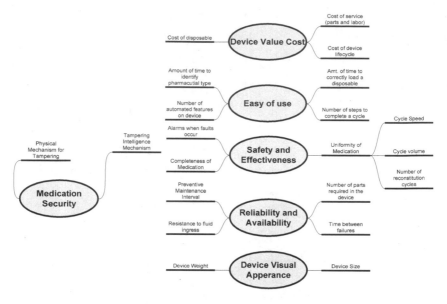

Figure 8.9   Auto 3D affinity diagram.

From QFD house of quality phase 1, the critical-to-satisfaction requirements were determined to be:

- Uniformity of medication
- Completeness of medication
- Tampering intelligence mechanism
- Number of automated features on the device
- Amount of time required to load a disposable device correctly
- Number of steps needed to complete a cycle
- Time between failures
- Resistance to fluid ingress
- Number of parts required in the device
- Preventive maintenance interval
- Cost of device life cycle
- Cost of disposable
- Cost of service (parts and labor)
- Device size
- Device Weight

Strong ● 9
Moderate ○ 3
Weak ▼ 1

Whats		Importance	1 Uniformity of Medication	2 Completeness of Medication	3 Tampering Intelligence Mechanism	4 Number of automated features on device	5 Amt. of time to correctly load a disposable	6 Number of steps to complete a cycle	7 Time between failures	8 Resistance to fluid ingress	9 Number of parts required in the device	10 Preventive mainteneance interval	11 Cost of device lifecycle	12 Cost of disposable	13 Cost of service (parts and labor)	14 Device Size	15 Device Weight	Competitor 1	Competitor 2	Competitor 3
1	Safety and effectivness	5	9	9	3	3	3			3								5	5	5
2	Medication security	4			9	3				3								3	5	2
3	Device ease of use	3			3	9	9	9										2	2	2
4	Device reliability and Availabilty	1			3	1	3	3	9	9	9	9						2	3	1
5	Device value cost	1											9	9	9	3	3	2	2	1
6	Device visual apperance	1	3	3												9	9	1	1	1

Hows; Competitive Benchmark "Importance Value on Whats"

		1	2	3	4	5	6	7	8	9	10	11	12	13	14	15
Technical Importance		48	48	63	55	45	30	9	36	9	9	9	9	9	12	12
Competitive Benchmark "Technical Importance Value on Hows"	Competitor 1															
	Competitor 2															
	Competitor 3															
Targets and Limits	Metric	Siemens (mS)	% transferd	% caught	Count	Seconds	Count	Months	% Leaked	Count	Months	$	$	$	in^3	Ibs
	USL	440	N/A	99%	10	26	6	36	99%	11	18	2000	3.2	110	50	22
	Target		95%	N/A	7	15	3	24	N/A	7	12	1600	2.5	90	40	18
	LSL	350	90%	95%	N/A	N/A	N/A	N/A	95%	N/A	N/A	N/A	N/A	N/A	N/A	N/A

(a)

Correlation:
Enter a value from '-5' to '5'
'-5' implies large negative correlation.
'5' implies large positive correlation.
'0' implies no correlation.

LIB= larger is better
NIB= nominal is best
SIB= samll is better

Hows		Direction	1 Uniformity of medication	2 Completeness of medication	3 Tampering Intelligence mechanism	4 Number of automated features on device	5 Amt. of time to correctly load a disposable	6 Number of steps to complete a cycle	7 Time between failures	8 Resistance to fluid ingress	9 Number of parts required in the device	10 Preventive maintenance interval	11 Cost of device lifecycle	12 Cost of disposable	13 Cost of service (parts and labor)	14 Device Size	15 Device weight
			HIB	HIB	NIB	NIB	SIB	SIB	LIB	LIB	SIB	LIB	SIB	SIB	SIB	NIB	NIB
1	Uniformity of medication	HIB															
2	Completeness of medication	HIB	0														
3	Tampering intelligence mechanism	NIB	0	0													
4	Number of automated features on device	NIB	0	0	0												
5	Amt. of time to correctly load a disposable	SIB	0	0	0	0											
6	Number of steps to complete a cycle	SIB	0	0	0	0	0										
7	Time between failures	LIB	0	0	0	0	0	0									
8	Resistance to fluid ingress	LIB	0	0	0	0	0	0	5								
9	Number of parts required in the device	SIB	0	0	0	0	0	0	-5	0							
10	Preventive maintenance interval	LIB	0	0	0	0	0	0	5	5	-5						
11	Cost of device lifecycle	SIB	-3	-3	-5	-3	0	0	-5	-3	-5	-5					
12	Cost of disposable	SIB	0	0	0	0	0	0	0	0	0	0	-5				
13	Cost of service (parts and labor)	SIB	0	0	0	0	0	0	-5	0	-3	-5	-5	0			
14	Device size	NIB	0	0	0	0	0	0	0	0	0	0	-5	0	0		
15	Device wei ght	NIB	0	0	0	0	0	0	0	0	0	0	-5	0	0	-5	

(b)

Figure 8.10 Auto 3D house of quality: (a) rooms 1 to 7; (b) room 8 (conflict).

8.11 SUMMARY

QFD is a planning tool used to translate customer needs and wants into focused design actions. This goal is best met using cross-functional teams and is a key in preventing problems from occurring once the design is operationalized. The structured linkage allows for a rapid design cycle and effective utilization of resources while achieving six sigma levels of performance.

To be successful with QFD, the team needs to avoid "jumping" right to solutions and must process HOQ 1 and HOQ 2 thoroughly and properly before performing detailed design. The team will also be challenged to keep the functional requirements solution neutral in HOQ 2.

It is important to have the correct voice of customer and the appropriate benchmark information. Also, a strong cross-functional team willing to think outside the box is required to obtain truly six sigma–capable products or processes. From this point the QFD is process driven, but it is not the charts that we are trying to complete—it is the total concept of linking the voice of the customer throughout the design effort.

9

DFSS AXIOMATIC DESIGN METHOD

9.1 INTRODUCTION

Axiomatic design is a prescriptive engineering design theory and methodology that provides a systematic and scientific basis for making design decisions. In addition to the corollaries and theorems derived from them, axioms give design teams a solid basis for formalizing design problems, conceptualizing solution alternatives, eliminating bad design ideas during the conceptual stages, choosing the best design among those proposed, and improving existing designs. An axiom is a proposition regarded as being self-evident without proof. The term *axiom* is a slightly archaic synonym for *postulate*. Axioms are comparable to hypotheses, both of which connote apparently true statements (e.g., Archimedes' axiom, Newton's laws, probability axioms, field axiom).

The verb *design*[1] refers to the process of developing an entity. *Engineering design* is the process of developing a product, service, or process to meet desired customer needs. Design entities share one common attribute,

---

[1]The term *Design* is defined by the National Research Council as "the process by which human intellect, creativity, and passion are translated into useful artifacts. *Engineering design* is a subset of this broad design process in which performance and quality objectives and the underlying science are particularly important. Engineering design is a loosely structured, open-ended activity that includes problem definition, learning processes, representation and decision making." See the National Academy of Engineering, 2002, *Approaches to Improve Engineering Design*, available on the Web at http://www.nap.edu/books/NI000469/html/.

Medical Device Design for Six Sigma: A Road Map for Safety and Effectiveness,
By Basem S. El-Haik and Khalid S. Mekki
Copyright © 2008 John Wiley & Sons, Inc.

hierarchy, which indicates the levels of complexity in both the magnitude of development effort and the end-result ease of operation. In the context of our book, design is an iterative decision-making process in which the physical, mathematical, and engineering sciences are applied to convert resources optimally to meet stated customer needs. Among the fundamental activities of the design process are the establishment of project objectives, synthesis, analysis, construction, testing, and launch.

Human technology evolution continually takes revolutionary steps from ancient civilizations to the twenty-first century. During the twentieth century, technology created by engineering design advanced at an exponential rate; new forms of communications, medical science, new means of travel, and the refinement and distribution of computer technology are just few examples.[2] Today's design teams have unprecedented technology at their disposal. Modern engineers rely heavily on technology, design tools, and proven design processes. Ancient civilizations could rely only on simple tools, although these tools were often truly innovative and far ahead of their time. In fact, when we compare today's design practices with ancient practices, we discover that the principles of design used to support the design process in tunes past continue to evolve. What has changed is the sophistication of the means at both the process and technology levels.

A *design principle* is a fundamental idea on which a design process can be based. For example, the principle of *concurrent engineering* calls for the continuous participation of design and manufacturing teams in almost all aspects of design activities, beginning as early as possible. A design principle helps drive efficient and effective design project management, faster development cycle time, lower cost of development, and improved customer satisfaction. A common set of design principles provides the medical device industry with a common foundation, enabling them to interpret and apply their design and development process from a common point of understanding and to make the right development and business decisions. Design principles need not be mixed with design axioms. In the context of this book, a principle can be promoted to an axiom when it possesses universal applicability (i.e., acceptance in all design domains). A principle is mostly domain specific (e.g., software versus hardware).

Design decision making has a significant impact on lead time, function and form, quality, and the cost of the end result. Studies suggest that decisions made during the early stages of the design phase commit 80% of the total costs associated with developing and manufacturing the product (Fredrikson, 1994). Furthermore, when manufacturing systems and processes are designed poorly, the productivity decreases substantially throughout. (Several case studies show that two serially clustered machine system can have a much lower throughput rate than the slowest machine by itself.) Despite the fundamental importance of proper design, several medical device companies do not have

---

[2]See Bill Jacobs paper at http://www.bandisoftware.com/Incose20010.pdf.

a rational design practice, producing poor-quality products and prolonging the development cycle. This problem can only be solved if the design teams understand what constitutes good design and how to produce such designs.

9.2 AXIOMATIC METHOD FUNDAMENTALS

The axiomatic design method establishes a scientific theoretical basis that gives structure to the medical device design process. Axiomatic design offers perspectives that most conventional algorithmic design approaches fail to achieve. Algorithmic methods such as design for assembly and design for manufacturability are goal oriented in that the design activities are devised around existing best practices and their integration in an algorithmic process setup. New design problems dictate the creation of new algorithms, or in the best case, modified algorithms. Algorithmic methods are most successful in conventional and simple design situations, mostly incremental design type. The practice of engineering using design algorithms is both time consuming and problem dependent. When a design problem is complex (i.e., a large number of functional requirements with numerous hierarchical levels), it might be difficult to fit the problem into an algorithmic format. In algorithmic design methods, the selection of a solution entity for a function from its pool of possible physical embodiment alternatives is usually motivated by economic considerations.

Axiomatic design introduces a different perspective to design theory. The new view offered by DFSS is not limited to the medical device conceptualizing stage (Figure 1.1) but is extended to include the detail design and manufacturing process domain. Axiomatic design delivers these premises via the concepts of *generalization* and *abstraction*.

Many designs have some degree of *coupling*, a design vulnerability that results in a diminishing degree of controllability of the device by both the design team and the customer in usage environments. Many designs require complicated processes with many decision points in order to fulfill the many voices of the customer. Axiomatic design provides a prescriptive methodology to assess coupling and seek to resolve it as well as to reduce design complexity in the early stages of the design cycle.

Axiomatic design is a design theory that constitutes knowledge of basic and fundamental design elements. In this context, a scientific theory is defined as a theory comprising fundamental knowledge areas in the form of perceptions and understandings of different entities and the relationship between these fundamental areas. To produce consequences that can be, but are not necessarily, predictions of observations, the theorist combines these perceptions and relations. Fundamental knowledge areas include mathematical expressions, mapping, categorizations of phenomena or objects, and models, and are more abstract than observations of real-world data. Such knowledge and relations between knowledge elements constitute a theoretical system. A theoretical system may be one of two types: axioms or hypotheses, depending on how the fundamental knowledge areas are treated. Fundamental knowledge that is generally accepted as true, yet cannot be tested, is treated as an axiom. If the fundamental knowledge areas are being tested, they are treated as hypotheses (Nordlund, 1996). In this regard, axiomatic design is a scientific design method, but with the premise of a theoretical system based on two axioms.

Motivated by the absence of scientific design principles, Suh (1984, 1990, 1995a,b, 1996, 1997, 2001) proposed the use of axioms as the scientific foundation of design. The following are two axioms that a design must satisfy:

Axiom 1: The Independence Axiom   Maintain the independence of the functional requirements.

Axiom 2: The Information Axiom   Minimize the information content in a design.

In the context of axiomatic deployment, the independence axiom will be used to address the conceptual design vulnerabilities, while the information axiom will be tasked with operational design vulnerabilities (El-Haik, 2005). Operational vulnerability is usually minimized and cannot be totally eliminated. Reducing the variability of the design functional requirements and adjusting their mean performance to desired targets are two steps toward achieving such minimization. Such activities will also result in reducing design information content, a measure of design complexity that follows from Axiom 1. The customer relates information content to the probability of successfully producing the design as intended and maintaining it afterward.

The design process involves three mappings among four domains (Figure 9.1). The reader may already notice the similarity with QFD phases in Chapter 8. The first mapping involves the mapping between *customer attributes* (CAs) and *functional requirements* (FRs). In Chapter 8 we learned that up to two

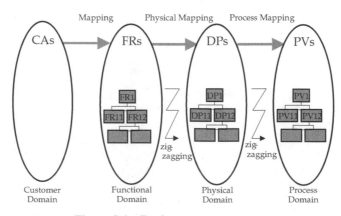

Figure 9.1   Design mapping process.

phases of quality function deployment may be necessary to correctly define the minimum set of FRs necessary to characterize the device design. In other words, the CA terminology is equivalent to the critical-to requirements (CTs) terminology in Chapter 8. This mapping is very important, as it yields the definition of the high-level minimum set of FRs needed to accomplish the design intent. Once the minimum set of FRs is defined, the *physical mapping* may be started. This mapping involves the FR domain and the *design param-eter (DP) codomain*. It represents the medical device development activities and can be depicted by design matrices; hence, the term *mapping* is used. This mapping is conducted over the design hierarchy as the high-level set of FRs, defined earlier, is cascaded down to the lowest hierarchical level. Design matrices reveal coupling, a conceptual vulnerability. Matrices provide a means to track the chain of effects of design changes as they propagate across the design mapping.

The *process mapping* is the last mapping of axiomatic design and involves the DP domain and the process variables (PV) codomain. This mapping can be represented formally by matrices as well and provides the process elements needed to translate the DPs to PVs in the manufacturing and production domains.

The mapping equation FR = f(DP) or, in matrix notation, $\{FR\}_{m \times 1} = [A]_{m \times p}$ $\{DP\}_{p \times 1}$, is used to reflect the relationship between the domain, array $\{FR\}$ and the codomain, array $\{DP\}$, in the physical mapping where the array $\{FR\}_{m \times 1}$ is a vector with m requirements, $\{DP\}_{p \times 1}$ is the vector of design parameters with p characteristics, and A is the design matrix (see Appendix 9A). According to Axiom 1, the ideal case is to have a one-to-one mapping so that a specific DP can be adjusted to satisfy its corresponding FR without affecting the other requirements. However, perfect deployment of the design axioms may not be feasible, due to technological and cost limitations. Under these circumstances, different degrees of conceptual vulnerabilities are established in the measures (criteria) related to the unsatisfied axiom. For example, a degree of *coupling* may be created because of Axiom 1 violation, and this design may function adequately for some time in the use environment. However, a conceptually weak system may have limited opportunity for continuous success even with the aggressive implementation of an operational vulnerability improvement phase.

When matrix A is a square diagonal matrix [see Figure 9.2(a)], the design is called *uncoupled* (i.e., each FR can be adjusted or changed independent of the other FRs). An uncoupled design is a one-to-one mapping. Another design that obeys Axiom 1, although with a known design sequence [see Figure 9.2(b)] is called *decoupled.* In a decoupled design, matrix A is a *lower* or *upper triangular matrix*. The decoupled design may be treated as an uncoupled design when the DPs are adjusted in some sequence conveyed by the matrix. Uncoupled and decoupled design entities possess conceptual robustness (i.e., the DPs can be changed to affect specific requirements without affecting other FRs unintentionally). A coupled design definitely results in a design matrix

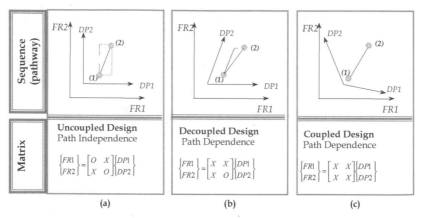

Figure 9.2   Design categories according to Axiom 1.

with a number of requirements, m, greater than the number of DPs, p [see Figure 9.2(c)]. Square design matrices ($m = p$) may be classified as a coupled design when the off-diagonal matrix elements are nonzeros. Graphically, the three design classifications are depicted in Figure 9.2 for the 2×2 design matrix case. Notice that we denote the nonzero mapping relationship in the respective design matrices by "X"; "0" denotes the absence of such a relationship.

Consider the uncoupled design in Figure 9.2(a). The uncoupled design possesses the path independence property; that is, the design team could set the design to level (1) as a start point and move to setting (2) by changing DP1 first (moving east to the right of the page or parallel to DP1) and then changing DP2 (moving toward the top of the page or parallel to DP2). Due to the path independence property of the uncoupled design, the team could start from setting (1) to setting (2) by changing DP2 first (moving toward the top of the page or parallel to DP2) and then changing DP1 second (moving east or parallel to DP1). Both paths are equivalent; that is, they accomplish the same result. Notice also that the FRs independence is depicted as orthogonal coordinates as well as perpendicular DPs axes that parallel its respective FR in the diagonal matrix.

Path independence is characterized, mathematically, by a diagonal design matrix (uncoupled design). Path independence is a necessary property of an uncoupled design and implies full control of the design team and ultimately the customer (user) over the design. It also implies a high level of design quality and reliability since interaction effects between the FRs are minimized. In addition, a failure in one (FR,DP) combination of the uncoupled design matrix is not reflected in the other (FR,DP) mappings within the same design hierarchical level of interest.

For the decoupled design, the path independence property is somehow fractured. As depicted in Figure 9.2(b), decoupled design matrices have design settings sequences that need to be followed for the FRs to maintain their independence. This sequence is revealed by the matrix as follows: First, we need to set FR2 using DP2, fix DP2, and second set FR1 by leveraging DP1. Starting from setting (1), we need to set FR2 at setting (2) by changing DP2, and then change DP1 to the desired level of FR1.

The discussion above is a testimony to the fact that uncoupled and decoupled designs have conceptual robustness; that is, coupling can be resolved with the proper selection of DPs, path sequence application, and employment of design theorems (Suh, 2001; El-Haik, 2005).

The coupled design matrix in Figure 9.2(c) indicates the loss of the path independence due to the off-diagonal design matrix entries (on both sides), and the design team has no easy way to improve controllability, reliability, and quality (measured by Z-score; see Chapter 3) of their design. The design team is left with compromise practices (e.g., optimization) among the FRs as the only option since a component of the individual DPs can be projected on all orthogonal directions of the FRs. The uncoupling or decoupling step of a coupled design is a conceptual activity that follows the design mapping (El-Haik, 2005).

9.3 INTRODUCTION TO AXIOM 1

Axiom 1: The Independence Axiom   Maintain the independence of the functional requirements.

In the context of axiomatic design, the array of FRs is the minimum set of independent requirements that completely characterizes the design objective, the customer attributes (CAs). *Design* is defined as the creation of a synthesized solution to satisfy perceived needs through the mapping between the FRs in the functional domain and the DPs in the physical domain, and through the mapping between the DPs and the PVs in the process domain. A violation of the independence axiom occurs when an FR is mapped to a DP that is coupled with another FR. Such practice creates a design vulnerability called *coupling*, which implies the lack of controllability and adjustability by both the design team and customer.

The mapping process can be written mathematically as the following matrix equations:

$$\{FR\}_{m\times1} = [A]_{m\times p}\{DP\}_{p\times1} \tag{9.1}$$

$$\{DP\}_{p\times1} = [B]_{p\times n}\{PV\}_{n\times1} \tag{9.2}$$

or, equivalently,

$$\{FR\}_{m\times1} = [C]_{m\times n}\{PV\}_{n\times1} \tag{9.3}$$

where $\{FR\}_{m\times 1}$ is the vector of independent functional requirements with m elements, $\{DP\}_{p\times 1}$ is the vector of design parameters with p elements, $\{PV\}_{n\times 1}$ is the vector of process variables with n elements, $A_{m\times p}$ is the physical design matrix, $B_{p\times n}$ is the process design matrix, and $[C]_{m\times n} = [A][B]$ is the overall design matrix. In general and throughout the book, we use physical mapping for illustration and derivation purposes. Nevertheless, the formulation, derivations, and conclusions are equally applicable to process mapping.

Before proceeding further, we would like to define the following terminology relative to Axiom 1, and to ground readers in the terminology and concepts that we have already used in previous sections.

- *Functional requirements* (FRs) are a minimum set of independent requirements that completely characterize the functional needs of a design solution in the functional domain within the constraints of safety, economy, reliability, and quality.

How should functional requirements be defined? In the context of the first mapping in Figure 9.1, customers define the medical device using some features or attributes that are saturated by some or all types of linguistic uncertainty. For example, in an automotive product design, customers use the terms *quiet, stylish, comfortable*, and *easy to drive* in describing the features of their dream car. The challenge is how to translate these features into functional requirements and then into solution entities. Quality function deployment (QFD) is the tool adopted here to accomplish an actionable set of FRs.

In defining their wants and needs, customers often use vague and fuzzy terms that are hard to interpret or to attribute to specific engineering terminology: in particular, the FRs. In general, FRs are technical terms extracted from the voice of the customer. Customer expressions are not dichotomous or crisp in nature but something in between. As a result, uncertainty may lead to inaccurate interpretation and therefore vulnerable or unwanted design. There are many classifications for customers' linguistic inexactness. In general, two major sources of imprecision in human knowledge, *stochastic uncertainty* and *linguistic inexactness* (Zimmermann, 1985), are usually encountered. Stochastic uncertainty is well handled by probability theory. Imprecision can arise from a variety of sources: incomplete knowledge, ambiguous definitions, inherent stochastic characteristics, measurement problems, and so on.

This brief introduction to linguistic inexactness is warranted to enable design teams to appreciate the task at hand, assess their understanding of the voice of the customer, and seek clarification where needed. Ignorance of such facts may cause several failures to the design project and their efforts altogether. The severest failure among them is the possibility of propagating inexactness into design activities, including analysis and synthesis of incorrect requirements.

- *Design parameters* (DPs) are the elements of the design solution in the physical domain that are chosen to satisfy the FRs specified. In general terms, standard and reusable DPs (grouped into design modules within the physical structure) are often used and generally have a higher probability of success, thus improving the quality and reliability of the design.
- *Constraints* (Cs) are bounds on acceptable solutions.
- *Process variables* (PVs) are the elements of the process domain that characterize the process that satisfies the DPs specified.

The design team will conceive a detailed description of what functional requirements the design entity needs to perform to satisfy customer needs, a description of the physical entity that will realize those functions (the DPs), and a description of how this object will be produced (the PVs).

9.4 INTRODUCTION TO AXIOM 2

Axiom 2: The Information Axiom   Minimize the information content in a design.

The second axiom of axiomatic design stated above provides a selection metric based on design information content. The selection problem between alternative design solution entities (concepts) of the same design variable (project) will occur in many situations. Even in the ideal case, a pool of uncoupled design alternatives, the design team still needs to select the best solution. The selection process is criteria-based, hence Axiom 1. Axiom 2 states that the design that results in the highest probability of FR success [Prob(FR1), Prob(FR2), ... , Prob(FRm)] is the best design. Information and probability are tied together via entropy, H (El-Haik, 2005). Entropy may be defined as

$$H = -\log_v(\text{Prob}) \tag{9.4}$$

Note that the probability [Prob in (9.4)] takes a Shannon entropy (1948) form of a discrete random variable supplying the information, the source. Note also that the logarithm is to the base v, a real nonnegative number. If $v = 2e$, where e is the base of the natural logarithm, H is measured in *bits (nats)*. The expression of information and hence design complexity in terms of probability hints to the fact that FRs are random variables themselves and have to be met within some tolerance accepted by the customer. The array {FR} also consists of functions (the physical mapping) of random variables, and the array {DP}, functions (the process mapping) of another vector of random variables, the array {PV}: hence, the transferred variation phenomenon.

The PVs' downstream variation can be induced by several sources, such as manufacturing process variation, including tool degradation and environmental factors, the noise factors. This fact facilitates mathematical formulation of the DFSS process and these enables several venues of design vulnerability treatment (however, with an axiomatic flavor). For example, assuming statistical independence, the overall (total) design information content of a given design hierarchical level is additive since its probability of success is the multiplication of the individual FR probability of success at that level. That is, to reduce complexity, we need to address the largest contributors to the total (the sum). When the statistical independence assumption is not valid, the system probability of success is not multiplicative; rather, it is conditional.

A solution entity is characterized as *complex* when the probability of success of the total design (all hierarchical levels) is low. Complex design solution entities require more information to manufacture. That is, complexity is a design vulnerability that is created in the design entity due to violation of Axiom 1. Note that complexity here has two arguments: the number of FRs as well as their probability of success.

Information content is related to tolerances and process capabilities since probabilities are. The *probability of success* may be defined as the probability of meeting design specifications: the area of intersection between the *design range* (voice of the customer) and the *system range* (voice of the process). The overlap between the design range (DR) and the system range (SR) is called the *common range* (CR) (see Figure 9.3). The probability of success is the area ratio of the common range to the system range, CR/SR. Substituting this definition in (9.4), we have

$$H = \log_v \frac{\text{SR}}{\text{CR}} \qquad (9.5)$$

An example of design coupling is presented in Figure 9.4, where two possible arrangements of a generic water faucet (Swenson and Nordlund, 1996)

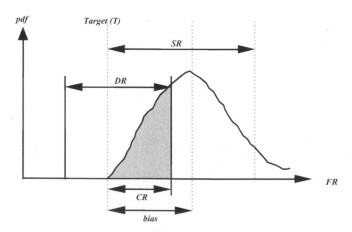

Figure 9.3   Probability of success definition.

are displayed. There are two functional requirements: water flow and water temperature. Figure 9.4(a) faucet has two design parameters, the water valves (knobs), one for each water line. When the hot-water valve is turned, both flow and temperature are affected. The same happens when the cold-water valve is turned. That is, the FRs are not independent, and the coupled design matrix below the schematic reflects that fact. From a consumer perspective, optimization of the temperature will require reoptimization of the flow rate until a satisfactory compromize among the FRs as a function of the DP settings is obtained over several iterations.

Figure 9.4(b) exhibits an alternative design with a one-handle system delivering the FRs, but with a new set of design parameters. In this design, flow is adjusted by lifting the handle, while moving the handle sideways will adjust the temperature. In this alternative, adjusting the flow does not affect the temperature, and vice versa. This design is better, since the functional requirements maintain their independence (i.e., obey Axiom 1). The uncoupled design will give the customer path independence to set either requirement without affecting the other. Note also that in the uncoupled design case, design changes to improve a FR can be done independently as well, a valuable design attribute.

The importance of design mapping has many perspectives. Chief among them is the identification of coupling among the functional requirements, due to the physical mapping process with the design parameters in the codomain. Knowledge of coupling is important because it provides the design team with clues from which to find solutions, make adjustments or design changes in

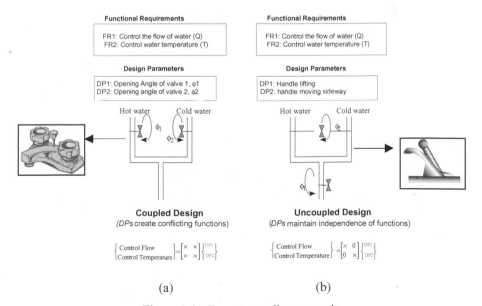

Functional Requirements

FR1: Control the flow of water (Q)
FR2: Control water temperature (T)

Design Parameters

DP1: Opening Angle of valve 1, $\phi 1$
DP2: Opening angle of valve 2, $\phi 2$

Hot water   Cold water

Coupled Design
(DPs create conflicting functions)

$$\begin{Bmatrix} \text{Control Flow} \\ \text{Control Temperature} \end{Bmatrix} = \begin{bmatrix} \times & \times \\ \times & \times \end{bmatrix} \begin{Bmatrix} \text{DP1} \\ \text{DP2} \end{Bmatrix}$$

Functional Requirements

FR1: Control the flow of water (Q)
FR2: Control water temperature (T)

Design Parameters

DP1: Handle lifting
DP2: handle moving sideway

Hot water   Cold water

Uncoupled Design
(DPs maintain independence of functions)

$$\begin{Bmatrix} \text{Control Flow} \\ \text{Control Temperature} \end{Bmatrix} = \begin{bmatrix} \times & 0 \\ 0 & \times \end{bmatrix} \begin{Bmatrix} \text{DP1} \\ \text{DP2} \end{Bmatrix}$$

(a)   (b)

Figure 9.4 Faucet coupling example.

proper sequence, and maintain their effects over the long term with minimal negative consequences.

The design matrices are obtained in a hierarchy, and result from employment of the *zigzagging* method of mapping depicted in Figure 9.5 (Suh, 1990). The zigzagging process requires a solution-neutral environment, where the DPs are chosen after the FRs are defined, and not vice versa. When the FRs are defined, we have to *zig* to the physical domain, and after proper DPs selection, we have to *zag* back to the functional domain for further decomposition or cascading, though at a lower hierarchical level. This process is in contrast with traditional cascading processes that utilize only one domain at a time, treating the design as the sum of functions or the sum of processes.

At lower levels of hierarchy, entries of design matrices can be obtained mathematically from basic process engineering quantities, enabling the definition and detailing of transfer functions, a DFSS optimization vehicle. In some cases, these relationships are not readily available and some effort needs to be paid to obtain them empirically or via modeling. Lower levels represent the roots of the hierarchical structure, where six sigma concepts can be applied with some degree of ease.

Similar to CTs, FRs, and DPs, the design specifications need to be cascaded. The specifications describe the limits that are acceptable by the customer to accomplish a design solution from their own perspective. The specification determines each limit required of a critical-to (CT) and then by mapping to FRs, DPs, and PVs. That is, the specification cascading start as a CT specification and then flowed-down to functional requirements, design parameters and process variables by methods such as quality function deployment and axiomatic design. For example, in a service software design, an "easy-to-use" CT cascaded (by mapping) could morph into the specification for application programs, file layouts, data elements, reports, tables, screens, or technical communication protocols that are required to accomplish the originating CT.

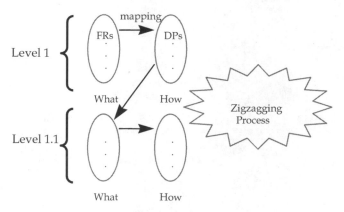

Figure 9.5   Zigzagging process.

The specification is written either to modify an existing FR, DP, or PV, or introduce a new FR, DP, or PV. The technical specification in a design mapping should also describe the concept and reasons for the change, or any new functionality, as well as providing the detailed effort necessary to achieve the result desired.

9.5 AXIOMATIC DESIGN THEOREMS AND COROLLARIES

The study of most famous examples (e.g., Euclidean geometry, Newton's laws, thermodynamics, the axiomatic branch of modern mathematics[3]) of the axiomatic disciplines reveals several common threads. For example, Euclid's axiomatic geometry opens with a list of definitions, postulates, then axioms, before proving propositions. The aim is to present geometrical knowledge as an ordered list of proven facts, a historical paradigm of disciplines with axiomatic origin. Newton's laws were deliberately set up to emulate the Euclidean style. The laws open with a list of definitions and axioms, before proving propositions. Although the axioms are justified empirically, consequences of the axioms are meant to be drawn deductively. Modern mathematics and empirical knowledge are two streams that can be observed in disciplines that emerge from an axiomatic origin.

In axiomatic design, the goal is to systematize our design knowledge regarding a particular subject matter by showing how particular propositions (derived theories and corollaries) follow the axioms, the basic propositions. To prove a particular proposition, we need to appeal to other propositions that justify it. But our proof is not done if those other propositions themselves need justification. Ultimately, to avoid infinite regression, we will have to start our proofs with propositions that do not themselves need justification. What sorts of propositions are not in need of justification? Answer: the axioms. Therefore, differentiation of axioms from other postulates is needed. The label *axiom* is used to name these propositions that are not in need of justification. Nevertheless, historically, various distinctions have been made between axioms and postulates. We encounter two ways of drawing the distinction, one based on logical status and the other based on status relative to the subject matter of the theory. Axioms are self-evident truths. For example, the independence and information axioms are axioms entertained in axiomatic design. They are self-evident and have been learned from a large pool of observations. Whereas the postulate is a synthetic proposition, the contradiction of which, though difficult to imagine, nevertheless remains conceivable, the axiom would be an analytic proposition, the denial of which is not accepted. As such, a science

---

[3]Axiomatic theories in modern mathematics include modern axiomatic geometry (Euclidean and non-Euclidean geometries), Peano's axioms for natural numbers, axioms for set theory, axioms for group theory, order axioms (linear ordering, partial ordering), and axioms for equivalence relations—not the sort of axiomatic theory we consider in this book.

must start from indemonstrable principles; otherwise, the steps of demonstration would be endless.

"One of the major causes for the dismal state of design is simply mental block: the notion that design, unlike the natural sciences, cannot stand on a scientific basis. This hypothesis is both unnecessary and incorrect." (Suh, 1990). The use of design principles is a vehicle capable of gearing design activities to fruitful systematic results while providing the design scientific basis desired. The two design axioms suggested by Suh (1990) are prominent examples of empirical design principles proven to be beneficial, as evidenced by application growth and industrial coverage. The employment of axioms in design seems to be promising because history tells us that knowledge based on axioms will continue to evolve through theorems and corollaries as long as the axioms are maintained. A subset of axiomatic design corollaries and theories, mostly developed by Suh, that are described in this book are given below. The rest can be found in a book by Suh (2001). Additional theorems are also developed in the present book by the authors.

Axiomatic Design Corollaries[4]

Corollary 1: Decoupling of Coupled Designs   Decouple or separate parts or aspects of a solution if FRs are coupled or become interdependent in the designs proposed.

Corollary 2: Minimization of FRs   Minimize the number of FRs and constraints.

Corollary 3: Integration of Physical Parts   Integrate design features in a single physical part if FRs can be satisfied independently in the solution proposed.

Corollary 4: Use of Standardization   Use standardized or interchangeable parts if use of the parts is consistent with FRs and constraints.

Corollary 5: Use of Symmetry   Use symmetrical shapes and/or components if they are consistent with the FRs and constraints.

Corollary 6: Largest Design Tolerance   Specify the largest allowable tolerance in stating FRs.

Corollary 7: Uncoupled Design with Less Information   Seek an uncoupled design that requires less information than do coupled designs in satisfying a set of FRs.

---

[4]A corollary is an immediate consequence of a result already proved. Corollaries usually state a more complicated theorem in a language simpler to use and apply.

Corollary 8: Effective Reangularity of a Scalar The effective reangularity[5], R, for a scalar coupling matrix element is unity.

Axiomatic Design Theorems[6] of General Design

Theorem 1: Coupling Due to Insufficient Number of DPs When the number of DPs is less than the number of FRs, either a coupled design results or the FRs cannot be satisfied.

Theorem 2: Decoupling a Coupled Design When a design is coupled due to the greater number of FRs than DPs (i.e., $m > p$), it may be decoupled by the addition new DPs so as to make the number of FRs and DPs equal to each other if a subset of the design matrix containing $p \times p$ elements constitutes a triangular matrix.

Theorem 3: Redundant Design When there are more DPs than FRs, the design is either a redundant design or a coupled design.

Theorem 4: Ideal Design In an ideal design, the number of DPs is equal to the number of FRs, and the FRs are always maintained independent of each other.

Theorem 5: Need for a New Design When a given set of FRs is changed by the addition of a new FR by substitution of one of the FRs with a new one or by selection of a completely different set of FRs, the design solution given by the original DPs cannot satisfy the new set of FRs. Consequently, a new design solution must be sought.

Theorem 6: Path Independence of an Uncoupled Design The information content of an uncoupled design is independent of the sequence by which the DPs are changed to satisfy the given set of FRs.

Theorem 7: Path Dependency of Coupled and Decoupled Design[7] The information contents of coupled and decoupled designs depend on the sequence by which the DPs are changed to satisfy the given set of FRs.

---

[5]R is a measure of coupling vulnerability and is defined as the orthogonality between the DPs in terms of the absolute value of the product of the geometric sines of all the angles between the different DP pair combinations of the design matrix.

[6]A *theorem* can be defined as a statement that can be demonstrated to be true by accepted mathematical operations and arguments. In general, a theorem is an embodiment of some general principle that makes it part of a larger theory. The process of showing a theorem to be correct is called a *proof*. See El-Haik (2005) and Suh (2002) for theorems other than those included here.

[7]See El-Haik (2005) for more details.

9.6   APPLICATION: MEDICATION MIXING MACHINE

Pharmaceutical companies must observe quality-affecting computerized systems in accordance with the FDA's ruling under 21 CFR Part 11. The high level of control required for compliance with good manufacturing practice makes automated control systems one of the most critical applications of this requirement. In this example a computer-based machine needs to be designed to mix medications in pharmacies. This case study was performed for a major pharmaceutical manufacturer headquartered in the United States that specializes in the manufacture of medical devices and pharmaceutical products. Here we list a partial decomposition. The highest-level functional requirement is

FR0 = design a mixing medication machine
DP0 = computer-based multimedia unit

$$\{FR0\} = [X]\{DP0\} \tag{9.6}$$

The machine should satisfy the following constraint:

C0 = has a manufactured per-unit cost under $4000

The level 2 FRs are as follows:

FR01 = PC-based software-controlled logic
FR02 = interact with pharmacist to conduct mixing

with the following DPs:

DP01 = run software
DP02 = pharmacy ac-powered unit

and the following design equation:

$$\begin{Bmatrix} FR01 \\ FR02 \end{Bmatrix} = \begin{bmatrix} X & 0 \\ X & X \end{bmatrix} \begin{Bmatrix} DP01 \\ DP02 \end{Bmatrix} \tag{9.7}$$

The level 3 FRs are as follows for DP01 decomposition:

FR011 = need computer module to run software
FR012 = need to provide 10-megabyte program storage
FR013 = ability to load various programs to hard disk

with the following DPs:

DP011 = at least 486 16-MHz computer module
DP012 = 60-megabyte hard disk
DP013 = compact disk

and the following design matrix:

$$
\begin{Bmatrix} FR011 \\ FR012 \\ FR013 \end{Bmatrix} = \begin{bmatrix} X & & \\ & X & \\ & & X \end{bmatrix} \begin{Bmatrix} DP011 \\ DP012 \\ DP013 \end{Bmatrix}
\tag{9.8}
$$

For DP02 decomposition:

FR021 = communicate visually with the pharmacist
FR022 = communicate verbally with the pharmacist
FR023 = product written as information to the pharmacist
FR024 = receive communication from the pharmacist
FR025 = need power

with the following DPs:

DP021 = use a monitor
DP022 = digitized voice capability
DP023 = use special type of printer
DP024 = use touch selection input
DP025 = use 120 volts/60 Hz

and the following design equation:

$$
\begin{Bmatrix} FR021 \\ FR022 \\ FR023 \\ FR024 \\ FR025 \end{Bmatrix} = \begin{bmatrix} X & & & & \\ & X & & & \\ & & X & & \\ & & & X & \\ & & & & X \end{bmatrix} \begin{Bmatrix} DP021 \\ DP022 \\ DP023 \\ DP024 \\ DP025 \end{Bmatrix}
\tag{9.9}
$$

9.7 APPLICATION: AXIOMATIC DESIGN APPLIED TO DESIGN CONTROLS[8]

The design controls section 820.30 of the QS regulation (21 CFR) applies to the design of products and processes and changes in existing designs and

[8]Adapted from Worona (2006).

processes. Changes should be made in existing designs in accordance with design control requirements even if the original design was not subject to these requirements. Design controls are not retroactive to completed portions of ongoing design programs.

Medical device companies should consider treating the design control development process with the same level of rigor that is used for product design. Doing so will enable device manufacturers to take the company beyond compliance and move toward business excellence.

Medical device manufacturers have some leverage in developing a design control system as long as they exceed the minimum criteria delineated in the quality systems regulation (QSR). The QSR states that procedures must be established for design input, design output, design review, design planning, design verification, design validation, design transfer, and design changes. The specific requirements for each are listed in 21 CFR 820.30. However, the definitions are broad and do not describe methods for implementing controls. For example, consider the following requirements regarding design changes: "820.30(i) Design Changes. Each manufacturer shall establish and maintain procedures for the identification, documentation, validation, or where appropriate verification, review, and approval of design changes before their implementation."

The creator of the design control procedures is often the quality manager or product development manager who is charged with passing audits. If a deficiency is noted through internal audits or design failures, a quick correction is added to the system to cover that particular weakness. Alternatively, sometimes, because of internal politics, the design control procedures are labeled difficult to comply with, and a round of procedure redesign and simplification removes detail and work instructions. The result of such hasty changes can be design control procedures that no longer meet the regulations.

To satisfy the design control functional requirements, a creator of a design change procedure might use data input fields in Microsoft (MS) Word format that prompt the user for specific information that was identified earlier. The fields in the MS Word document should be a design parameter used to fulfill the functional requirements. In design change procedures, manufacturers can meet a functional requirement (FR1) with a specified design parameter (DP1):

FR1 = have complete information available to the auditor that enables the organization to defend the design at the field change order stage

DP1 = provide a field change order form that contains information of concern to an auditor

The design equation is given by

$$\{FR1\} = [X]\{DP1\} \qquad (9.10)$$

At this stage, the procedures are still defined broadly and will need more detail at a later stage. Examples of lower-level requirements and design parameters include the following:

FR11 = means to describe the change fully

DP11 = have a segment of the field change order form for information such as the nature of the change, the scope of the change, and the specific change (e.g., list products and subassemblies affected, with part numbers)

FR12 = means to describe the reason for the change

DP12 = have a segment of the field change order to describe the reason for the change and clarify whether the change is due to a safety concern

FR13 = means to link the change to CAPA-type systems that initiated the change for reference

DP13 = have a segment of the field change order to define the links to other CAPA systems by quoting a reference number for nonconforming material or complaints

FR14 = means to describe how the change fixes the problem

DP14 = have a segment of the field change order to identify the problem the change is trying to fix, the root cause of the problem, and how the change corrects the problem

The design equation is given by

$$
\begin{Bmatrix} FR11 \\ FR12 \\ FR13 \\ FR14 \end{Bmatrix} = \begin{bmatrix} X & & & \\ X & X & & \\ X & X & X & \\ X & X & X & X \end{bmatrix} \begin{Bmatrix} DP11 \\ DP12 \\ DP13 \\ DP14 \end{Bmatrix} \tag{9.11}
$$

The relationship between functional requirements and design parameters is made using the concept of zigzagging. Zigzagging is used very naturally during product design. When designers identify a high-level user requirement, they also identify a high-level design parameter (or technology) that will fulfill the requirement. For example, the functional requirement "control the operation of an electromechanical device" could be fulfilled by the design parameter of an industrial PC or a microcontroller. Each selection will have its own implications and limitations when implementing lower-level control requirements, such as the number of sensor inputs, monitoring frequency, or others.

Accordingly, the high-level technology must also be considered when identifying lower-level requirements and when ensuring that those requirements are met. This process is the strength of the zigzagging concept. Once the high-level requirement and the high-level technology to be used to fulfill the requirements are defined, create lower-level functional requirements and then identify how they will be fulfilled individually (keeping in mind the microcontroller or industrial PC). If at any point the lower-level requirements cannot be met because of the limitations of the higher-level technology selection, a new technology will need to be selected. Only by keeping that high-level design parameter in mind can designers successfully identify lower-level functional requirements.

Once DP1 for the design change process (as described earlier) is established as a form that contains information, it becomes easier to visualize the lower-level functional requirements and design parameters as fields in a form that meets different functions. Lower-level requirements will then define the specific fields that need to be included in the form.

9.8   SUMMARY

DFSS methodology hinges on the axiomatic design, a prescriptive engineering design method. Axiomatic design is a design theory that constitutes basic and fundamental design elements knowledge. It is a scientific design method, but with the premise of a theoretical system based on two axioms.

APPENDIX 9A: MATRIX REVIEW[9]

A matrix can be considered a two-dimensional array of numbers. They take the form

$$A = \begin{bmatrix} a_{11} & a_{12} & a_{13} \\ a_{21} & a_{22} & a_{23} \\ a_{31} & a_{32} & a_{33} \end{bmatrix}$$

Matrices are very powerful and form the basis of all modern computer graphics, the advantage of them being that they are so fast. We define a matrix with an uppercase boldface letter. Look at the example above. The dimension of a matrix is its height followed by its width, so the matrix above has dimension 3×3. Matrices can be of any dimensions, but in terms of computer graphics, they are usually kept to 3×3 or 4×4. There are a few types of special matrices: the column matrix, row matrix, square matrix, identity matrix, and zero matrix. A *column matrix* has a width of 1 and a height greater than 1. A *row matrix* has a width greater than 1 and a height of 1. In a *square matrix*, the dimensions are the same. For instance, the example above is a square

[9]Adapted from http://www.gamedev.net/reference/articles/article1832.asp, by Phil Dadd.

matrix, because the width equals the height. An *identity matrix* is a special type of matrix that has values in the diagonal from the top left to the bottom right as 1 and the rest as 0. The identity matrix is known by the letter I, where

$$I = \begin{bmatrix} 1 & 0 & 0 \\ 0 & 1 & 0 \\ 0 & 0 & 1 \end{bmatrix}$$

An identity matrix can be any dimension, as long as it is also a square matrix. A *zero matrix* is a matrix that has all its elements set to 0. The elements of a matrix are all the numbers in it. They are numbered by the row and column position, so a_{13} indicates the matrix element in row 1 and column 3.

10

DFSS INNOVATION FOR MEDICAL DEVICES

10.1 INTRODUCTION

As we design devices, there are many contradictions or trade-offs that must be resolved. When the design is operationalized, we often discover that the design will not achieve the desired level of performance because of the unresolved or suboptimized resolution of the contradictions or coupling, as introduced in Chapter 9. What if a tool existed that allows for effective resolution of these contradictions, expands the DFSS team's knowledge, and allows for safe and effective innovation? Wouldn't a DFSS team be interested in such a tool?

Well, there is such a tool, the theory of inventive problem solving (TRIZ or TIPS), introduced in the United States about 1991. The purpose of this chapter is to familiarize the reader with the basics of TRIZ, some practical applications, and with references to where to become more practiced. TRIZ is a tool that can be used heavily in the DFSS road map characterize phase (see Figure 7.1). Moving forward, opportunities for TRIZ application are vital in other phases.

10.2 HISTORY OF THE THEORY OF INVENTIVE PROBLEM SOLVING

The history of TRIZ is interesting and mirrors the life of its inventor, Genrich S. Altshuller. Altshuller was born on October 15, 1926 in Tashkent,

Medical Device Design for Six Sigma: A Road Map for Safety and Effectiveness,
By Basem S. El-Haik and Khalid S. Mekki
Copyright © 2008 John Wiley & Sons, Inc.

Uzbekistan. While in the ninth grade he obtained his first patent (Author's Certificate), for underwater diving apparatus. In the tenth grade he developed a boat propelled by a carbide-fueled rocket engine. In 1946 he invented a method for escaping an immobilized submarine, and this led to his employment in the patent office of the Caspian Sea Military Navy. The head of this department challenged Altshuller to solve a difficult problem, and he was successful. A series of events, meetings, and letters led to his imprisonment four years later. He was driven to invent and assist others to invent. He was troubled by the common thought that invention was the result of accidental enlightenment or genealogy. He began a journey to discover a methodology for inventing. He called upon a former schoolmate, Rafael Shapiro, also a passionate inventor, to work with him to discover the methodology of invention. By now, Altshuller believed that invention was no more than the removal of technical contradictions with the help of certain principles. Shapiro was excited about the discovery and they researched all the existing patents and took part in inventing competitions in their search for new methods of invention. They received a National Competition Award for the design of a flame- and heat-resistant suit. As recognition they were invited to Tbilisi, Georgia's present capital, where upon arrival they were arrested, interrogated, and sentenced to 25 years in Siberia. It turns out that all of the letters that Alshuller had written to Stalin had him pegged as an intellectual, and there was only one place for intellectuals in the new Russia. Altshuller used his TRIZ model to survive, minimizing harmful functions and optimizing useful functions. In Siberia, he worked 12 hours a day logging and decided it was better to be put in solitary confinement. Later he was transferred to the Varkuta coal mines, where he had to toil for 8 to 10 hours per day. In 1954, a year and a half after Stalin's death, Altshuller was released from prison. In 1956 the first paper by Altshuller and Shapiro, "Psychology of Inventive Creativity," was published. In 1961, their first book, *How to Learn to Invent*, was published and 50,000 readers paid around 25 cents for the First 20 Inventive Principles. In 1959 he wrote his first letter to the highest patent organization in the former Soviet Union, VOIR, requesting a chance to prove his theory. After hundreds of letters, nine years later they promised a meeting no later than December 1968. When the meeting was held, he met for the first time many people who considered themselves to be his students. In 1969 he wrote a new book, *Algorithm for Inventing*, in which he delivered the mature 40 Principles and the first algorithm to solve complex inventive problems.

For a period from 1970 through 1980, many TRIZ schools were opened throughout Russia and hundreds of students were trained. During this period Altshuller traveled to conduct seminars. This stage ended in 1980 when the first TRIZ specialist conference took place in Petrozavodsk, Russia.

In the period from 1980 through 1985, TRIZ received publicity in the former USSR. During this time, many people became devotees of TRIZ and of Altshuller; the first TRIZ professionals and semiprofessionals appeared. Altshuller was highly efficient at developing his TRIZ model, due to the large number of seminars conducted, the various TRIZ schools established, and individual followers who joined the ranks, allowing for the rapid testing of ideas and tools. TRIZ schools in St. Petersburg, Kishinev, Minsk, Novosibirsk, and others became very active under Altshuller's leadership.

In 1986, the situation changed dramatically. Altshuller's illness limited his ability to work on TRIZ and control its development. Also, for the first time in the history of TRIZ, Russian *Perestroika* allowed it to be applied commercially. The Russian TRIZ Association was founded in 1989 with Altshuller as president. The period of 1991 and beyond saw the rapid deterioration of the economic situation in the former USSR, causing many capable TRIZ specialists, most of whom had established their own businesses, to move abroad. Many of the TRIZ specialists immigrated into the United States and started promoting TRIZ individually. Others found international partners and established TRIZ companies. Today there are many consultants and firms offering training, consultation, and software tools. The Altshuller Institute and www.trizjournal.com have become a force in disseminating worldwide knowledge and information regarding the development and application of TRIZ.

10.3   TRIZ FUNDAMENTALS

Contradictions and trade-offs are constraints that often create design issues for which neither QFD nor other tools in the DFSS tool kit provide a means of resolution. In our DFSS methodology, we have axiomatic design as an efficient tool for contradiction and coupling identification. Contradiction is a conflict or a coupling (i.e. opposite interests). For this reason, TRIZ is a welcome improvement on past innovation tools.

10.3.1   Overview

When Genrich Altshuller completed his research of the world patent base, he had identified four key observations:

1. *There are five levels of invention:*
   - *Level 5:* discovery of new phenomena
   - *Level 4:* invention outside a design paradigm, requiring new technology from a different field of science
   - *Level 3:* invention inside a design paradigm, which requires resolution of a physical contradiction
   - *Level 2:* improvement by invention, which requires resolution of a technical contradiction
   - *Level 1:* apparent solution (no innovation) results in simple improvement

2. *Inventive problems contain at least one contradiction.* Altshuller recognized that the same design problem that includes contradiction had been addressed by a number of inventions in different industries. He also observed the repetition of using the same fundamental solutions, often separated by several years. Altshuller concluded that if the latter designer had knowledge of the earlier solution, his or her task would have been simpler. He sought to extract, compile, and organize such information, leading him to observations 3 and 4 below.

3. *The same principles are used in many inventive designs and can therefore be considered solution patterns.* An inventive principle is a best practice that has been used in many applications and has been extracted from several industries. For example, the "nested doll principle" offers the most efficient use of internal cavities of objects such as holes and dents: to store material. These hollow spaces may enclose objects of interest to the design, a packaging benefit. A footwear designer from Great Britain, Helen Richard, invented a method to help women following youthful fashion eliminate carrying a purse. Richard designed a number of models where the cavity in the shoe is used as a depository for necessary little things through a special cover door in a shoe's heel (Figure 10.1).

4. *There are standard patterns of evolution.* To create a product , a medical device for example, it is necessary to forecast and make analogies with the future situation for similar concepts in terms of design functionality. The past evolution of a design is examined and the analogy is then applied to predict the future of the design of interest. For example, when searching for variants of attaching a detachable soap dish to a wall, one may use an analogy with a load-handling fixture, as in Figure 10.2.

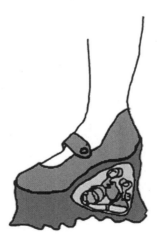

Figure 10.1 Nested doll TRIZ principle applied to shoe design. (From Shpakovsky and Novitskaya, 2002a.)

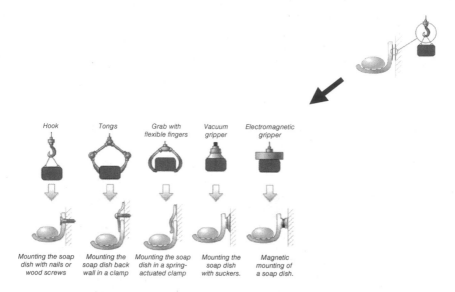

Figure 10.2   Design evolution by analogy. (From Novitskaya, 2002.)

Exhaustive study of the world's patents reveals that the same principles have been used in innovative solutions to problems in different industries and fields, sometimes with many years elapsing between applications. Access to this information is one of the contributions of TRIZ. For example, Figure 10.3 shows multiple applications of radio transmission. In 1897, Marconi obtained a patent for radio transmission. In 1901, he transmitted a message across the Atlantic Ocean. In 1922, the British Broadcast Corporation (BBC) was founded. In 1989, 200 patents were issued with *radio* in the abstract and it has ramped up to 1194 patents issued in 2002. Radio waves have been used in television broadcasting and then in remote controls for television sets (noninfrared types). Wireless telephone, wireless speakers, wireless internet connection, magnetic resonance imaging, and RFID tags on products for inventory control all demonstrate how one invention can be applied to multiple industries to enable unique solutions.

Defining function is the very basis of TRIZ methodologies. In fact, TRIZ is obsessed with functional definition. For example, the main useful function of a device is "to maintain the health of a patient's stem cells." The device is a technical system that contains two elements: a container and the biohuman material itself, with added preservatives (if any). The function of the container is "to enclose the biohuman material." A coffee vending machine performs its main useful function, to make and sell coffee. Part of this technical system is a Styrofoam cup, which contains the coffee.

A cup and coffee are two elements of the design parameters (structure) delivering the function "to enclose liquid." A cup with coffee, a device con-

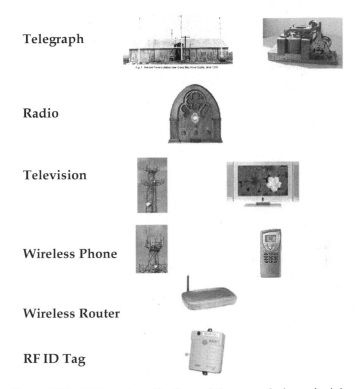

Telegraph

Radio

Television

Wireless Phone

Wireless Router

RF ID Tag

Figure 10.3   Different applications of the same design principles.

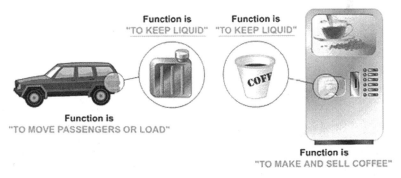

Figure 10.4   Different applications with similar functions. (From Novitskaya, 2002.)

tainer with biohuman material, and a vehicle fuel tank have a similar function and to some degree similar design parameters: "shell and filler" (see Figure 10.4). With such a function definition approach, it is possible to analyze a selected system and search for solutions.

A quick survey of our environment reveals that the same patterns of evolution exist in very diverse products. One such pattern is the introduction of modified substances. Look at the variety of soft drinks in a store today: regular, diet, cherry, vanilla, and so on. Another pattern is mono–bi–poly, in which a system moves from a mono system such as a camera with one lens to a camera with two lenses (one lens for far distances and the other for near distances), and now a camera with zoom capability, a system with an infinite number of lenses. In the business world we have observed the evolution from mainframe computers handling "batch" processes to distributed personal computers that have the same functionality. In the business arena, we have also observed the need for centralized specialties such as forms providers and marketing brochures that evolve to distribute desktop publishing. TRIZ offers eight patterns of evolution containing 280 lines, from which tomorrow's products, including medical devices, can be designed today.

Using the TRIZ methodology, it is possible to generate concepts for reducing negative effects and improving the performance of existing designs. TRIZ includes four analytical tools used to structure the innovative problem and six knowledge-based tools used to point in the direction of solution concepts.

10.3.2   Analytical Tools

Within TRIZ there is a set of analytical steps forming a methodology to focus on the correct problem or opportunity.

1. *Clarify the opportunity:* gathers all the relevant data for analysis and ensures focus on the correct opportunity, not just on symptoms.

2. *Functional analysis:* takes a single problem statement and, through the use of linked cause-and-effect statements, generates an exhaustive list of more explicit problems. The objective of functional analysis is simplification. A trend in design development in which the number of the design parameters decreases but cannot be less than the number of functional requirements (Chapter 9). In this case, the cost of the design decreases while its functionality remains within permissible specifications. Trimming, a functional analysis role-based technique is used to simplify the design mapping.

3. *Algorithm for inventive problem solving:* an alternative way to structure problem definitions for more difficult problems. This is used by experienced TRIZ practioners and requires over 80 hours of training to use properly.

4. *Substance-field analysis:* models a problem into three components for breakthrough thinking with regard to system structure and energy sources.

10.3.3   Knowledge-Based Tools

The knowledge-based tools listed here represent the key observations which Altshuller made that improve the efficiency and effectiveness of resolving contradictions and generating inventive breakthrough concepts.

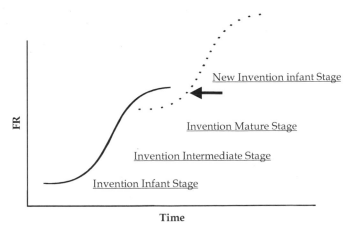

Figure 10.5 S-curve of design evolution.

Patterns/Predictions of Evolution   These are descriptions of the sequence of designs possible for a current design. One prediction, for example, describes the evolution of a system from a macro level to a micro level. Examples of this can be a hospital to a walk-in clinic to home diagnosis and treatment (WebMD). To create a competitive product, it is necessary to forecast the future situation for similar functional designs. This is usually made through the method of analogy and exploration. The past evolution of a design functional requirement is examined and plotted on a S-shaped evolution curve as in Figure 10.5. Then a conclusion is made about probable conceptual alternatives of its evolution, with proper consideration given to evolution trends and the design parameter differences.

TRIZ evolution studies are specific to certain design hierarchy (components, subsystems, or systems) within a design concept. It should be noted that some S-curves describe the evolution of a total system. To predict the evolution of a current design, use an analogy with a specific design element. A specific solution depends on the structure of the design mappings to be transformed as well as on the parameters to be improved and resources available.

Inventive Principles and Contradiction Table   The following performance parameters are used in TRIZ:

1. Weight of moving object
2. Weight of stationary object
3. Length of moving object
4. Length of stationary object
5. Area of moving object
6. Area of stationary object

7. Volume of moving object
8. Volume of stationary object
9. Velocity
10. Force
11. Stress or pressure
12. Shape
13. Stability of object's composition
14. Strength
15. Duration of action generalized by moving object
16. Duration of action generalized by stationary object
17. Temperature
18. Brightness
19. Energy consumed by moving object
20. Energy consumed by stationary object
21. Power
22. Energy loss
23. Substance loss
24. Information loss
25. Waste of time
26. Quantity of a substance
27. Reliability
28. Accuracy of measurement
29. Manufacturing precision
30. Harmful actions affecting the design object
31. Harmful actions generated by the design object
32. Manufacturability
33. User friendliness
34. Repairability
35. Flexibility
36. Complexity of design object
37. Difficulty to control or measure
38. Level of automation
39. Productivity

Design contradictions between two parameters may be resolved by using one or more from among 40 inventive principles, described in Section 10.8. Principles used successfully for 1201 contradictions are presented in a matrix (see Appendix 10A). For example, let's look at improving the productivity (principle 39) of an organization by creating specialists. This creates a contradiction of loss of strength (principle 14), in that if one specialists is out sick, how does the DFSS team cover for the specialist? Appendix 10A gives us possible solutions of principle 10: preliminary actions, principle 18: mechanical vibration, principle 28: mechanical interaction substitution, and principle 29: pneumatics and hydraulics. We get several suggested solutions for each principle. It is easy to translate these TRIZ suggestions into practical suggestions. Translation of these four follows.

- *Principle 10: Preliminary action.* Ensure that incoming information is accurate and complete; have customers fill in information; have tools and forms available.
- *Principle 18: Mechanical vibration.* Have specialists rotate jobs to maintain breadth of experience.
- *Principle 28: Mechanical interactions substitution.* Use sensory means of detection instead of manual effort; auto-check for completeness of fields, validate zip codes, and so on.
- *Principle 29: Pneumatics and hydraulics.* Use voice or data transmission instead of hard copy; use a central database (hydraulic reservoir).

Separation Principles: Inherent (or Physical) Contradictions   The simultaneous occurrence of two mutually exclusive conditions can be resolved using separation principles. For example, a frying pan has a very simple design with the following design parameters: a bottom metal disk, an annular board, a handle, and a cover. Historically, the pan has been improved by using better materials: for instance, nonstick coatings or changing the handle shape or cover design. While frying, food must be turned from time to time. Over the years, one improvement proposed replaced the conventional conical shape of the board with a toric. A chop is pushed up on the board surface and then turns over following the geometry. However, there is a contradiction. It is very difficult to extract the chop from the frying pan because of the board's shape, but it is easy to turn the chop on such a frying pan. This contradiction can be resolved by space separation principles. For this purpose the board is made traditional (i.e., conical) on one side of the frying pan and toric on the other side, as in Figure 10.6.

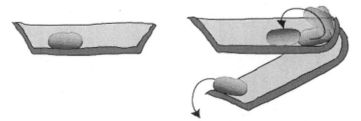

Figure 10.6 Frying pan TRIZ separation example. (From Shpakovsky and Novitskaya, 2002b.)

76 Standard Solutions   These are generic system modifications for the model developed using substance-field analysis. These solutions can be grouped into five major categories:

1. *Improving the systems with no or little change:* 13 standard solutions
2. *Improving the system by changing the system:* 23 standard solutions
3. *System transitions:* 6 standard solutions
4. *Detection and measurement:* 17 standard solutions
5. *Strategies for simplification and improvements:* 17 standard solutions

For example, in recycling household wastes, we used to place all waste into a single trash container; then we had paper, metal/plastic, and other waste; today, many municipalities require separation of wastes into specialized categories. This is one of the standard solutions suggested as segmentation flow into many parts.

Effects   Effect is a physical action of an object that produces a field or another action as a consequence. As a rule, these are phenomena related generally to product design. Physical, chemical, geometric, and other effects offer "free" resources commonly forgotten and sometimes even incompatible with the system as designed.

1. Material resources
   a. System elements
   b. Inexpensive materials
   c. Modified materials
   d. Waste
   e. Raw materials
2. Time resources
   a. Parallel operations
   b. Pre and post work
   c. Information resources
   d. Field resources
   e. Energy in system
   f. Energy in environment
3. Space resources
   a. Empty space
   b. Another dimension
   c. Nesting
4. Function resources
   a. Harmful functions that can be converted to good
   b. Enhance secondary effects of functions

System of Operators When analyzing a function model after the "clarify the opportunity" step, we can approach the model from three perspectives or strategies: (1) eliminate harmful effects; (2) eliminate excessive action; and (3) enhance useful actions. Universal operators are recommendations which are potentially applicable to any situation, such as excessive action (e.g., e-mailing every employee or customer when the message is only relevant to a small subgroup). General operators are recommendations applicable toward improving functionality and eliminating undesired effects, such as elimination of a harmful action (e.g., separation or transfer to a subsystem). Specialized operators are used to improve specific parameters or features of a product or process; that is, improve useful actions (examples include those for increasing speed, accuracy, or reliability). All of the TRIZ knowledge-based tools yield concepts that require conversion to practical solutions to satisfy the needs of the current problem.

10.4 TRIZ PROBLEM-SOLVING PROCESS

The application of TRIZ needs to follow a logical flow since the methodology can solve many different issues or provide enhancements within the DFSS design project. Figure 10.7 shows one such flow. This flow emulates the structure of TechOptimizer software. The flow begins with the DFSS team's practical issue and must end with a practical solution or set of solutions. Once the DFSS team enters the realm of TRIZ, the first step is to clarify the opportunity. In this step the model is created with true functions, covered in

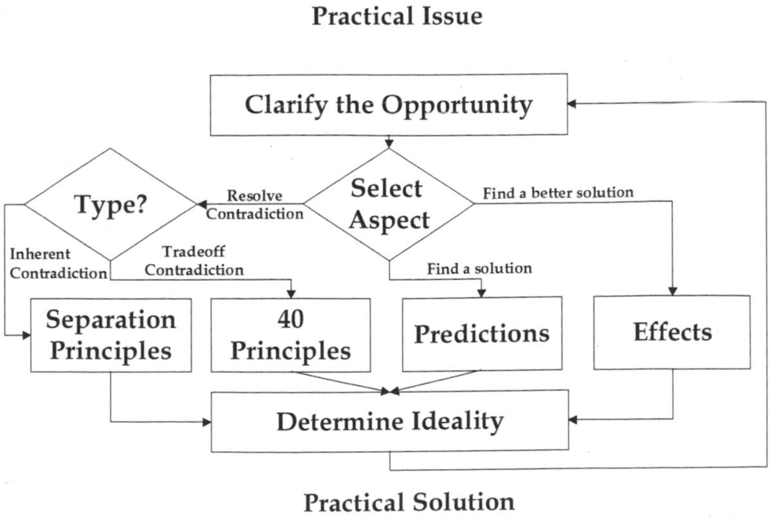

Figure 10.7 TRIZ flowchart.

Section 10.6, and the super system, the device and its environment, that interacts with the model. The ideal final result should be formulated at this point to assist in the last step to determine the ideality of any solution determined.

Next we look at the model and decide which aspect to resolve. There are three options at this point. We either have contradictions that need to be resolved or we need a solution or an improved solution. If we know that we have a contradiction, we need to determine the type of contradiction. It is either a trade-off contradiction or an inherent or design contradiction.

In *trade-off contradictions*, sometimes referred to as *technical contradictions*, we try to improve one attribute, and this leads to deterioration in another attribute. We can often see these contradictions in the roof of an HOQ when we have both plus and minus signs (Chapter 8).

Inherent contradictions, sometimes referred to as *physical contradictions*, are more difficult to resolve. In these contradictions the same object requires having two opposite properties.

If we are simply in search of a solution, we can use the prediction element of TRIZ patterns/predictions of evolution covered in Section 10.11, whereas if we need to improve a solution, we can use the TRIZ effects and standard solutions generator. Each time we apply the methodology and discover a solution to our issue, we need to determine how good the solution is against our standard of the ideal final result, which is explained in Section 10.5.

10.5 IDEAL FINAL RESULT

The ideal final result (IFR) is the situation that suits us best, when the action required is performed by design objects themselves without additional cost or effort. In solving an inventive problem, the notion of IFR creates a solution ideality that the design team should target. An IFR describes (defines) an ideal system that delivers benefit without harm. It is often gauged against goals such as the following:

- It occupies no space.
- It has no weight.
- It requires no labor.
- It takes no time.
- It requires no maintenance.

There are three methods for defining an IFR: itself, ideality checklist, and ideality equation.

10.5.1 Itself Method

Using the *itself method*, teams can look at functions and define them in a ideal state for use in developing concept solutions. To perform this method, we express an IFR as itself, then reexpress it in terms of actual circumstances of the problem. For example, an ideal computer is one that is absent while its functions are performed:

- "Patient treats himself or herself." How? Certain home therapies allow this solution to be performed.
- "Grass mows itself." Grass keeps itself at an attractive height. How can grass do that? How do other biological systems do it? In southern parts of the United Sates, grasses such as Zoysia, Bermuda, and St. Augustine, which are slow-growing, creeping grasses are used. Homeowners also spray their grass with a growth inhibitor, which slows the growth rate. That is, two solutions are used to achieve close to the ideal result "grass keeps itself at an attractive height."
- "Data enters itself." How? Data stay accurate, current, and in correct form. This example is the basis of many Web-enabled self-service solutions.

10.5.2   Ideality Checklist

When any concept is created, the design team can test the concept against the *ideality checklist*:

1. Eliminates the deficiencies of the original system
2. Preserves the advantages of the original system
3. Does not make a system more complicated (uses free or available resources)
4. Does not introduce new disadvantages

Anytime that there is a "no" answer to the checklist, the concept should be reevaluated for usefulness.

10.5.3   Ideality Equation

Using the *ideality equation*, we define benefits in terms of useful functions and look at the associated costs as well as any harmful effects or functions required with the delivery of the useful function. This evaluation can yield the following equation:

$$\text{ideality} = \frac{\sum \text{benefits}}{\sum \text{cost} + \sum \text{harm}} \tag{10.1}$$

The objective is to maintain or maximize the benefits while minimizing or eliminating the cost and harmful effects. The IFR is obtained when the denominator in (10.1) is zero. Some TRIZ software packages automatically create the ideality equation through interactive modeling and dialogue boxes. This method allows for baselining improvement toward the goal of ideal.

10.6 BUILDING SUFFICIENT FUNCTIONS

One of the key requirements of using TRIZ is that we focus on the correct problem or opportunity. To do this we have to be careful of the words we use to describe the functions to which we refer. Too often we use high-level descriptions that cover several specific functions. The key to determining if we have a sufficient function is that a function requires an object A which does something to object B that changes object B somehow. In medical device design, objects can be design parameters, process variable resources in the design environment. The change can be in space, time, or some intrinsic change such as temperature or knowledge. Take the example "thermometer measures temperature"; in itself, this is not a true TRIZ function but a contraction of several functions. One set of functions may be "body heats thermometer," "thermometer informs patient." What are the true functions in this statement? If we focus on an intranet search, a person enters search information into an application, the application searches databases, and the application informs the person.

10.7 ELIMINATING HARMFUL FUNCTIONS

In a design there are two types of functions: useful functions and harmful or undesirable functions. Harmful functions are such things as damages and injuries. Consider a medical latex glove system. Occasionally, a glove user may experience discomfort in the hands during or after wearing latex gloves. People allergic to natural rubber products with contact urticaria from the natural proteins in rubber, causing atopic disorders, including allergic rhinitis, asthma, and oreczema. An eluted latex allergen can more easily penetrate eczematous skin, with symptoms varying from mild itching to severe systemic reactions such as generalized urticaria, facial swelling, gastrointestinal and oto-rhino-laryngeal symptoms, asthma, or even anaphylaxis. The primary function of the glove is to protect patient and caregiver. Consider the functional diagram shown in Figure 10.8. The solid line between the two objects indicates the useful function "protects," and the dashed line indicates the harmful function "harm." Useful and harmful functions coexist between the glove and both the nurse and the patient. Functional analysis is used to model design problem situations. The design problem definition can be reformulated as: glove needs to eliminate allergies without reducing the level of protection or adding any harmful functions.

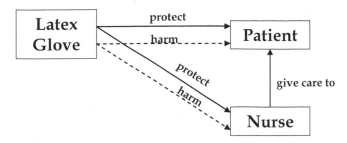

Figure 10.8   Functional diagram example.

Altshuller understood the importance of a functional approach in design development since the earliest days of TRIZ. For example, his concept of the ideal final result of a design says that the ideal design performs its function but does not exist, which means that it performs its function for free and with no harm. However, the need for integration of function analysis into TRIZ was recognized after developing methods to solve generic problems in innovation. Function analysis plays the key role in problem formulation.

10.8   INVENTIVE PRINCIPLES

The 40 inventive principles provide innovators with systematic and significant means of breaking out of current paradigms into often exciting and beneficial new ones.

Principle 1: Segmentation

   a. Divide an object into independent parts.
   b. Make an object easy to disassemble.
   c. Increase the degree of fragmentation or segmentation.

Principle 2: Taking Out   Separate an interfering part or property from an object, or single out the only necessary part (or property) of an object.

Principle 3: Local Quality

   a. Change an object's structure from uniform to nonuniform; change an external environment (or external influence) from uniform to nonuniform.
   b.   Make each part of an object function in the conditions that are most suitable for its operation.
   c. Make each part of an object fulfill a different and useful function.

Principle 4: Asymmetry

   a. Change the shape of an object from symmetrical to asymmetrical.

   b. If an object is asymmetrical, change its degree of asymmetry.

Principle 5: Merging

   a. Bring closer together (or merge) identical or similar objects; assemble identical or similar parts to perform parallel operations.

   b. Make operations contiguous or parallel; bring them together in time.

Principle 6: Universality

   a. Make an object or structure perform multiple functions; eliminate the need for other parts.

Principle 7: "Nested Dolls"

   a. Place one object inside another; place each object, in turn, inside the other.

   b. Make one part pass through a cavity in the other.

Principle 8: Anti-Weight

   a. To compensate for the weight (downward tendency) of an object, merge it with other objects that provide lift.

   b. To compensate for the weight (downward tendency) of an object, make it interact with the environment (e.g., use global lift forces).

Principle 9: Preliminary Anti-Action

   a. If it will be necessary to do an action with both harmful and useful effects, this action should be replaced with anti-actions to control harmful effects.

   b. Create beforehand, stresses in an object that will oppose later known undesirable working stresses.

Principle 10: Preliminary Action

   a. Perform, before it is needed, the required change of an object (either fully or partially).

   b. Prearrange objects such that they can come into action from the most convenient place and without losing time for their delivery.

Principle 11: Beforehand Cushioning

    a. Prepare emergency means beforehand to compensate for the relatively low reliability of an object.

Principle 12: Equipotentiality

    a. In a potential field, limit position changes (e.g., change operating conditions to eliminate the need to raise or lower objects in a gravity field).

Principle 13: "The Other Way Around"

    a. Invert the action(s) used to solve the problem (e.g., instead of cooling an object, heat it).

    b. Make movable parts (or the external environment) fixed, and fixed parts movable.

    c. Turn the object (or process) upside down.

Principle 14: Spheroidality (Curvature)

    a. Instead of using rectilinear parts, surfaces, or forms, use curvilinear ones; move from flat surfaces to spherical ones; move from parts shaped as a cube (parallelepiped) to ball-shaped structures.

    b. Use rollers, balls, spirals, or domes.

    c. Go from linear to rotary motion, use centrifugal forces.

Principle 15: Dynamics

    a. Allow (or design) the characteristics of an object, external environment, or process to change to be optimal or to find an optimal operating condition.

    b. Divide an object into parts capable of movement relative to each other.

    c. If an object (or process) is rigid or inflexible, make it movable or adaptive.

Principle 16: Partial or Excessive Actions

    a. If 100 percent of an objective is hard to achieve using a given solution method, using slightly less or slightly more of the same method, may make the problem considerably easier to solve.

Principle 17: Another Dimension

   a. Move an object in two- or three-dimensional space.
   b. Use a multistory arrangement of objects instead of a single-story arrangement.
   c. Tilt or reorient the object; lay it on its side.
   d. Use another side of a given area.

Principle 18: Mechanical Vibration

   a. Cause an object to oscillate or vibrate.
   b. Increase the object's frequency (even up to the ultrasonic).
   c. Use an object's resonant frequency.
   d. Use piezoelectric vibrators instead of mechanical ones.
   e. Use combined ultrasonic and electromagnetic field oscillations; use external elements to create oscillation or vibration.

Principle 19: Periodic Action

   a. Use periodic or pulsating action instead of continuous action.
   b. If an action is already periodic, change the periodic magnitude or frequency.
   c. Use pauses between impulses to perform a different action.

Principle 20: Continuity of Useful Action

   a. Carry on work continuously; make all parts of an object work at full load all the time.
   b. Eliminate all idle or intermittent actions or work.

Principle 21: Skipping

   a. Conduct a process, or certain stages (e.g., destructive, harmful, or hazardous operations), at high speed.

Principle 22: "Blessing in Disguise" or "Turn Lemons into Lemonade"

   a. Use harmful factors (particularly, harmful effects of the environment or surroundings) to achieve a positive effect.
   b. Eliminate the primary harmful action by adding it to another harmful action to resolve the problem.
   c. Amplify a harmful factor to such a degree that it is no longer harmful.

Principle 23: Feedback

a. Introduce feedback (referring back, cross-checking) to improve a process or action.
b. If feedback is already being used, change its magnitude or influence.

Principle 24: Intermediary

a. Use an intermediary carrier article or intermediary process.
b. Merge one object temporarily with another (which can be easily removed).

Principle 25: Self-Service

a. Make an object serve itself by performing auxiliary helpful functions.
b. Use waste (or lost) resources, energy, or substances.

Principle 26: Copying

a. Instead of an unavailable, expensive, fragile object, use simpler, inexpensive copies.
b. Replace an object or process with optical copies.
c. If optical copies are used, move to infrared or ultraviolet (use an appropriate way out of the ordinary illumination and viewing situation).

Principle 27: Cheap, Short-Lived Objects

a. Replace an expensive object with multiple inexpensive objects, compromising certain qualities.

Principle 28: Mechanics Substitution

a. Replace a mechanical means by a sensory (optical, acoustic, taste, or smell) means.
b. Use electric, magnetic, and electromagnetic fields to interact with the object.
c. Change from static to movable fields, from unstructured fields to those having structure.
d. Use fields in conjunction with field-activated (e.g., ferromagnetic) particles.

Principle 29: Pneumatics and Hydraulics

   a. Use gas and liquid parts of an object instead of solid parts (e.g., inflatable, filled with liquids, air cushion, hydrostatic, hydroreactive).

Principle 30: Flexible Shells and Thin Films

   a. Use flexible shells and thin films instead of three-dimensional structures.
   b. Isolate the object from the external environment using flexible shells and thin films.

Principle 31: Porous Materials

   a. Make an object porous or add porous elements (inserts, coatings, etc.).
   b. If an object is already porous, use the pores to introduce a useful substance or function.

Principle 32: Color Changes

   a. Change the color of an object or its external environment.
   b. Change the transparency of an object or its external environment.

Principle 33: Homogeneity

   a. Make objects interact with a given object of the same material (or material with identical properties).

Principle 34: Discarding and Recovering

   a. Make portions of an object that have fulfilled their functions go away (discard by dissolving, evaporating, etc.) or modify them directly during operation.
   b. Conversely, restore consumable parts of an object directly in operation.

Principle 35: Parameter Changes

   a. Change an object's physical state (e.g., to a gas, liquid, or solid).
   b. Change the concentration or consistency.
   c. Change the degree of flexibility.
   d. Change the temperature.

Principle 36: Phase Transitions

    a. Use phenomena occurring during phase transitions (awareness of macroscale business phenomena).

Principle 37: Thermal Expansion

    a. Use thermal expansion (or contraction) of materials.
    b. If thermal expansion is being used, use multiple materials with different coefficients of thermal expansion.

Principle 38: Strong Oxidants ("Boosted Interactions")

    a. Replace common air with oxygen-enriched air (enriched atmosphere)
    b. Replace enriched air with pure oxygen (highly enriched atmosphere).
    c. Expose air or oxygen to ionizing radiation.
    d. Use ionized oxygen.
    e. Replace ozonized (or ionized) oxygen with ozone (atmosphere enriched by unstable elements).

Principle 39: Inert Atmosphere

    a. Replace a normal environment by an inert environment.
    b. Add neutral parts or inert additives to an object.

Principle 40: Composite Structures

    a. Change from uniform to composite (multiple) structures.

After reading this list, the DFSS team will be asking how this applies to their environment. It is really the same as taking these concepts and thinking what the analogous situation would be in a medical device project.

10.9 DETECTION AND MEASUREMENT CONCEPTS

Although the ideal final result in six sigma is automatic control without detection or measurement, many contradictions require enhanced measurement or detection before evolving to this state. *Detection* is defined as observing whether something or not occurred, pass or fail, or other binary conditions. *Measurement* is the ability to measure along a continuous scale with precision and accuracy. Use these concepts to improve or resolve the need to measure or detect. Measurement and detection concepts in TRIZ fall into three main categories:

1. Introduction of marks
   - *Into the object.* The DFSS team tries to detect the feature parameter of an object by introducing a mark into the object.
   - *Onto the object.* The DFSS team tries to detect the feature parameter of an object by introducing a mark onto the object.
   - *Into the environment.* The DFSS team tries to detect the feature parameter of an object by introducing a mark into the surroundings of the object.
2. Introduction of modified marks
   - *Into the object.* The DFSS team tries to detect the feature parameter of an object by introducing a modified mark into the object.
   - *Onto the object.* The DFSS team tries to detect the feature parameter of an object by introducing a modified mark onto the object.
   - *Into the environment.* The DFSS team tries to detect the feature parameter of an object by introducing modified mark into the surroundings of the object.
3. Changes in detection and measurement
   - *Roundabout.* Instead of detecting the feature parameter of the object, remove the need for detection.
   - *Discrete detecting.* Instead of measuring the parameter of the object continuously, detect discrete changes(s). Use phase changes, instabilities, or other changes that occur at specific conditions.
   - *Indirect measuring.* Instead of measuring the parameter of the object directly, measure another feature or features connected with the parameter.
   - *Measuring derivatives.* Instead of measuring absolute values of the parameter of the object, measure relative changes in the parameter (e.g., speed of changes or acceleration).

10.10 TRIZ ROOT CAUSE ANALYSIS

TRIZ also relies on traditional root-cause analysis tools to ensure that the DFSS team is working on the root cause and not addressing symptoms or science projects. One popular method is to ask "why?" until the DFSS team doesn't know the answer; this is usually the point of impact on which to focus. The other method is to ask "who?", "what?", "when?", "where?", "why?", "how many?", "how large?": the 5W and 2H method.

Other published methods that can help provide focus are six sigma, the Koepner–Tregoe method, or the global TOPS 8D (team-oriented problem solving) method. Also, a cause-and-effect diagram (or Ishakawa diagram or fishbone chart) can help a team focus on the true root causes. Whatever method is chosen, the team should feel confident that they are working on the correct opportunity.

10.11   EVOLUTION TRENDS IN TECHNOLOGICAL SYSTEMS

Technological systems are driven by demand and technology life cycles. The saying "necessity is the mother of invention" is a driving force in these life cycles. When there is a demand for solutions, many people enter into the development of new and innovative designs, and the rate of invention follows an S-curve when plotted over time. Early on, only a few inventors create novel inventions. When demand increases, many people cluster around the market and rush to create innovative applications by resolving the contradictions that have not yet been conquered. This flurry of activity drives the number of inventions. As demand tapers off, based either on saturation of market demand or as a result of dramatically new technological solutions (via R&D), the pace of invention dwindles. Along this S-curve of evolution lie 19 definite patterns of invention. These patterns are:

1. Introduction: New substances
   - Internal
   - External
   - In the environment
   - Between objects
2. Introduction: Modified substances
   - Internal
   - External
   - In the environment
   - Between objects
3. Introduction: Voids
   - Internal
   - External
   - In the environment
   - Between objects
4. Introduction: Fields
   - Internal
   - External
   - In the environment
   - Between objects
5. Mono–bi–poly: Similar objects
   - Introduction of similar objects

- Introduction of several similar objects
- Combining similar objects into a common system

6. Mono–bi–poly: Varying objects
   - Introduction of varying objects
   - Introduction of several varying objects
   - Combining varying objects into a common system

7. Segmentation: Substances
   - Monolith
   - Segmented
   - Liquid or powder
   - Gas or plasma
   - Field

8. Segmentation: Space
   - Introduction of a void
   - Segmentation of a void
   - Creating pores and capillaries
   - Activating pores and capillaries

9. Segmentation: Surface
   - Flat surface
   - Protrusions
   - Roughness
   - Activating surface

10. Segmentation: Flow
    - Into two parts (paths)
    - Into several parts (paths)
    - Into many parts (paths)

11. Coordination: Dynamism
    - Immobile
    - Joint (partial mobility)
    - Many joints (degrees of freedom)
    - Elastic (flexible)
    - Liquid or gas (transition to molecular)
    - Field (transition to field)

12. Coordination: Rhythm
    - Continuous action
    - Pulsating action
    - Pulsation in the resonance mode

- Several actions
- Traveling wave
13. Coordination: Action
    - None
    - Partial
    - Full
    - Interval
14. Coordination: Control
    - Manual
    - Semiautomatic
    - Automatic
15. Geometric evolution: Dimensions
    - Point
    - Line
    - Surface
    - Volume
16. Geometric evolution: Linear
    - Line
    - Two-dimensional curve
    - Three-dimensional curve
    - Compound three-dimensional
17. Geometric evolution: Surface
    - Plane
    - Single curvature of plane
    - Double curvature of plane
    - Combined surface
18. Geometric evolution: Volumetric
    - Prism
    - Cylindrical
    - Spheroidal
    - Combined object
19. Trimming
    - Complete system
    - System with objects eliminated
    - Partially trimmed system
    - Fully trimmed system

It would be unusual to find a modern invention that relied on only one of these patterns. Cameras, for example, started out monolithic: with a single lens.

Later they became hinged and had two lenses, one for near and one for far distance. Today, a compact digital camera has a liquid crystal display (gas or plasma) and a zoom lens (a combined poly system) as well as a jointed flash.

Organizations and processes follow similar patterns. Paper forms, for example, have evolved to electronic forms, a journey from immobility to a field (electrons).

The important application of this topic is that a DFSS team can actually tell where the solution the team selects lies along the S-curve. The team doesn't want to rely on a declining technology nor do they want to be at the bleeding edge of invention, in particular for next-generation devices. Recall the multigenerational planning discussed in Chapter 6.

10.12   TRIZ FUNCTIONAL ANALYSIS AND ANALOGY

In this section we introduce a tool that is based on the substance-field analysis model of TRIZ. Earlier we discussed a function model where object A acts on object B. For this model to function, object A has to change something in object B, implying that energy has to be transferred between the objects. To fulfill the transfer of energy, three elements are required: (1) a source of energy, (2) transmission of energy, and (3) guidance and control. A worksheet similar to that in Figure 10.9 is used to create the full analysis.

Identifying the starting point in a problem is the first step, so we fill in the column "My Problem Starting." Next you search the TRIZ knowledge databases for innovations that appear to be similar to what you are looking for. We search every field (chemical, electrical, business, psychology, sociology, etc.) for physical and scientific effects, then use the research results to complete the columns "Example Starting" and "Example Improved." Finally, we use the model to complete the transition and fill in the column "My Problem Improved."

Element	Example Starting	Example Improved	My Problem Starting	My Problem Improved
Object B (acted on)				
Object A (Acting)				
Source of energy				
Transmission of energy				
Guidance and Control				

Figure 10.9   Functional analogy worksheet.

TABLE 10.1 Functional Analogy Example

Element	Example Starting	Example Improved	My Problem Starting	My Problem Improved
Object B (acted on)	Message	Message	Paper invoice	Electronic invoice
Object A (acting)	Letter	Fax machine	Accounts payable organization	Accounts payable system
Source of energy	Mail deliverer/ mail vehicle	Electrical	Mail delivery	Electrical
Transmission of energy	Mail deliverer/ mail vehicle	Telecommunication system	Invoice is carried along in vehicle	Telecommunication system
Guidance and control	Mail deliverer	Telephone company	Post office	Internet service provider

We often see an invention reapplied in a different field, the result of discovery and application. Sometimes this happens because people are in the right place at the right time. What we are proposing here is a methodology that allows for discovery of these effects in order to improve the basic functions that formulate the team DFSS concept. The way to perform this research varies. It may be done through benchmarking, Internet searches, patent searches, or through the use of a TRIZ software package.

Table 10.1 shows a completed example where the method of delivering messages went from land mail to fax and then to e-mail. An invoice was mailed to customers can now be sent electronically. This example is contrived to demonstrate use of the analogy worksheet. In most cases you will be working a much more elementary (lower-level) function, and it will be easier to see the connections.

10.13 APPLICATION: USING TRIADS TO PREDICT AND CONCEIVE NEXT-GENERATION PRODUCTS[1]

The main function of a defibrillator is to restart the heartbeat of a heart-attack victim through application of an electrical shock (Figure 10.10). The passive object is the heart. The active object is the defibrillator system. The enabling object is an emergency team member. The essential functions are:

1. A defibrillator shocks the heart electrically.
2. An emergency team member activates the defibrillator.

[1]Adapted from Mueller (1999).

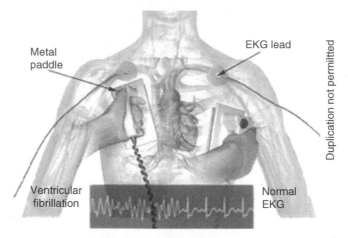

Metal paddle

EKG lead

Ventricular fibrillation

Normal EKG

Figure 10.10   External defibrillator application.

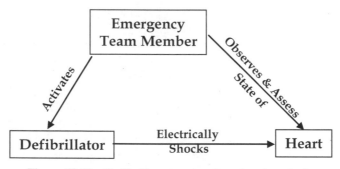

Figure 10.11   Defibrillator system functional analysis.

3. An emergency team member observes and assesses the state of the heart.

These three objects (the heart, a defibrillator, and an emergency team member), and their interactions, form the triad shown in Figure 10.11.

If one of the objects of the triad is "pruned" (i.e., eliminated), that object's functions need to be considered. For example, suppose that we decide to prune the emergency team member (Figure 10.12).

Eight key questions emerge from this decision:

1. Is the defibrillator really necessary from the point of view that it needs to be activated by an emergency team member? Under what circumstances would the defibrillator not be necessary?
2. Is it necessary for the defibrillator to be activated? Under what circumstances might it not have to be activated?

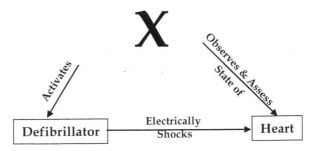

Figure 10.12   Pruned defibrillator system functional analysis (case 1).

3. Can the patient himself, or his own heart, activate the defibrillator? What could this mean in terms of a new design?
4. Can the defibrillator activate itself? What could this mean in terms of a new design?
5. Is the heart really necessary—from the point of view that its state (or the patient's state) needs to be observed and assessed? Under what circumstances would the heart or patient not be necessary from this point of view?
6. Is it necessary for the state of the heart or patient to be observed and assessed by the emergency team member? Under what circumstances would that not be necessary?
7. Can the patient, or the patient's heart, observe and assess its (his) own state? What could this mean in terms of a new design?
8. Can the defibrillator observe and assess the state of the heart or patient? What could this mean in terms of a new design?

The answers to these eight questions are not easy. Some of them may appear to be ridiculous. Others may, in fact, actually be ridiculous. Nevertheless, as a collection, they lead to next-generation revival systems—in a manner that also leads to the ideal final system.

Eight different questions arise if we decide to prune the defibrillator (Figure 10.13):

9. Is the heart really necessary from a "providing an electrical shock to the heart" point of view? Under what circumstances would the heart not be necessary from this point of view?
10. Is it necessary for the heart to be shocked electrically? Under what circumstances might it not have to be shocked?
11. Can the emergency team member, in the absence of a defibrillator, somehow shock the heart electrically? What could this mean in terms of a new design?

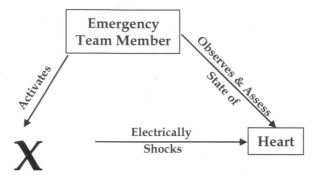

Figure 10.13   Pruned defibrillator system functional analysis (case 2).

12. Can the heart (or the patient), in the absence of a defibrillator, electrically shock itself (himself)? What could this mean in terms of a new design?

13. Is the emergency team member really necessary if the defibrillator is pruned? Under what circumstances would the emergency team member not be necessary?

14. Is it necessary for the defibrillator to be activated at all? Under what circumstances would that not be necessary?

15. Can the emergency team member, in the absence of a defibrillator, somehow activate an electrical shock to the heart of the patient? What could this mean in terms of a new design?

16. Can the heart itself (or the patient), in the absence of a defibrillator, somehow activate an electrical shock to itself (himself)? What could this mean in terms of a new design?

If we consider the 16 questions listed above as a whole, certain creative paths, and features of creative solutions, come to mind. The following is a list of potential solution features.

1. The defibrillator can be activated remotely by a third party of from an auxiliary device. Design this feature in.

2. When there is a patient heartbeat, the defibrillator will not deliver an electrical shock, but it will deliver an electrical shock when there is no heartbeat. This feature should be designed into the defibrillator.

3. The patient sends out a signal to the defibrillator to activate an electrical shock. This signal decision may come directly from the patient's heart or from a device that is monitoring the patient's heart. The defibrillator is designed to receive such a signal and to deliver an electrical shock automatically when signaled.

4. A self-activating defibrillator is designed. When an electrical shock is required for a patient, the defibrillator itself activates that requirement. No human being (i.e., emergency team member) is necessary to activate it.

5. Some other part of the patient (i.e., other than the heart) is assessed or observed to determine the patient's state of health. This observation or assessment does not require an emergency team member.

6. The state of the heart (patient) can be observed or assessed by means other than by the emergency team member (i.e., by a sensor or monitor worn by the patient which is programmed to determine the need for an electrical shock).

7. The heart or patient has its own "micro" version of an emergency team member attached to it. This device is electrosensory, recording one or more of the patient's vital signs or signals and transposing them into a signal which is transmitted to a miniaturized defibrillator also attached to the patient.

8. The defibrillator is equipped with a receiver that senses the patient's state and determines appropriate action.

9. A heartbeat is started by doing something to another organ, to the nervous system, or other entity, via another medical device system.

10. Another way to reinstate a heartbeat is found or designed other than through an electrical shock or other than from a defibrillator.

11. The emergency team member's vehicle, equipped to deliver the required power–time profile electrically to the patient is used.

12. The patient wears an electrical shock device that also senses the patient's state and decides if the patient needs the shock.

13. The defibrillator is self-activating (see 4 above).

14. The defibrillator is always activated, and therefore never needs to reactivated, as long as the patient has no heartbeat.

15. The emergency team member has an alternative way of reviving the patient.

16. See 7 above.

It is easy to miss important results that can be gathered by the steps that we just went through, even though we have not yet completed the entire procedure. We start with a generic description of the procedure used, referring to the defibrillation system case study for clarification.

1. We began with the selection of an actual system for accomplishing some performance function. The specific system chosen was a defibrillation system, used to restart the heart of a heart attack victim.

2. The next step we took was to construct a triad of three objects that describe the function. The triad actually is the function, because without any

one of the three objects, there would be no function. Therefore, the objects in the triad are essential parts of the system selected, called "restarting the heart of a heartattack victim."

    a. There are always three objects in a triad. One of the objects is the passive object, the object to which something is being "done" or "accomplished."

    b. A second object is the active object, the object that does something to the passive object. It's also the object that accomplishes what is being accomplished.

    c. The third object, the enabling object, is not always easy to identify. It is the object without which the active and passive objects would not interact as desired.

3. Once we have the triad in place, we examine the interactions in the triad to determine the functional relationships between the objects. Generally speaking, the functional relationship between the active and passive objects is easy to understand. The relationships between the enabling object and the other two objects, however, are not always easy to understand.

If we have gone this far in analyzing a problem situation, we are already pretty far along. We usually have three interactions to examine. Each of these can be improved in various ways, and there are several tools of the TRIZ approach that can assist us in improving these interactions. For example, we could apply the laws of development of technical systems to the objects and actions in this triad. Or, we could look at the interactions between any two objects, develop the problem further in terms of a conflict, and use Altshuller's conflict matrix (Appendix 10A) to locate inventive principles that we can apply to the objects and actions of the interaction. Or, we can follow the entire TRIZ procedure for a particular interaction in the triad; usually, TRIZ is spplied to an interaction between the active and passive objects.

All of these "ways leading to creative solutions" are admissible, but there is a way that leads us to the ideal final result not only ultimately, but quite rapidly. This way involves pruning (i.e., removing) a part, or the whole, of one of the objects in the triad. Pruning leads us rapidly toward the ideal final result. The system is also simplified (not made more complex). By pruning a system, one or more measures of ideality of the system are increased.

If one of the objects in a triad is pruned, we have a problem: We no longer have a function, because there is no triad. The minimum requirement for any function to exist is that there have to be three objects (active, passive, and enabling). So after pruning occurs, we truly have a conflict: *The object must be pruned, in order to simplify the system and move towards ideality, and the object must not be pruned, so that we retain the function.*

We continue the "triads plus pruning" procedure with step 4.

4. Choose one of the objects for pruning, using your intuition and knowl-edge of the constraints on the system. It may be good not to choose the passive object first, although it is probably a good idea to explore the ramifications of pruning each of the three objects in the system, one at a time. For the defibril-lator system, we decided to prune the operator, the emergency team member who applies the defibrillator to the heart attack victim.

5. Examining the remaining parts of the triad, ask the following question: When the object chosen is pruned, what interactions are affected? Identify the interaction or interactions that are affected. For example, if we prune the emergency team member, two interactions are affected: "Emergency team member activates defibrillator," and "Emergency team member observes and assesses the state of the patient's heart."

6. Identify the interactions in which the object being pruned is the active object. For each interaction where the object being pruned is the active object, consider the following questions:

a. Is it possible that some other object in the system (including any parts remaining from the object being pruned) can assume the functions of the object being pruned? What design configurations will make this happen? Identify those design configurations.

b. Are there design configurations where for the sake of the interaction under consideration the passive object (or the part or parts of it that are involved in the interaction) is not required? Identify those design con-figurations (keeping in mind that the active object, or certain parts of it, have been pruned).

c. Are there design configurations where the interaction or action itself is not required? Identify those design configurations, keeping in mind that the active object of that interaction has been pruned.

In the defibrillator example this is about as far as we have gone in the process of forming a triad and then pruning. If you recall, the team generated 16 generic solutions, some of which appeared to be very similar to each other. Then they considered each generic solution, and through the application of abstract thinking, generated specific solutions. Let's attempt to summarize the features of specific designs that are generated by our procedure.

Features of Next-Generation Reviving Systems

1. *Elimination of human involvement.* The system under consideration involves human beings other than the heart attack victim, for two purposes: assessing the victim's state of health, and activating the defibrillator. Inventive prompts from the triads plus pruning process suggest that designs of the future

will eliminate these aspects of human involvement. Instead, the defibrillator itself will assess the victim and decide to deliver what is necessary to the victim. This requires sensory, feedback, decision-making, and activating features in new defibrillator designs. Implied in these features are connections between the new defibrillator and the victim.

2. *Remote, third-party, or automatic involvement.* Intelligent sensing, decision making, and activation can be provided remotely at any time, around the clock. This implies an intimate connection between the next-generation defibrillator and the victim, as well as sensory, feedback, decision-making, and activation features at a distance from the victim.

3. *Intelligent sensing and decision making.* Next-generation designs will have some sort of programmed intelligence concerning the information communicated from intelligent sensors already in touch with (i.e., monitoring) the victim's body (perhaps before the oncome of a heart attack). These intelligent sensors may be monitoring the victim's heart directly, or they may be monitoring other patient characteristics indirectly (i.e., other vital signs of the patient), which may be able to be monitored more remotely (and with less invasiveness or patient inconvenience). Sensing devices can be described as being electrosensory, recording one or more of the patient's vital signs or signals and transposing them into a signal which is transmitted to a miniaturized defibrillator attached to the patient.

4. *Patient "wears" certain system parts.* Sensors with feedback capability and means of delivering shocks or signals can be worn in advance by a patient (or implanted in advance in the patient). The implication is that advance shocks could be far milder than conventional defibrillator shock (e.g., more like a pacemaker). In the case of a conventional defibrillator, future design requirements call for far lighter and far more intelligent defibrillators, capable of being worn by patients who might require defibrillation sometime in the future (as determined by their physicians).

5. *Reviving victims through means other than electric shock.* Next-generation designs will feature means to revive heart attack victims other than through the conventional method of delivering an electrical shock with a fixed power–time profile. A next-step design configuration will probably include a pulsed power–time profile, delivering the same profile shape but with significantly less energy. New revivification techniques will follow. These may involve organs and bodily systems other than the heart alone or instead of the heart.

6. *Modifications to the "engine" of current defibrillators.* In the near term we can expect to see some system merging involving the use of other available systems to be the source of power for defibrillators, thereby allowing defibrillators to be lighter and more effective. For example, motorized vehicle power units can be equipped to provide defibrillator power to victims reached by mobile emergency teams.

These characteristics of next-generation defibrillator devices are only a few, among many, that can be realized by using all the tools of TRIZ. They are, however, major characteristics and features that move current defibrillators closer to the ideal final design.

It is also possible to use the triads and pruning procedure to defibrillators (or to any product or process) on a micro level. For example, one of the problems associated with defibrillators is "chest area burns" associated with the energy absorbed during shock delivery. Medical research dictates that the shape of the electrical power–time profile delivered has to have a certain shape for maximizing the probability of reviving the patient. The area under the power–time curve is energy, and unfortunately, this excessive energy causes the harmful side effects mentioned above.

The passive object of this triad is the heart. The active object is an electrical shock having a certain power–time profile shape. The enabling object is an electrical power supply system. Let us divide the electrical power–time profile into two parts, a useful one and a harmful one. If the harmful part of the electrical shock profile (the one that contributes to patient burns) is pruned, we are left with the useful part (the essential part of the electrical shock profile that revives the patient).

This is where the tools of TRIZ can be used. Let's express the physical contradiction as follows: *The profile shape of the electrical shock has to be unchanged to maximize the probability of reviving the victim, and the profile shape of the electrical shock has to be changed to reduce the area (energy) under the power–time curve.* This conflict can be resolved in several ways, including the following:

- Deliver a rapid burst of many shorter-in-time power–time profiles, each having the shape required.
- Deliver the same profile shape except that the power is pulsed. That is, the overall shape looks the same in time and in power, but on a more microscopic scale, the shock is delivered in short pulses with no electrical delivery between the pulses. In this way the power–time profile shape is the same, but the total energy delivered is only a fraction of what was delivered to the victim previously. Drawings of the problem and the solution (i.e., before and after a triad was applied) are shown below. Notice in Figure 10.14(a) that the energy is maximum under a continuous profile, whereas in Figure 10.14(b) the energy is significantly reduced but the profile shape is the same.

Let's look at what was accomplished. We first formed a triad. Then the original power–time profile was pruned and replaced by a pulsed power–time profile having the same shape. A modification of existing system resources was used to solve the problem.

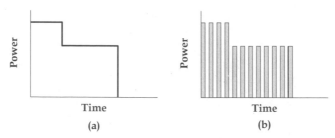

Figure 10.14 Defibrillator energy profile: (a) problem; (b) solution.

10.14 SUMMARY

Altshuller was an inventor's inventor, and what he has provided designers and DFSS teams throughout the world is a priceless tool to help us see the true design opportunity and provide us with principles to resolve, improve, and optimize designs. TRIZ is a useful innovation and problem-solving tool. It mirrors the philosophy of Taguchi in the ideality equation and effective problem-solving methodologies such as six sigma and TOPS 8D upon which it is based. It relies on a set of principles that guide inventive activity by defining contradictions and resolving them or by removing harmful effects or using predictions to choose superior useful functions. Applying the TRIZ thinking tools of inventive problem solving in engineering successfully replaces the trial-and-error method in the search for solutions in the everyday life of engineers and developers. The majority of product development decisions made by designers and managers, however, are still based on their personal intuition and experience. TRIZ is just as applicable in this environment to provide systematic, innovative, and low-risk solutions. This is part of the reason for the growing demand from management people for systematic and powerful design and innovation tools, which assist teams processing the information and making the right decisions in time.

TRIZ-based thinking for management tasks helped to identify the technology tools that come into play:

- TRIZ tools such as innovation and separation principles for resolving organizational contradictions and conflicts.
- Operators for revealing and utilizing system resources as a basis for effective and cost-saving decisions.
- Patterns of evolution of technical systems to support optimum selection of the most relevant solution.

APPENDIX 10A: CONTRADICTION MATRIX

A contradiction matrix or table is one of the earliest TRIZ tools to aid designers. It is a 39 × 39 matrix that deals with about 1263 common technical contradictions (i.e., one parameter improves while the other degrades). The 39 parameters in the rows and columns are the same. The rows represent what needs to be improved, while the columns represent the parameters that degrade. In the cell of any (row, column) intersection, the reference numbers of the applicable inventive principles given in Section 10.8 are listed. For example, in Figure 10A.1 if we want to improve the strength of an object, its weight becomes heavy. To solve this contradiction, inventive principle 40 (composite structures), inventive principle 26 (copying), inventive principle 27 (cheap, short-lived objects), and inventive principle 1 (segmentation) can be used.

Using Altshuller's contradiction matrix is as simple as following five steps:

1. Convert your design problem statement into one of a contradiction between two performance considerations, parameters, or design requirements.
2. Match these two requirements to any two of the 39 parameters.
3. Look up solution principles to the conflict of these two requirements using the contradiction matrixes shown in Figures 10A.2 to 10A.5. That is, the two requirements have numbers associated with them. Look at the corresponding row and column numbers' cell, which will have a list of numbers in the cell. These numbers are the inventive principle numbers given in Section 10.8.
4. Look up the applicable principles in Section 10.8.
5. Convert these general solution principles into a working solution for your design problem.

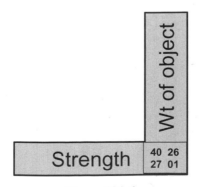

Figure 10A.1

	1	2	3	4	5	6	7	8	9	10	11	12	13	14	15	16	17	18	19	20
1			15, 8, 29, 34		29, 17, 38, 34		29, 2, 40, 28		2, 8, 15, 38	8, 10, 18, 37	10, 36, 37, 40	10, 14, 35, 40	1, 35, 19, 39	28, 27, 18, 40	5, 34, 31, 35		6, 29, 4, 38	19, 1, 32	35, 12, 34, 31	
2				10, 1, 29, 35		35, 30, 13, 2		5, 35, 14, 2		8, 10, 19, 35	13, 29, 10, 18	13, 10, 29, 14	26, 39, 1, 40	28, 2, 10, 27		2, 27, 19, 6	28, 19, 32, 22	19, 32, 35		18, 19, 28, 1
3	15, 8, 29, 34				15, 17, 4		7, 17, 4, 35		13, 4, 8	17, 10, 4	1, 8, 35	1, 8, 10, 29	1, 8, 15, 34	8, 35, 29, 34	19		10, 15, 19	32	8, 35, 24	
4		35, 28, 40, 29				17, 7, 10, 40		35, 8, 2, 14		28, 10	1, 14, 35	13, 14, 15, 7	39, 37, 35	15, 14, 28, 26		1, 40, 35	3, 35, 38, 18	3, 25		
5	2, 17, 29, 4		14, 15, 18, 4				7, 14, 17, 4		29, 30, 4, 34	19, 30, 35, 2	10, 15, 36, 28	5, 34, 29, 4	11, 2, 13, 39	3, 15, 40, 14	6, 3		2, 15, 16	15, 32, 19, 13	19, 32	
6		30, 2, 14, 18		26, 7, 9, 39						1, 18, 35, 36	10, 15, 36, 37		2, 38	40		2, 10, 19, 30	35, 39, 38			
7	2, 26, 29, 40		1, 7, 35, 4	1, 7, 4, 17	1, 7, 4, 17				29, 4, 38, 34	15, 35, 36, 37	6, 35, 36, 37	1, 15, 29, 4	28, 10, 1, 39	9, 14, 15, 7	6, 35, 4		34, 39, 10, 18	2, 13, 10	35	
8		35, 10, 19, 14	19, 14	35, 8, 2, 14						2, 18, 37	24, 35	7, 2, 35	34, 28, 35, 40	9, 14, 17, 15		35, 34, 38	35, 6, 4			
9	2, 28, 13, 38		13, 14, 8		29, 30, 34		7, 29, 34			13, 28, 15, 19	6, 18, 38, 40	35, 15, 18, 34	28, 33, 1, 18	8, 3, 26, 14	3, 19, 35, 5		28, 30, 36, 2	10, 13, 19	8, 15, 35, 38	
10	8, 1, 37, 18	18, 13, 1, 28	17, 19, 9, 36	28, 10	19, 10, 15	1, 18, 36, 37	15, 9, 12, 37	2, 36, 18, 37	13, 28, 15, 12		18, 21, 11	10, 35, 40, 34	35, 10, 21	35, 10, 14, 27	19, 2		35, 10, 3, 21		19, 17, 10	1, 16, 36, 37
11	10, 36, 37, 40	13, 29, 10, 18	35, 10, 36	35, 1, 14, 16	10, 15, 36, 28	10, 15, 36, 37	6, 35, 10	35, 24	6, 35, 36	36, 35, 21		35, 4, 15, 10	35, 33, 2, 40	9, 18, 3, 40	19, 3, 27		35, 39, 19, 2		14, 24, 10, 37	
12	8, 10, 29, 40	15, 10, 26, 3	29, 34, 5, 4	13, 14, 10, 7	5, 34, 4, 10		14, 4, 15, 22	7, 2, 35	35, 15, 34, 18	35, 10, 37, 40	34, 15, 10, 14		33, 1, 18, 4	30, 14, 10, 40	14, 26, 9, 25		22, 14, 19, 32	13, 15, 32	2, 6, 34, 14	
13	21, 35, 2, 39	26, 39, 1, 40	13, 15, 1, 28	37	2, 11, 13	39	28, 10, 19, 39	34, 28, 35, 40	33, 15, 28, 18	10, 35, 21, 16	2, 35, 40	22, 1, 18, 4		17, 9, 15	13, 27, 10, 35	39, 3, 35, 23	35, 1, 32	32, 3, 27, 15	13, 19	27, 4, 29, 18
14	1, 8, 40, 15	40, 26, 27, 1	1, 15, 8, 35	15, 14, 28, 26	3, 34, 40, 29	9, 40, 28	10, 15, 14, 7	9, 14, 17, 15	8, 13, 26, 14	10, 18, 3, 14	10, 3, 18, 40	10, 30, 35, 40	13, 17, 35		27, 3, 26		30, 10, 40	35, 19	19, 35, 10	35
15	19, 5, 34, 31		2, 19, 9		3, 17, 19		10, 2, 19, 30		3, 35, 5	19, 2, 16	19, 3, 27	14, 26, 28, 25	13, 3, 35	27, 3, 10			19, 35, 39	2, 19, 6	28, 6, 35, 18	
16		6, 27, 19, 16		1, 40, 35				35, 34, 38					39, 3, 35, 23				19, 18, 36, 40			
17	36, 22, 6, 38	22, 35, 32	15, 19, 9	15, 19, 9	3, 35, 39, 18	35, 38	34, 39, 40, 18	35, 6, 4	2, 28, 36, 30	35, 10, 3, 21	35, 39, 19, 2	14, 22, 19, 32	1, 35, 32	10, 30, 22, 40	19, 13, 39	19, 18, 36, 40		32, 30, 21, 16	19, 15, 3, 17	
18	19, 1, 32	2, 35, 32	19, 32, 16		19, 32, 26		2, 13, 10		10, 13, 19	26, 19, 6		32, 30	32, 3, 27	35, 19	2, 19, 6		32, 35, 19		32, 1, 19	32, 35, 1, 15
19	12, 18, 28, 31		12, 28		15, 19, 25		35, 13, 18		8, 15, 35	16, 26, 21, 2	23, 14, 25	12, 2, 29	19, 13, 17, 24	5, 19, 9, 35	28, 35, 6, 18		19, 24, 3, 14	2, 15, 19		
20		19, 9, 6, 27								36, 37	27, 4, 29, 18		35					19, 2, 35, 32		

Figure 10A.2 Contradiction matrix 1 through 20 × 1 through 20.

	1	2	3	4	5	6	7	8	9	10	11	12	13	14	15	16	17	18	19	20
21	8,36,38,31	19,26,17,27	1,10,35,37		19,38	17,32,13,38	35,6,38	30,6,25	15,35,2	26,2,36,35	22,10,35	29,14,2,40	35,32,15,31	26,10,28	19,35,10,38	16	2,14,17,25	16,6,19	16,6,19,37	
22	15,6,19,28	19,6,18,9	7,2,6,13	6,38,7	15,26,17,30	17,7,30,18	7,18,23	7	16,35,38	36,38			14,2,39,6	26			19,38,7	1,13,32,15		
23	35,6,23,40	35,6,22,32	14,29,10,39	10,28,24	35,2,10,31	10,18,39,31	1,29,30,36	3,39,18,31	10,13,28,38	14,15,18,40	3,36,37,10	29,35,3,5	2,14,30,40	35,28,31,40	28,27,3,18	27,16,18,38	21,36,39,31	1,6,13	35,18,24,5	28,27,12,31
24	10,24,35	10,35,5	1,26	26	30,26	30,16		2,22	26,32						10	10		19		
25	10,20,37,35	10,20,26,5	15,2,29	30,24,14,5	26,4,5,16	10,35,17,4	2,5,34,10	35,16,32,18		10,37,36,5	37,36,4	4,10,34,17	35,3,22,5	29,3,28,18	20,10,28,18	28,20,10,16	35,29,21,18	1,19,21,17	35,38,19,18	1
26	35,6,18,31	27,26,18,35	29,14,35,18		15,14,29	2,18,40,4	15,20,29		35,29,34,28	35,14,3	10,36,14,3	35,14	15,2,17,40	14,35,34,10	3,35,10,40	3,35,31	3,17,39		34,29,16,18	
27	3,8,10,40	3,10,8,28	15,9,14,4	15,29,28,11	17,10,14,16	32,35,40,4	3,10,14,24	2,35,24	21,35,11,28	8,28,10,3	10,24,35,19	35,1,16,11		11,28	2,35,3,25	34,27,6,40	3,35,10	11,32,13	21,11,27,19	36,23
28	28,32,13,18	28,35,25,26	28,26,5,16	32,28,3,16	26,28,32,3	26,28,32,3	32,13,6		28,13,32,24	32,2	6,28,32	6,28,32	32,35,13	28,6,32	28,6,32	10,26,24	6,19,28,24	6,1,32	3,6,32	
29	28,32,13,18	28,35,27,9	10,28,29,37	2,32,10	28,33,29,32	2,29,18,36	32,28,2	25,10,35	10,28,32	28,19,34,36	3,35	32,30,40	30,18	3,27	3,27,40		19,26	3,32	32,2	
30	22,21,27,39	2,22,13,24	17,1,39,4	1,18	22,1,33,28	27,2,39,35	22,23,37,35	34,39,19,27	21,22,35,28	13,35,39,18	22,2,37	22,1,3,35	35,24,30,18	18,35,37,1	22,15,33,28	17,1,40,33	22,33,35,2	1,19,32,13	1,24,6,27	10,2,22,37
31	19,22,15,39	35,22,1,39	17,15,16,22		17,2,18,39	22,1,40	17,2,40	30,18,35,4	35,28,3,23	35,28,1,40	2,33,27,18	35,1	35,40,27,39	15,35,22,2	15,22,33,31	21,39,16,22	22,35,2,24	19,24,39,32	2,35,6	19,22,18
32	28,29,15,16	1,27,36,13	1,29,13,17	15,17,27	13,1,26,12	16,40	13,29,1,40	35	35,13,8,1	35,12	35,19,1,37	1,28,13,27	11,13,1	1,3,10,32	27,1,4	35,16	26,27,18	28,24,27,1	28,26,27,1	1,4
33	25,2,13,15	6,13,1,25	1,17,13,12		1,17,13,16	18,16,15,39	1,16,35,15	4,18,39,31	18,13,34	28,13,35	2,32,12	15,34,29,28	32,35,30	32,40,3,28	29,3,8,25	1,16,25	26,27,13	13,17,1,24	1,13,24	
34	2,27,35,11	2,27,35,11	1,28,10,25	3,18,31	15,13,32	16,25	25,2,35,11	1	34,9	1,11,10	13	1,13,2,4	2,35	11,1,2,9	11,29,28,27	1	4,10	15,1,13	15,1,28,16	
35	1,6,15,8	19,15,29,16	35,1,29,2	1,35,16	35,30,29,7	15,16	15,35,29		35,10,14	15,17,20	35,16	15,37,1,8	35,30,14	35,3,32,6	13,1,35	2,16	27,2,3,35	6,22,26,1	19,35,29,13	
36	26,30,34,36	2,26,35,39	1,19,26,24	26	14,1,13,16	6,36	34,26,6	1,16	34,10,28	26,16	19,1,35	29,13,28,15	2,22,17,19	2,13,28	10,4,28,15		2,17,13	24,17,13	27,2,29,28	
37	27,26,28,13	6,13,28,1	16,17,26,24	26	2,13,18,17	2,39,30,16	29,1,4,16	2,18,26,31	3,4,16,35	36,28,40,19	35,36,37,32	27,13,1,39	11,22,39,30	27,3,15,28	19,29,25,39	25,34,6,35	3,27,35,16	2,24,26	35,38	19,35,16
38	28,26,18,35	28,26,35,10	14,13,17,28	23	17,14,13		35,13,16		28,10	2,35	13,35	15,32,1,13	18,1	25,13	6,9		26,2,19	8,32,19	2,32,13	
39	35,26,24,37	28,27,15,3	18,4,28,38	30,7,14,26	10,26,34,31	10,35,17,7	2,6,34,10	35,37,10,2		28,15,10,36	10,37,14	14,10,34,40	35,3,22,39	29,28,10,18	35,10,2,18	20,10,16,38	35,21,28,10	26,17,19,1	35,10,38,19	1

Figure 10A.3 Contradiction matrix 21 through 39 × 1 through 20.

	21	22	23	24	25	26	27	28	29	30	31	32	33	34	35	36	37	38	39
1	12.36. 18.31	6.2.34. 19	5.35.3. 31	10.24. 35	10.35. 20.28	3.26. 18.31	3.11.1. 27	28.27. 35.26	28.35. 26.18	22.21. 18.27	22.35. 31.39	27.28. 1.36	35.3.2. 24	2.27. 28.11	29.5. 15.8	26.30. 36.34	28.29. 26.32	26.35. 18.19	35.3. 24.37
2	15.19. 18.22	18.19. 28.15	5.8.13. 30	10.15. 35	10.20. 35.26	19.6. 18.26	10.28. 8.3	18.26. 28	10.1. 35.17	2.19. 22.37	35.22. 1.39	28.1.9	6.13.1. 32	2.27. 28.11	19.15. 29	1.10. 26.39	25.28. 17.15	2.26. 35	1.28. 15.35
3	1.35	7.2.35. 39	4.29. 23.10	1.24	15.2. 29	29.35	10.14. 29.40	28.32. 4	10.28. 29.37	1.15. 17.24	17.15	1.29. 17	15.29. 35.4	1.28. 10	14.15. 1.16	1.19. 26.24	35.1. 26.24	17.24. 26.16	14.4. 28.29
4	12.8	6.28	10.28. 24.35	24.26	30.29. 14		15.29. 28	32.28. 3	2.32. 10	1.18		15.17. 27	2.25	3	1.35	1.26	26		30.14. 7.26
5	19.10. 32.18	15.17. 30.26	10.35. 2.39	30.26	26.4	29.30. 6.13	29.9	26.28. 32.3	2.32	22.33. 28.1	17.2. 18.39	13.1. 26.24	15.17. 13.16	15.13. 10.1	15.30	14.1. 13	2.36. 26.18	14.30. 28.23	10.26. 34.2
6	17.32	17.7. 30	10.14. 18.39	30.16	10.35. 4.18	2.18. 40.4	32.35. 40.4	26.28. 32.3	2.29. 18.36	27.2. 39.35	22.1. 40	40.16	16.4	16	15.16	1.18. 36	2.35. 30.18	23	10.15.6. 17.7
7	35.6. 13.18	7.15. 13.16	36.39. 34.10	2.22	2.6.34. 10	29.30. 7	14.1. 40.11	25.26. 28	2.16	22.21. 27.35	17.2. 40.1	29.1. 40	15.13. 30.12	10	15.29	26.1	29.26. 4	35.34. 16.24	10.6.2. 34
8	30.6		10.39. 35.34		35.16. 32.18	35.3	2.35. 16		35.10. 25	34.39. 19.27	30.18. 35.4	35		1			2.17. 26		35.37. 10.2
9	19.35. 38.2	14.20. 19.35	10.13. 28.38	13.26		10.19. 29.38	11.35. 27.28	28.32. 1.24	10.28. 32.25	1.28. 35.23	2.24. 32.21	35.13. 8.1	32.28. 13.12	34.2. 28.27	15.10. 26	10.28. 4.34	3.34. 27.16	10.18	
10	19.35. 18.37	14.15	8.35. 40.5		10.37. 36	14.29. 18.36	3.35. 13.21	35.10. 23.24	28.29. 37.36	1.35. 40.18	13.3. 36.24	15.37. 18.1	1.28.3. 25	15.1. 11	15.17. 18.20	26.35. 10.18	36.37. 10.19	2.35	3.28. 35.37
11	10.35. 14	2.36. 25	10.36. 37		37.36. 4	10.14. 36	10.13. 19.35	6.28. 25	3.35	22.2. 37	2.33. 27.18	1.35. 16	11	2	35	19.1. 35	2.36. 37	35.24	10.14. 35.37
12	4.6.2	14	35.29. 3.5		14.10. 34.17	36.22	10.40. 16	28.32. 1	32.30. 40	22.1.2. 35	35.1	1.32. 17.28	32.15. 26	2.13.1	1.15. 29	16.29. 1.28	15.13. 39	15.1. 32	17.26. 34.10
13	32.35. 27.31	14.2. 39.6	2.14. 30.40		35.27	15.32. 35		13	18	35.23. 18.30	35.40. 27.39	35.19	32.35. 30	2.35. 10.16	35.30. 34.2	2.35. 22.26	35.22. 39.23	1.8.35	23.35. 40.3
14	35.28	35	35.28. 31.40		29.3. 28.10	29.10. 27	11.3	3.27. 16	3.27	18.35. 37.1	15.35. 22.2	11.3. 10.32	32.40. 28.2	27.11. 3	15.3. 32	27.3. 15.28	27.3. 15.40	15	29.35.
15	19.10. 35.38		28.27. 3.18	10	20.10. 28.18	3.35. 10.40	11.2. 13	3	3.27. 16.40	22.15. 33.28	21.39. 16.22	27.1.4. 27	12.27	29.10. 27	1.35. 13	10.4. 29.15	19.29. 39.35	6.10	10.14
16	16	21.17. 35.38	27.16. 18.38	10	28.20. 10.16	3.35. 31	34.27. 6.40	10.26. 24		17.1. 40.33	22	35.10	1	1	2		25.34. 6.35	1	20.10. 16.38
17	2.14. 17.25	19.16. 1.6	21.36. 29.31	1.6	35.28. 21.18	3.17. 30.39	3.10	32.19. 24	24	22.33. 35.2	22.35. 2.24	26.27	26.27	4.10. 16	2.18. 27	2.17. 16	3.27. 35.31	23.2. 19.16	15.28
18	32		13.1		19.1. 26.17	1.19		11.15. 32	3.32	15.19	35.19. 32.39	19.35. 28.26	28.26. 19	15.17. 13.16	15.1. 19	6.32. 13	32.15	2.26. 10	15.28
19	6.19. 37.18	12.22. 15.24	35.24. 18.5		35.38. 19.18	34.23. 16.18	19.21. 11.27	3. 1.32		1.35.6. 27	2.35.6	28.26. 30	19.35	1.15. 17.28	15.17. 13.16	2.29. 27.28	35.38	32.2	12.28. 35
20			28.27. 18.31			3.35. 31	10.36			10.2. 22.37	19.22. 18	1.4					19.35. 16.25		1.6

Figure 10A.4 Contradiction matrix 1 through 20 × 21 through 39.

Figure 10A.5 Contradiction matrix 21 through 39 × 21 through 39.

	21	22	23	24	25	26	27	28	29	30	31	32	33	34	35	36	37	38	39
21		10,35,38	28,27,18,38	10,19	35,20,10,6	4,34,19	19,24,26,31	32,15,2	32,2	19,22,31,2	2,35,18	26,10,34	26,35,10	35,2,10,34	19,17,34	20,19,30,34	19,35,16	28,2,17	28,35,34
22	3,38		35,27,2,37	19,10	10,18,32,7	7,18,25	11,10,35	32		21,22,35,2	21,35,2,22	19,35	35,32,1	2,19		7,23	35,3,15,23	2	28,10,29,35
23	28,27,18,38	35,27,2,31			15,18,35,10	6,3,10,24	10,29,39,35	16,34,31,28	35,31,10,24	33,22,30,40	10,1,34,29	15,34,33	32,28,2,24	2,35,34,27	15,10,2	35,10,28,24	35,18,10,13	35,10,18	28,35,10,23
24	10,19	19,10			24,26,28,32	24,28,35	10,28,23			22,10,1	10,21,22	32	27,22				35,33	35	13,23,15
25	35,20,10,6	10,5,18,32	35,18,10,39	24,26,28,32		35,38,18,16	10,30,4	24,34,28,32	32,26,28,18	35,18,34	35,22,18,39	35,28,34,4	4,28,10,34	32,1,10	35,28	6,29	18,28,32,10	24,28,35,30	
26	35	7,18,25	6,3,10,24	24,28,35	35,38,18,16		18,3,28,40	13,2,28	33,30	35,33,29,31	3,35,40,39	29,1,35,27	35,29,10,25	2,32,10,25	15,3,29	3,13,27,10	3,27,29,18	8,35	13,29,3,27
27	21,11,26,31	10,11,35	10,35,29,39	10,28	10,30,4	21,28,40,3		32,3,11,23	11,32,1	27,35,2,40	35,2,40,26	27,17,40	1,11	13,35,8,24	13,35,1	27,40,28	11,13,27	1,35,29,38	1,35,10,38
28	3,6,32	26,32,27	16,34,31,28		24,34,28,32	2,6,32	5,11,1,23			28,33,23,26	3,33,39,10	6,35,25,18	1,13,17,34	1,32,13,11	13,35,2	27,35,10,34	26,24,32,28	28,2,10,34	10,34,28,32
29	32,2	13,32,2	35,31,10,24		32,26,28,18	32,30	11,32,1			26,28,10,36	4,17,34,26			25,10				26,28,18,23	10,18,32,39
30	19,22,31,2	21,22,35,2	33,22,19,40	22,10,2	35,18,34	35,33,29,31	27,24,2,40	28,33,23,26	26,28,10,18			24,2	2,25,28,39	35,10,2	35,11,22,31	22,19,29,40	22,19,29,40	33,3,34	22,35,13,24
31	2,35,18	21,35,2,22	10,1,34	10,21,29	1,22	3,24,39,1	24,2,40,39	3,33,26	4,17,34,26					4,17,34,26		19,1,31	2,21,27,1	2	22,35,18,39
32	27,1,12,24	19,35	15,34,33	32,24,18,16	35,28,34,4	35,23,1,24	1,35,12,18			24,2			2,5,13,16	35,1,11,9	2,13,15	27,26,1	6,28,11,1	8,28,1	35,1,10,28
33	35,34,2,10	2,19,13	28,32,2,24	4,10,27,22	4,28,10,34	12,35	17,27,8,40	25,13,2,34	1,32,35,23	2,25,28,39		2,5,12		12,26,1,32	15,34,1,16	32,26,12,17		1,34,12,3	15,1,28
34	15,10,32,2	15,1,32,19	2,35,34,27		32,1,10,25	2,28,10,25	11,10,1,16	10,2,13	25,10	35,10,2,16	1,16,7,4	1,13,2,4	1,12,26,15		7,1,4,16	35,1,13,11	1	34,35,7,13	1,32,10
35	19,1,29	18,15,1	15,10,2,13		35,28	3,35,15	35,13,8,24	35,5,1,10		35,11,32,31		2,13,15	27,17,40	1,16,7,4		15,29,37,28	27,4,1,35	27,34,35	35,28,6,37
36	20,19,30,34	10,35,13,2	35,10,28,24		6,29	13,3,27,10	13,35,1	2,26,10,34	26,24,32	22,19,29,40	19,1	27,26,1,13	27,9,26,24	1,13	29,15,28,37		15,10,37,28	15,1,24	12,17,28
37	19,1,16,10	35,3,15,19	35,10,28,24	35,33	18,28,32,9	3,27,29,18	27,40,28,8	26,24,32,28		22,19,29,28	2,21	5,28,11,29	2,5	12,26	1,15	15,10,37,28		34,21	35,18
38	28,2,27	23,28	35,10,18,5	35,33	24,28,35,30	35,13	11,27,32	28,26,10,34	28,26,18,23	2,33	2	1,26,13	1,12,34,3	1,35,13	27,4,1,35	15,24,10	34,27,25		5,12,35,26
39	35,20,10	28,10,29,35	28,10,35,23	13,15,23		35,38	1,35,10,38	1,10,34,28	18,10,32,1	22,35,13,24	35,22,18,39	35,28,2,24	1,28,7,19	1,32,10,25	1,35,28,37	12,17,28,24	35,18,27,2	5,12,35,26	

239

11

DFSS RISK MANAGEMENT PROCESS

11.1 INTRODUCTION

In general, safety and effectiveness can only be considered in relative terms. Safety is, by definition, the freedom from unacceptable risk, where risk is a combination of likelihood of harm and the severity of that harm. Subsequently, a *hazard* is the potential for an adverse event, a source of harm. Like any other engineered systems, all medical devices carry a certain degree of risk and could cause problems in a definite situation. Many medical device problems cannot be detected until extensive market experience is gained. For example, an implantable device may fail in a manner that was not predictable at the time of implantation, where the failure may reflect distinctive conditions to certain patients. For other devices, a failure can also be random. The current approach to device safety is to manage all potential risks of a device becoming a hazard that could result in safety problems and harm. This approach to risk management affects broad categories of risk, such as project risks, technical risks, environmental risks, health risks, and many others. In this chapter we elected to combine all risks pertaining to environment and health into a category named *safety risks* and all the other risks into a category named *business risks*, and then used the design for six sigma methodology to manage both types of risks.

Medical device manufacturers are generally required to have a quality management system as well as processes for addressing device-related risks.

Medical Device Design for Six Sigma: A Road Map for Safety and Effectiveness,
By Basem S. El-Haik and Khalid S. Mekki
Copyright © 2008 John Wiley & Sons, Inc.

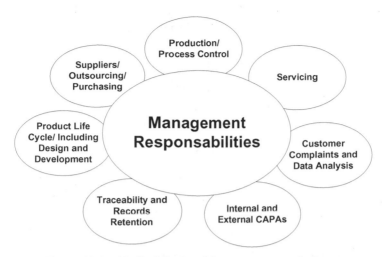

Figure 11.1 Medical device risk management elements.

Figure 11.1 illustrates integration of the risk management process into a medical device quality management system. Also shown in Figure 11.2 is a design process model with medical device design controls, including risk management, reproduced from Figure 1.2.

A medical device risk management begins with *planning* for the device based on the quality system objectives to include the risk acceptability criteria defined by management, then followed by *risk analysis* to identify all potential hazards associated with the medical device, followed by *risk evaluation* to estimate the risk for each hazard. Risk evaluation is based on experience, evidence, testing, calculation, or even subjective judgment. Risk assessment is complex, as it can be influenced by personal perception and other factors, such as political climates, economic conditions, and cultural background. It is highly recommended that risk assessment of medical devices be based on expert's knowledge and safety-centric engineering. The causal relationship among the harm, the hazard, and the cause of the hazard plays a great role in risk management, where causes may occur in the absence of failures or as a result of one or more failure modes. Naturally, hazards are inherent in products, and many unplanned attempts to overcorrect a hazardous event tend to increase the potential risk of creating new hazards. Therefore, the focus should be on the cause of the hazard, not on the actual harm itself. Figure 11.3 depicts the risk management elements discussed in detail in this chapter.

11.2 PLANNING FOR RISK MANAGEMENT ACTIVITIES IN DESIGN AND DEVELOPMENT

Business risk can be defined as a potential threat to achieving business objectives for the device under development. These risks are related to, but not

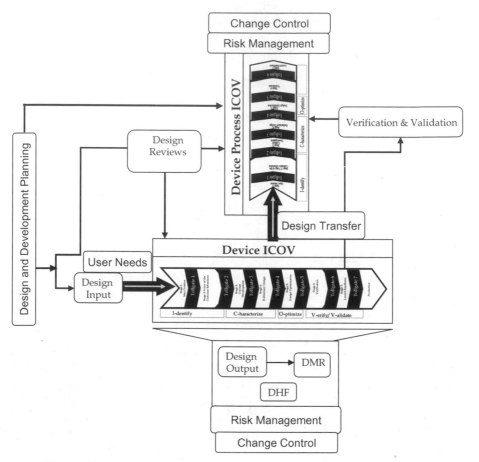

Figure 11.2 Design process model with medical device design controls.

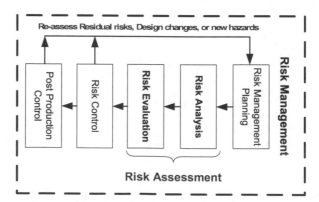

Figure 11.3 Risk management elements. (Adapted from ISO 14971.)

limited to, technology maturity, product complexity, product reliability and availability, performance and robustness, and finally, the project time line. *Safety risk* is defined as a potential threat to health and environment for the product under development; these risks are related to, but not limited to, product failure, process failure, customer misuse and abuse, physical systems interaction, and social or cultural systems interaction. When considering safety risks, it is apparent that it can be classified as business risk due to the criteria mentioned above. It is isolated in category by itself for its profound effect on the patient or end user. The emphasis on decoupling safety risk from business risk is to manage the complexity of the rigor applied to reduce or eliminate safety risk as a result of the regulatory expectations for risk management. A structured approach to risk management, as described throughout this chapter, is required by a medical device producer when safety risk and regulatory compliance are affected. Contrasting rigor is required when dealing with business risks only.

The risk management process starts early in the voice-of-the-customer stage (see Chapter 7 for a DFSS project road map) by identifying potential hazards and establishing risk assessment criteria. A risk management plan defines the process for ensuring that hazards resulting from errors in clinical use, product foreseeable misuses, and product development and production failures are addressed. As stated by various standards and regulatory authorities[1] (discussed in Chapter 2), a risk management plan must include the following:

1. The scope of the plan in the context of the product development life cycle, as applicable
2. A verification plan, allocation of responsibilities, requirements for activities review
3. Criteria for risk acceptability

Risk management plans are performed on projects (or device platforms) where activities are reviewed for effectiveness either as part of a standard design review process or in independent stand-alone reviews. Sometimes the nature of hazards and their causes is unknown, so the plan may change as knowledge of the device is accumulated. Eventually, hazards and their controls will be linked to verification and validation plans.

At the design input stage, which is equivalent to the DFSS identify phase, risk estimation establishes linkage between requirements and hazards and ensures that safety requirements are complete. Then risk assessment is performed on the device as a design activity. Subsequently, risk mitigation, includ-

---

[1] 21 CFR 820.30, 820.100, and 820.198; ISO 14971:2001; ISO 13485; ISO 9001:2000; and IEC 60601-1.

ing risk elimination and/or reduction measures, ensures that effective traceability between hazards and requirements is established during verification and validation. Risk acceptability and residual risks are reviewed at applicable milestones of the product design (see Chapter 7 for DFSS tollgates in the ICOV process). The knowledge of risk and safety is transferred as part of the design transfer. Existing and potential new hazards and risks are reassessed according to the design change control. It is very important for management to determine responsibilities, establish competent resources, and review risk management activities and results to ensure that an effective management process is in place. This should be ongoing process in which design reviews and DFSS gate reviews are decision-making milestones.

A risk management report summarizes all results from risk management activities, such as a summary of risk assessment techniques, risk versus benefit analysis, and overall residual risk assessment. The results of all risk management activities will be recorded and maintained in a risk management file.

11.3   RISK ASSESSMENT TECHNIQUES

Risk assessment starts with a definition of the intended use of a device and its potential hazards, followed by a detailed analysis of the characteristics that cause each potential hazard, and finally, a well-defined rating scale is used to evaluate the potential risk under both normal and fault conditions. In risk evaluation, the design team decides whether risk reduction is needed. Risk assessment includes both risk analysis and risk evaluation. Brainstorming is a useful tool for identifying hazards. Requirement documents are another source of hazard identification, since there are many hazards associated with the nonfulfillment or partial fulfillment of each requirement. For example, in infusion medicine instruments, there may be requirements for medication delivery and hazards associated with over- or underdelivery. Estimating the risks associated with each hazard usually concludes the risk analysis part of the process. The next step is risk evaluation and assessment.

As defined earlier in the chapter, risk is a combination of the likelihood of harm and the severity of that harm. Risk evaluation can be *qualitative* or *quantitative*, depending on when in the device life cycle the risk estimation is occurring and what information is available at that point in time. If the risk cannot be established or predicted using objective (quantitative) data, expert judgment may be sought. Many risk analysis tools can be used for risk assessment; in this chapter we discuss the most common tools used in the medical device industry, such as preliminary hazard analysis, hazard and operability analysis, failure mode and effects analysis, and fault tree analysis. We then touch base on other risk analysis tools used by other industries as a gateway to the medical device industry.

11.3.1 Preliminary Hazard Analysis

Preliminary hazard analysis (PHA) is a qualitative risk assessment method used to identify hazards and estimate risk based on the intended use of the device. In this approach, risk is estimated by assigning severity ratings to the consequences of hazards and the likelihood of occurrence ratings to causes. PHA helps to identify risk reduction or elimination measures early in the design life cycle to help establish safety requirements and test plans.

11.3.2 Hazard and Operability Study

The hazard and operability study (HAZOP) technique can be defined as the application of a systematic examination of complex facilities, processes, and/or designs to find actual or potentially hazardous procedures and operations so that they may be eliminated or mitigated (CCPS, 1992). The methodology may be applied to any process or project, although most practitioners and most expertise originates in chemical and offshore industries. This technique is usually performed using a set of key words (e.g., "more," "less," "as well as"). From these key words, a scenario that may result in a hazard or an operational problem is identified. Consider the possible flow problems in a process line; the guide word *more* will correspond to a high flow rate, and *less* will correspond to a low flow rate. The consequences of the hazard and measures to reduce the frequency with which the hazard will occur are evaluated.

11.3.3 Failure Mode and Effects Analysis

Failure mode and effects analysis (FMEA) (introduced in the late 1940s with the introduction of the U.S. Military Procedure MIL-P-1629) is a systematic method used to analyze products and processes by qualitatively determining their failure modes, causes of failure, and potential effects, then quantitatively classifying their risk estimate to better prioritize corrective and preventive actions and risk reduction measures required by the analysis.

When FMEA is extended by a criticality analysis, the resulting technique is then called failure mode and effects criticality analysis (FMECA). Failure mode and effects analysis has gained wide acceptance by most industries. In fact, the technique has adapted itself in many other forms, such as concept FMEA, robust design FMEA [Mekki (2006); see also Yang and El-Haik (2003) and El-Haik and Roy (2005)], process (manufacturing and service) FMEA, software FMEA, and use FMEA.

FMEAs, especially design FMEA, have gone through a metamorphosis of sorts in the last decade, as a focus on severity, and occurrence has replaced risk priority number (RPN)–driven activities. In large part this is due to measurement risk outcomes resulting from associated RPNs being misinterpreted, as so many practitioners of FMEAs believe that the RPN is the most important outcome. However, the FMEA methodology must consider taking actions as soon as it is practical.

An FMEA can be described as complementary to the process of defining what a design or process must do to satisfy the customer. In our case the process of defining what a design or a process must do to satisfy the customer is what we entertain in the device DFSS project road map discussed in Chapter 7. The DFSS team may visit an existing datum FMEA, if applicable, for further enhancement and updating. In all cases, the FMEA should be handled as a living document.

The fundamentals of a robust design FMEA inputs are depicted in Appendix 11A. Process FMEA, service FMEA, and software FMEA are discussed by El-Haik and Roy (2005).

11.3.4   Fault Tree Analysis

Fault tree analysis (FTA) is a technique for performing safety evaluation of a system. It is a process that utilizes logical diagrams for identifying the potential causes of a hazard or undesired event based on a method of breaking down chains of failures. FTA identifies a combination of faults based on two main types: (1) several items must fail together to cause another item to fail (called an "and" combination), and (2) only one of a number of possible faults needs to happen to cause another item to fail (called an "or" combination). FTA is used when the effect of a failure or fault is known and the team needs to find how the effect can be caused by a combination of failures. The probability of the top event can be predicted using estimates of failure rates for individual failure. It helps in identifying single point failures and failure path sets to facilitate improvement actions and other measures of making the product under analysis more robust.

FTA can be used as a qualitative or quantitative risk analysis tool. The difference is that the earlier is less structured than the later analysis and does not require use of the same rigorous logic. The FTA diagram shows faults as a hierarchy controlled by gates, as they prevent the failure event above them from occurring unless their specific conditions are met. The symbols that may be used in FTA diagrams are shown in Table 11.1.

Many other tree analysis techniques, such as event tree analysis (ETA), are used in risk assessment. ETA is a method for illustrating graphically the sequence of outcomes that may arise after the occurrence of a selected initial event. This technique provides an inductive approach to risk assessments, as they are constructed using forward logic. ETA and FTA are closely linked. Fault trees are often used to quantify system events that are part of event tree sequences. The logical processes employed to evaluate an event tree sequence and quantify the consequences are the same as those used in FTA.

TABLE 11.1 Symbols Used in FTA Diagrams

Symbol	Name	Meaning
	AND gate	Event above happens only if all events below happen.
	OR gate	Event above happens if one or more of events below are met.
Condition	Inhibit gate	Event above happens if event below happens and conditions described in oval happen.
Event	Combination gate	Event that results from combination of events passing through gate below it.
Event	Basic event	Event that does not have any contributory events.
Event	Undeveloped basic event	Event that does have contributory events, but which are not shown.
Event	Remote basic event	Event that does have contributory events, but which are shown in another diagram.
Out / In	Transferred event	A link to another diagram or to another part of the same diagram.
	Switch	Used to include or exclude other parts of the diagram which may or may not apply in specific situations.

Cause–consequence analysis (CCA) is a mixture of FTA and ETA. This technique combines cause analysis, described by fault trees, and consequence analysis, described by event trees. The purpose of CCA is to identify chains of events that can result in undesirable consequences. With the probabilities of the various events in the CCA diagram, the probabilities of the various consequences can be calculated, thus establishing the risk level of the device or any subset of it.

The management oversight risk tree (MORT) is an analytical risk analysis technique for determining causes and contributing factors for safety analysis purposes, where it would be compatible with complex goal-oriented management systems. MORT arranges safety program elements in an orderly and logical fashion, and its analysis is carried out similar to FTA.

TABLE 11.2 Severity of Hazard Rating

Criteria	Description	Rating 1–5	Rating 1–10
Catastrophic	Death or serious injury.	5	9–10
Serious	Potential death or serious injury, enduring harm which diminishes the long-term quality of life or life expectancy. Major impact to environment.	4	7–8
Critical	Harm of limited extent and duration; medical intervention required. M oderate impact to environment.	3	5–6
Marginal	Harm not needing intervention of or treatment by medical personnel. Minor impact to environment.	2	3–4
Negligible	No impact on safety and environment.	1	1–2

11.4 RISK EVALUATION

Risk evaluation starts once the components of risk for each hazard or harm have been identified, then uses risk acceptability criteria, defined by the risk management plan, to rank-order the risk to complete risk evaluation. Given the various risk analysis techniques discussed above, the evaluation of risk is totally dependent on the medical device company's culture and internal procedures, as regulations and standards cannot dictate one's approach for risk evaluation, due to the difference in medical device applications within the medical device industry. Two of the most used standards for medical device risk management are ISO 14971:2007(E)[2] and IEC/TR 60513.[3] In addition, the Global Harmonization Task Force[4] (GHTF) drafted a risk management procedure in 2004. In this chapter we discuss risk evaluation criteria based on our own *hybrid* approach to the various standards listed above.

To quantify risk consistently, we need to estimate the severity for each hazard and the likelihood of occurrence associated with its cause against criteria set forth by the risk management plan defined at the product level. The *severity rating* is the rank associated with the possible consequences of a hazard or harm. Table 11.2 lists generic severity ratings based on two com-

[2]ISO 14971:2007 specifies a process for a manufacturer to identify the hazards associated with medical devices, including in vitro diagnostic medical devices, to estimate and evaluate the associated risks, to control these risks, and to monitor the effectiveness of the controls.

[3]This standard identifies fundamental considerations to be taken into account in developing standards to ensure the safety of medical electrical equipment. It follows closely recommendations of ISO/IEC Guide 51 and expands on matters that are unique to, or critical in, the application of medical electrical equipment.

[4]The Global Harmonization Task Force (GHTF) was conceived in 1992 in an effort to respond to the growing need for international harmonization in the regulation of medical devices. You can visit the GHTF Web site at www.GHTF.org.

monly used scales: 1 to 5 and 1 to 10. A risk management team can develop the severity rating that best suits their application.

The *likelihood of occurrence rating* is the rank associated with probability (or frequency) that a specific cause will occur and cause a potential hazard during a predetermined time period (typically, the product design life). Table 11.3 lists generic likelihood-of-occurrence ratings based on two commonly used scales: 1 to 5 and 1 to 10. A risk management team can develop a likelihood-of-occurrence rating that best suits their application.

Risk classification is a process of categorizing risk in various criteria as defined by the risk management plan. Risk classification criteria define the foundation for risk acceptance or highlight the need for risk reduction. Table 11.4 lists the various risk classification criteria.

Risk acceptance is a relative term, as the product is deemed acceptable if it is risk-free or if the risks are *as low as reasonably practicable* (ALARP) and the benefits associated with the product outweigh the residual risk. However, intolerable risks are not acceptable and must be reduced at least to the level

TABLE 11.3   Likelihood of Occurrence Rating

Criteria	Description	Rating 1–5	Rating 1–10
Frequent	Hazard/harm likely to occur frequently.	5	9–10
Probable	Hazard/harm will occur several times during the life of the product.	4	7–8
Occasional	Hazard/harm likely to occur sometime during the life of the product.	3	5–6
Remote	Hazard/harm unlikely but possible to occur during the life of the product.	2	3–4
Improbable	Hazard/harm unlikely to occur during the life of the product.	1	1–2

TABLE 11.4   Risk Classification Criteria

	Severity of Hazard[a]				
Likelihood of Occurrence	1	2	3	4	5
	Negligible	Marginal	Critical	Serious	Catastrophic
5 Frequent	R_3	R_4	R_4	R_4	R_4
4 Probable	R_2	R_3	R_4	R_4	R_4
3 Occasional	R_1	R_2	R_3	R_3	R_4
2 Remote	R_1	R_1	R_2	R_2	R_4
1 Improbable	R_1	R_1	R_1	R_1	R_3

[a]R4, intolerable; risk is unacceptable and must be reduced. R3, risk should be reduced as much as reasonably practicable; benefits must rationalize any residual risks even at a considerable cost. R2, risk is unacceptable and should be reduced as much as reasonably practicable; benefits must rationalize any residual risks at a cost that represents value. R1, broadly acceptable; no need for further risk reduction.

of ALARP risks. If this is not feasible, the device must be redesigned from a fault prevention standpoint.

The concept of practicability in ALARP analysis involves both technical and economic considerations, part of what we defined earlier as business risk, where *technical* refers to the availability and feasibility of solutions that mitigate or reduce risk and *economic* refers to the ability to reduce risks at a cost that represents value.

Risk versus benefit determination must satisfy at least one of the following: (1) all practicable measures to reduce the risk have been applied, (2) risk acceptance has been met, and finally, (3) the benefit that the device provides outweighs the residual risk.

11.5   RISK CONTROL

Once the decision is made to reduce risk, control activities begin. Risk reduction should focus on reducing the hazard severity, the likelihood of occurrence, or both. Only a design revision or technology change can create a reduction in the severity ranking. Likelihood of occurrence reduction can be achieved by removing or controlling the cause (mechanism) of the hazard. Increasing design verification actions can reduce detection ranking.

Risk control should consist of an integrated approach in which medical device companies will use one or more of the following in the priority order listed: (1) inherent safety by design (designed-in safety lead to a more robust design); (2) protective design measures where the product will fail safe and/or sounds an alarm when risk presents; (3) protective manufacturing measures, which improve the process (e.g., mistake-proofing) and/or test capabilities; and (4) information for safety, such as labeling, instructions for use, and training.

11.6   POSTPRODUCTION CONTROL

Information gained about the medical device or similar devices in the postproduction phase (see beyond stage 8 in the medical device life cycle shown in Figure 1.1) performance should be reviewed and evaluated for possible relevance to safety for the following: (1) if new or previously unrecognized hazards or causes are present; (2) if the estimated risk arising from hazard is no longer acceptable; and (3) if the original assessment of risk is invalidated. If further action is necessary, a CAPA should be initiated to investigate the problem.

11.7   SUMMARY

The most significant aspects of building risk management into the flow of the design and development process is to embed the trade-off concept of the risk versus benefit analysis as part of the design and development process. The DFSS methodology helps in the data decision–based process and allows for logical trade-offs and quantifiable risk–benefit analysis. DFSS methodology provides traceability where relationships between hazards, requirements, and verification and validation activities are identified and linked.

Risk management itself is a process centered on understanding risks and evaluating their acceptability, reducing risks as much as possible, and then evaluating residual risk and overall device safety against the benefits derived. Integrating risk management into the design and development process requires keeping risk issues at the forefront of the entire process, from design planning to verification and validation testing. In this way, risk management becomes part of the product development process, evolves with the design, and provides a framework for decision making.

The design for six sigma process, the subject of this book, is utilized as a risk management toolkit, where it drives the data-driven approach behind decision making. It is well known that if we make decisions based on factual data, the chances of negative consequences are lessened. Finally, and most important, risk management reduces the potential for systematic errors in the development process and increases the likelihood that manufacturers will get it right the first time.

APPENDIX 11A   ROBUST DESIGN FAILURE MODE AND EFFECTS ANALYSIS

Robust design (see Chapter 15) failure mode and effects analysis (robust design FMEA) is an enhancement to the design FMEA currently in use by anticipating safety and reliability failure modes through the use of a parameter diagram (P-diagram), a robust design brainstorming tool used here to define FMEA inputs, which takes each failure mode into five dimensional failure–cause domains:

1. Total design and manufacturing variation
2. Changes over time
3. Customer misuse and abuse
4. External environment
5. System coupling and interaction

These five domains act as a mechanism of product failure and can be used as the basis for product design verification (Chapter 17) (see Mekki, 2006). Next, we describe the parameter diagram and its use in robust design FMEA.

11A.1 Parameter Diagram

The parameter diagram (Figure 11A.1) is a block diagram used to facilitate the formulation of a robust design study. It is a graphical illustration of the individual parameters that affect product design under analysis to produce desirable outputs, functional requirements, and undesirable outputs, the error states.

The P-diagram will be used as a structured tool to enhance the current design FMEA process. Information collected in developing a P-diagram will be transferred directly to robust design FMEA form. Figure 11A.1 also depicts an example that will be carried on to the robust design FMEA form as well.

There are five elements to a P-diagram:

1. *Input signal.* The input signal is the energy, material, and information that a product requires in delivering a desirable or undesirable output.

2. *Ideal functions.* An ideal function is the mathematical expression of the ideal energy transformation phenomenon in a system in the absence of noise factor effects. In other words, a desired output, the functional requirement, y, is a function of the signal, M. We learned in Chapters 8 and 9 that such requirements are stated in engineering terms that are unambiguous, complete, verifiable, and not in conflict with one another. Functional requirements are the foundation of the robust design FMEA work structure, so special emphasis and reasonable effort should be put into developing them.

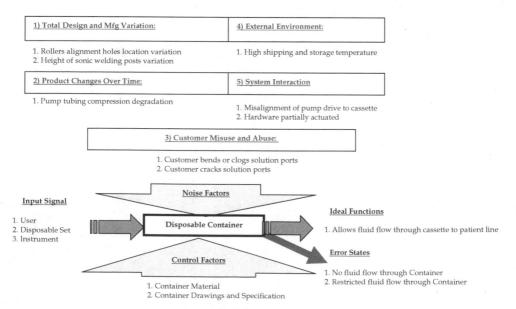

Figure 11A.1   P-diagram, including an example.

3. *Error states.* Error states are also called undesirable outputs or *failure modes.* They are the ways in which the device under analysis may fail to transform 100% of the signal into the functional requirement, the useful output. Failure modes or error states occur in one or all of the following four states:

a. No function
b. Degraded function
c. Intermittent function
d. Unintended function

4. *Noise factors.* Noise factors are also called potential causes and mechanism of failure. Noise factors are the sources of variation that can cause the error states or failure modes to occur. Noise factors are categorized in five categories. Any or all of the five categories described below may cause error states or failure modes to occur:

a. *Noise type 1: Total design and manufacturing variation*
   - *Total design variability* refers to the ability of a design to allow misuse (e.g., design asymmetry, improper installation, etc).
   - *Total manufacturing variability* refers to the special design characteristics (safety and reliability) that are sensitive to variation in the manufacturing or assembly environments (e.g., tube inner-diameter variation).
b. *Noise type 2: Changes over time.* Products may vary over time with regard to dimensions or strength (e.g., wearout, degradation, material properties changes).
c. *Noise type 3: Customer misuse and abuse.* For various reasons, the customer may misuse or abuse a product (e.g., overstressing a product to an extent considered acceptable by customers).
d. *Noise type 4: External environment.* External environmental conditions, such as temperature, humidity, altitude, and electromagnetic interference may affect product function.
e. *Noise type 5: System coupling and interaction.* The interaction of various subsystems and components within a system may lead to failures (e.g., heat generated from a component may affect a neighboring component).

5. *Control factors.* Control factors are design parameters used to optimize product performance in the presence of noise factors (e.g., material type and dimensions).

11A.2   Robust Design FMEA Elements

In a particular example, the following elements constitute the robust design FMEA, depicted in Figure 11A.2:

No	Item/Function	Potential Failure Mode	Potential Effect(s) Of Failure	SEV	Potential Cause(s) Mechanism(s) Of Failure	Current Design Controls — Prevention	Current Design Controls — Verification	OCC	DET	CLASS	Recommended Actions	SEV	OCC	DET	CLASS
1	Disposable Container/ Allows fluid flow through container to patient line	No fluid flow through container	Procedure does not start on time	4	Rollers alignment holes location variation	Design and Mfg review	Disposable container functional test (Protocol # Xxx 19.1)	3	3	R3	Define rollers alignment holes location as a potential reliability design characteristics / Initiate process FMEA and control plan to control rollers alignment holes location / Continue Design and Mfg reviews	4	2	2	R1
			Loss of disposable container		Customer bends or clogs solution ports	Design and Mfg review	None	3	5	R3	Establish a misuse warning in user manual for bending and clogging solution ports / Increase ports thickness to improve design durability / Develop a verification test to verify improved design against bending or clogging solution ports / Continue Design and Mfg reviews	4	2	2	R1
			Customer dissatisfaction		Misalignment of Pump drive to container	Worst case misalignment tolerance stack up study, Design and Mfg review	Disposable container functional test (Protocol # Xxx 19.1)	1	2	R1	None				R1
		Restricted fluid flow through container	Under fill patient	5	Height of Sonic welding posts variation	Worst case container tolerance stack up study, Design of experiment study on container dimensions, Design and Mfg review	Disposable container functional test (Protocol #Xxx 19.1)	2	2	R4	Safety mitigation included in SA-11736-001 at R02 SA029.180 / Continue Design and Mfg reviews	5	1	2	R1
			Patient does not receive full therapy / Possible dehydration		Pump tubing compression degradation	pump tubing material study, Design and Mfg review	Disposable container life test (Protocol # Xxx 87.1)	2	2	R4	Safety mitigation included in SA-11736-001 at R02 SA029.250 / Continue Design and Mfg reviews	5	1	2	R1
					Customer cracks solution ports	Design and Mfg review	None	3	5	R4	Establish a misuse warning in user manual for cracking solution ports. / Increase ports thickness to improve design durability / Develop a verification test to verify improved design against cracking solution ports / Safety mitigation included in SA-11736-001 at R02 SA029.70 / Continue Design and Mfg reviews	5	1	2	R1
					High shipping and storage temperature	Temperature compatibility study, Design and Mfg review	Disposable container temperature test (Protocol # Xxx 184.1)	2	2	R4	Safety mitigation included in SA-11736-001 at R02 SA029.21 / Continue Design and Mfg reviews	5	1	2	R1
					Hardware partially actuated	Hardware Robust design FMEA- FMXxx-05-005 Design and Mfg review	Hardware Functional test (Protocol # Xxx 71.1)	3	2	R4	Safety mitigation included in SA-11736-001 at R02 SA029.230 / Continue Design and Mfg reviews	5	1	2	R1

Figure 11A.2 Robust design FMEA form.

1. *Item/function(s)*

- The item corresponds to the device under analysis. The item under analysis in this example is an assembly of three molded-plastic components. These components undergo multiple welding and assembly steps. The assembly is then used in an instrument along with other assemblies. The assembly name is *disposable container*.
- Function(s) correspond to the ideal functions in the P-diagram (i.e., the functional requirement is "Allows fluid flow through container to patient line"). See Figure 11A.2.

2. *Potential failure mode(s)*. Potential failure modes correspond to the error states in a P-diagram. For the disposable container P-diagram example shown below, only two error states apply to the ideal function: "no function" and "degraded function"(i.e., first failure mode (FM1): "No fluid flow through container"; second failure mode (FM2): "Restricted fluid flow through container"). See Figure 11A.2.

3. *Potential effect(s) of failure.* Potential effects of failure are the effects of each failure mode on the function as perceived by the customer. Failure effects are forecasted based on the team's level of knowledge. It is recommended that all potential effects leading to the ultimate product user(s) be identified and forecast. The DFSS team with cross-functional representation is extremely valuable in defining potential effects of failure. The team should consist of representatives with expertise in design, human factors, manufacturing, testing, service, quality, reliability, clinical, regulatory, supplier, or other fields, as appropriate (i.e., effects for FM1: "Procedure does not start on time/Loss of disposable container/Customer dissatisfaction"; effects for FM2: "Under fill patient/Patient does not receive full therapy possibly causing dehydration"). See Figure 11A.2.

4. *Severity rating.* Severity is the rank associated with the most serious effects of a given failure. We can use severity of hazard/harm ratings from Table 11.1. This table lists severity ratings based on two commonly used scales: 1 to 5 and 1 to 10. For the sake of this example, we will use a 1 to 5 scale (i.e., severity of FM1 most serious effect, 4; severity of FM2 most serious effect, 5). See Figure 11A.2.

5. *Potential cause(s)/mechanism(s) of failure.* Potential causes and mechanisms of failure correspond to the noise factors in the P-diagram. Each failure mode under consideration should go through a step-by-step brainstorming of possible causes with regard to the five noise factor categories (i.e., noise factors for FM1: "Roller alignment hole location variation," "Customer bends or clogs solution ports," and "Misalignment of pump drive to cassette." For FM2: "Height of sonic welding post variation," "Pump tubing compression degradation," "Customer cracks solution ports," "High shipping and storage tempera-

ture," and "Hardware partially actuated"). Each of these noise factors or causes corresponds to an appropriate category of the five noise factor categories. See Figure 11A.2.

6. *Current design controls.* Current design controls, prevention and verification, are the activities that will assure and verify design adequacy against the failure mode and/or cause under consideration. These activities will prevent the cause/mechanism or failure mode/effects from occurring, or reduce the rate of occurrence. Prevention design controls can include proven modeling/ simulation (e.g., finite element analysis), tolerance stack-up study (e.g., geometric dimensional tolerance), material compatibility study (e.g., thermal expansion, corrosion), subjective design and manufacturing reviews, tolerance design studies, design of experiments studies, parameter design studies, software intelligence, and others. Verification design controls can include tests on preproduction samples or prototype samples, analytical tests, design verification plan tests, and others. Current design controls will act as a proof of design robustness, and a lack of control will define the need for more.

7. *Occurrence rating.* Occurrence rating is the probability or likelihood that a specific cause or noise factor will occur, subsequently causing the potential failure mode. [*Note:* The probability of occurrence is a function of the cause of failure mode, not a function of the cause of effect(s) of failure. FMEA practitioners tend to confuse the FMEA and hazard analysis at this point, which results in an underestimation of the rate of occurrence.]

The probability of occurrence can be qualitative or quantitative depending on when in the product life cycle the probability estimation is occurring and what information is available on the product. If the probability cannot be established or predicted using objective (quantitative) data, expert judgment may be used. Historical experience, existing preventions, and mitigation measures need to be factored when assigning values for the probability of occurrence.

Table 11.2 lists the likelihood of occurrence rating criteria based on two commonly used scales: 1 to 5 and 1 to 10. In the example shown in Figure 11A.2 we use a scale of 1 to 5.

8. *Detection rating.* Detection is the ability or likelihood that current design controls (verification controls) will detect a potential cause/mechanism or failure mode and lead to corrective actions. When considering detection, a design team should evaluate the design controls prior to the product being released for production and market. Detection should be evaluated before the fact, not when the product is in a customer's hands. Detection is a function of the verification portion of current design controls. The ultimate goal of the detection rating is to quantify the verification design controls' effectiveness for each design characteristic (potential causes or mechanisms of failure). As a result of any robust design FMEA exercise, project teams will clearly define the current product design's verification effectiveness, as well as opportunities

TABLE 11A.1   Probability of Detection

Detection	Criteria	Rating 1–5	Rating 1–10
Improbable	Current design controls will not and/ or cannot detect a potential cause/ mechanism and subsequent failure mode, or there are no current design controls.	5	9–10
Low	Low chance that the current design controls will detect a potential cause/mechanism and subsequent failure mode.	4	7–8
Moderate	Moderate chance that the current design controls will detect a potential cause/mechanism and subsequent failure mode.	3	5–6
High	High chance that the current design controls will detect a potential cause/mechanism and subsequent failure mode.	2	3–4
Almost certain	Current design controls will almost certainly detect a potential cause/ mechanism and subsequent failure mode.	1	1–2

required for further design verification improvements. Table 11A.1 lists the probability of detection by current design controls based on two commonly used rating scales, 1 to 5 and 1 to 10. For the sake of this example, we use a scale of 1 to 5. In the example shown in Figure 11A.2, we use a scale of 1 to 5.

9. *Classification.* Classification is used to categorize any special design characteristics, including safety and reliability characteristics of the system, key subsystems, and key components that require additional mitigation and/or recommended actions. It may also be used to highlight high-priority failure modes for assessment. Classification criteria are based on a combination of failure mode effects (the severity rating) and the probability of occurrence (the occurrence rating). There are four classification categories (see Table 11.3). The classification category can best be utilized as a project management tool to prioritize projects. Use of the classification category in robust design FMEA replaces prioritization of activities based on risk priority number. This approach helps to focus the project team(s) on product improvement activities.

10. *Recommended actions.* Recommended actions are the continuation of design control activities that will assure proper prevention and verification for

all special design characteristics. The intent of recommended actions is to reduce any or all of the severity, occurrence, and detection ratings. Only a design revision or technology change can bring a reduction in the severity ranking. Occurrence reduction can be achieved by removing or controlling the cause or mechanism of the failure mode, where detection reduction can be achieved by increasing the design verification actions. For the rollers' alignment hole location variation, Figure 11A.2 shows the following recommended actions:

- Define roller alignment hole location as potential key reliability design characteristics.
- Initiate a process FMEA and control plan to control roller alignment hole location variation.
- Continue design and manufacturing reviews.

Such activities will prove design robustness. All activities listed in the recommended actions column must be tracked via an issue-tracking system to assure proper implementation. The following criteria can be applied:

- *R4.* Risk is intolerable and must be reduced.
- *R3 and R2.* Risk should be reduced as much as reasonably practicable; benefits must rationalize any residual risks at a cost that represents value.
- *R1.* Risks is broadly acceptable; there is no need for further risk reduction.

11. *Action results.* Action results are the reassessment of the severity, occurrence, and detection ratings, along with classification based on implementing recommended action activities. Figure 11A.2 shows a complete robust design FMEA form, including an example.

12

MEDICAL DEVICE DESIGN FOR X

12.1 INTRODUCTION

This chapter, for the most part, has a product focus. This is attributed to evolution of the design for X (DFX) family of tools in manufacturing industries such as the medical device industry. We focus on the vital few members of the DFX family most relevant to medical device design. DFSS teams with projects can benefit from this chapter by drawing analogies between their device design project and the topics presented here. Many DFSS teams have found the concepts, tools, and approaches presented here very useful, acting in many ways as eye-openers by stimulating out-of-the-box thinking.

Concurrent engineering is a contemporary approach to DFSS. A DFSS green or black belt should revise the DFSS team membership continually to reflect the concurrent design, which means that both design and process members are important equal team members. DFX techniques are part of detail design and provide ideal approaches to improving the device life-cycle cost[1] and quality, enhancing design flexibility, and increasing efficiency and productivity using concurrent design concepts (Maskell, 1991). Benefits usually cited are competitiveness measures, improved decision making, and enhanced operational efficiency. The letter "X" in DFX is made up of two parts: life-

---

[1]Life-cycle cost is the real cost of the design. It includes not only the original cost of manufacture, but the associated costs of defects, litigations, buybacks, distributions support, warranty, and the implementation cost of all DFX methods employed.

Medical Device Design for Six Sigma: A Road Map for Safety and Effectiveness,
By Basem S. El-Haik and Khalid S. Mekki
Copyright © 2008 John Wiley & Sons, Inc.

cycle processes (x) and performance measure (ability) (i.e., $X = x +$ ability). In product development, for example, one of the first members of the DFX family is design for assembly (DFA). The DFX family is one of the most effective approaches to implement concurrent engineering. DFX focuses on vital business elements of concurrent engineering, maximizing use of the limited resources available to the DFSS team. In DFA, the focus is placed on such factors as size, symmetry, weight, orientation, form features, and other factors related to the device as well as such factors as handling, gripping, insertion, and other factors related to the assembly process. In effect, DFA focuses on the assembly business process as part of production by studying these factors and their relationships to ease device assembly.

The DFX family started with DFA but keeps increasing in number as fostered by the need for better decision-making up front, in particular those related to manufacturing. Manufacturing and production issues are often ignored or omitted in early design steps. This oversight cannot be generalized, due to the early work of Matousek (1957), Neibel and Baldwin (1957), Pech (1973), and several workshops organized by (Collège Internationale de Recherches pour la Production and Workshop Design–Konstruktion. Other efforts started in 1970s by a group of researchers in the UK and the United States resulted in two commercial DFA tools: the Boothroyd–Dewhurst (1983) and Lucas DFA (Miles, 1989). They employed worksheets, a data and knowledge base, and systematic procedures to overcome limitations of design guidelines, differentiating themselves from the old practices. The DFA approach is considered a revolution in design for assembly.

The Boothroyd–Dewhurst DFA moved out of research on automatic feeding and insertion to broader industrial applications, including manual assembly: in particular, locomotive engines. This success led to a new array of DFX, expanding the family to design for manufacturability, design for reliability, design for maintainability, design for serviceability, design for inspectability, design for environmentality, and design for recyclability, among others.

The DFX family of tools collect and present factuals about both the design entity and its production processes, analyze all relationships between them, measure performance as depicted by physical mappings, generate alternatives by combining strengths and avoiding vulnerabilities, provide a redesign recommendation for improvement, provide if–then scenarios, and do all that with many iterations. The objective of this chapter is to introduce the vital few members of the DFX family. It is up to the reader to seek more in-depth material using Table 12.1.

A DFSS team should take advantage of, and strive to design into, the existing capabilities of suppliers, internal plants, and assembly lines. It is cost-effective, at least for the near term. The idea is to create designs sufficiently robust to achieve six sigma product performance from current capability. Concurrent engineering enables this type of upside-down thinking. Such thoughts happen in the DFSS algorithm to improve design for manufacturing,

TABLE 12.1 DFX Citations

X	DFX	Reference
Product/process		
Assembly	Boothroyd–Dewhurst DFA	O'Grady and Oh, 1992
	Lucas DFA	Sacket and Holbrook, 1998
	Hitachi AEM	Huang, 1996
Fabrication	Design for dimension control	Haung, 1996
	Hitachi MEM	
	Design for manufacturing	Arimoto et al., 1993
		Boothroyd et al., 1994
Inspection and test	Design for inspectability	Haung, 1996
	Design for dimensional control	
Material logistics	Design for material logistics	Foo et al., 1990
Storage and distribution	Design for storage and distribution	Huang, 1996
Recycling and disposal flexibility	Design ease of recycling	Beitz, 1990
	Variety reduction program	Suzue and Kohdate, 1988
Environment	Design for environmentality	Navinchandra, 1991
Repair	Design for reliability and maintainability	Gardner and Sheldon, 1995
Service		
Cost	Design whole-life costs	Sheldon et al., 1990
Service	Design for serviceability	Gershenson and Ishii, 1991
Purchasing	Design for profit	Mughal and Osborne, 1995
Salcs and marketing	Design for marketability	Zaccai, 1994
	QFD	
Use and operation	Design for safety	Wang and Ruxton, 1993
	Design for human factors	Tayyari, 1993

improve design for assembly, and improve design for service. There are three the key "design for" activities to be tackled by the team:

1. Use DFX as early as possible in the DFSS algorithm.
2. Start with DFA and design for variety for device projects.
3. Based on the findings in activity 2, determine what DFX to use next. This is a function of DFSS team competence. Time and resources need to be provided to carry out the "design for" activities. The major challenge is implementation.

A danger lurks in the DFX methodologies that can curtail or limit the pursuit of excellence. Time and resource constraints can tempt DFSS teams to accept the unacceptable on the premise that the shortfall can be corrected in one of the subsequent steps: the second-chance syndrome. Just as wrong concepts cannot be recovered by brilliant detail design, bad first-instance detail designs cannot be recovered through failure mode analysis, optimization, or tolerance.

12.2 DESIGN FOR RELIABILITY

Reliability is a broad term that focuses on the ability of a device to perform its intended function. Mathematically speaking, assuming that a device is performing its intended function at time equals zero, reliability can be defined as the probability that the device will continue to perform its intended function without failure for a specified period of time under stated conditions.

There are a number of reasons that device reliability is an important device attribute, including risk to patient, reputation, customer satisfaction, warranty costs, repeat business, cost analysis, and competitive advantage.

Even though a device has a reliable design, when the device is manufactured and used in the field, its reliability may be below expectations. Although the device has a reliable design, it is effectively unreliable when fielded, which is actually the result of a substandard manufacturing process. As an example, cold solder joints could pass initial testing at the manufacturer but fail in the field as the result of thermal cycling or vibration. This type of failure did not occur because of improper design, but rather, is the result of an inferior manufacturing process. Just as a chain is only as strong as its weakest link, a highly reliable device is only as good as the inherent reliability of the device and the quality of the manufacturing process.

Evaluating and finding ways to attain high device reliability are all aspects of reliability engineering. A number of types of reliability analyses are typically performed as part of this DFX discipline. The reliability engineering activity should be an ongoing process starting at the charcterize phase of a DFSS design project and continuing throughout all phases of a device life cycle. The goal always needs to be able to identify potential reliability problems as early as possible in the device life cycle. Although it may never be too late to improve the reliability of a device, changes in a design are orders of magnitude less expensive in the early part of a design phase rather than once the product is manufactured and in service. Reliability engineering tools play a vital role in the development of all devices.

Reliability prediction can be performed in the characterize DFSS phase to get a "ballpark" estimate of the reliability expected for the device. A reliability prediction, which is simply the analysis of parts and components in an effort to predict and calculate the rate at which an item will fail, is one of the most common forms of reliability analyses for calculating failure rate and mean time between failures. If a critical failure is identified, a reliability block diagram analysis can be used to see if redundancy should be considered to mitigate the effect of a single point failure.

The assessment of reliability usually involves testing and analysis of stress strength and environmental factors and should always include improper use by the end user. A reliable design should anticipate all that can wrong. We view design for reliability as a means to maintain and sustain six sigma capability over time. It adapts the law of probability to predict failure and adopts (Yang and El-Haik, 2003):

- Measures to reduce failure rates in the physical entity by employing design axioms and reliability science concurrently.
- Techniques to calculate reliability of key parts and design ways to reduce or eliminate functional coupling and other design weaknesses.
- Derating, using parts below their specified nominal values.
- Design failure mode and effect analysis, which develops alternative ways for failures. A *failure* is an unplanned occurrence that causes a system or component not to meet its functional requirements under the operating conditions specified.
- Robustness practices, by making the design insensitive to all uncontrollable sources of variation (noise factors).
- Redundancy, where necessary, which calls for a parallel system to back up an important part or subsystem in case it fails.

Next, a life-cycle device cost assessment can be performed to judge whether it is more cost-effective to modify an existing design or to create a new one. A life-cycle cost analysis is a method of calculating the cost of a device over its entire life span. The analysis of a typical device could include such costs as all those involved in the DFSS ICOV process, production costs, maintenance costs, and disposal costs. This type of life-cycle assessment often uses values calculated from other reliability analyses, such as failure rate, cost of spares, repair times, and component costs. Software packages such as Relex (www. relax.com) automates a life-cycle cost analysis by making all of the values calculated available through its fully integrated interface.

As the design progresses, if there are particular safety concerns, a fault tree analysis can be used for the systematic identification of the most likely causes of a safety problem. In addition, an FMEA (Chapter 11) can show the effects of a failure of key pieces of the design. The results of either of these analyses may prompt another look at a reliability block diagram analysis to find a way to reduce the probability that a particular failure will occur.

As a design matures, there may be more information showing that certain failure events are dependent on other events, so a Markov[2] analysis would be

---

[2]Markov models are a flexible system modeling tool that enables an analyst to consider scenarios that are not traditionally supported by other classes of analyses. Markov models are used to consider systems where future performance is determined solely by its current state. They are particularly useful where a simulated answer to a complex problem is not acceptable. See www.relex. com/resources/markov.asp.

appropriate to guarantee accurate results. The ease and speed of performing routine maintenance on the device would require the use of preventive maintenance software and maintainability techniques. Also, since the optimum number of spare parts will be required for service, a device optimization and simulation analysis can be performed.

Once prototypes are built and testing begins in the verify/validate DFSS phase, the DFSS team may want to start collecting failure data using Weibull analysis to help identify trends. Once the product is fielded, issues can be tracked using corrective action techniques. Many companies employ a multipurpose closed-loop corrective action process to monitor products, systems, or services continually to improve quality and product reliability. These processes are generally known as a failure reporting, analysis, and corrective action system (FRACAS) or sometimes a data reporting, analysis, and corrective action system (DRACAS). The process typically provides a means of collecting test or field information, analyzing the data, then implementing and tracking corrective actions.

Design for reliability has to deal with a wide spectrum of issues that include human errors, technical malfunctions, environmental factors, inadequate design practices, and material variability. The DFSS team can improve the reliability of the design by:

- Minimizing damage from shipping, service, and repair
- Counteracting environmental and degradation factors
- Using Axiom 2 of Chapter 9 to reduce the design complexity
- Maximizing the use of standard components
- Determining all root causes of defects, not symptoms, using the DFMEA
- Controlling the significant and critical factors using SPC where applicable
- Tracking all yield and defect rates from both in-house and external suppliers, and developing strategies to address them

To minimize the probability of failure, it is first necessary to identify all possible modes of failures and the mechanism by which these failures occur. Detailed examination of design for reliability is developed after physical and process mappings followed by prototyping; however, considerations regarding reliability should be taken into account in the characterize phase when Axiom 1 of Chapter 9 is employed. The team should take advantage of existing knowledge and experience of similar entities and any advanced modeling techniques that are available.

Failure avoidance, in particular when related to safety, is critical. Various hazard analysis approaches are available. In general, these approaches start by highlighting hazardous elements and then proceed to identify all events that may transform these elements into hazardous conditions and their symptoms. The team then has to identify the corrective actions to eliminate or reduce these conditions. One of these approaches is fault tree analysis (FTA), which uses deductive logic gates to combine events that can produce the failure or the fault of interest (Chapter 11). Other tools that can be used in conjunction with FTA include DFMEA and PFMEA as well as the fishbone diagram.

12.3   DESIGN FOR PACKAGING (see Nolan, 2006)

In designing for packaging, the DFSS team should use intelligent strategies instead of simplified, often cost-intensive routine test programs to ensure the highest possible device safety. They should test, characterize, and evaluate, comprehensively and device specifically, its biological safety. This can be achieved by considering all available information on materials, devices, and processes; by utilizing sensitive, convincing tests; and by employing them according to current guidelines and standards, both FDA and international. Precondition for the design for packaging strategy is know-how beyond the simple application of guidelines and normative requirements which enables a well-founded justification of the procedure. A process such as the one depicted in Figure 12.1 is generally used. Notice that design for packaging is a little DFSS project within the device DFSS project itself. For example, step 5 can

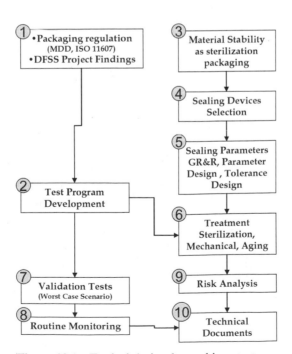

Figure 12.1 Typical design for packing strategy.

be done in the light of Chapters 15 and 16. Packaging risk analysis can be carried out using Chapter 11.

Design for packaging for medical devices plays a key role in delivering specialized treatment to patients safely. Most single-use sterilized medical devices can be opened with a high degree of confidence that it has remained sterile throughout storage, handling, and transportation. What makes packaging doubly important is that regulatory authorities recognize the critical nature of sterile barrier or primary package by considering them components or accessories to the medical device. This implies that packaging is almost as important as the device itself—and it is. If, for example, a package does not keep a pacemaker or catheter sterile, patients will be put at risk.

The design and development of packaging has rightfully come under closer scrutiny by international and domestic regulatory agencies. This scrutiny has placed a great deal of emphasis on standardizing package development. Some standardization comes in the form of the international standard ISO 11607, packaging for terminally sterilized medical devices.

According to Nolan (2006), the most common defect in medical packaging is loss of sterile integrity from fractured thermoforms, along with pinholes, slits, cuts, and tears in pouch packages. These defects come from handling (or mishandling) vibrations during transportation, storage, and impacts caused by dropping.

Tears are usually caused by manufacturing or assembly or while inserting pouches into cartons. Even "Information for Use" booklets can be hazardous because their sharp edges or staples can snag the packaging.

Sterile-barrier systems, formerly called primary packages, and *protective packages*, formerly referred to as shipping containers, may provide the solution to package defects from handling and shipping. The two-part system reduces the risks of puncturing, tearing, and fracturing the primary package.

Most people in manufacturing are unaware of the need to test their packaging, or even that the ISO 11607 standard exists and is used by the FDA and the European Union, so they try to validate the packaging cheaply without using sound scientific practices. In their haste to get a product to market, companies risk noncompliance with regulations, or worse yet, unknowingly let suspect devices reach patients.

The time to validate a full package system properly depends on a product's shelf life and its expiration date. For example, it usually takes three to six months to go from package concept to final qualification for a one-year shelf life. The validation schedule should also allow for unexpected events, such as finding pinholes in packaging after a test. Of course, this halts the validation.

Package validation should be on a parallel path with device development, so the product and package finish together. This is possible using prototype devices for package compatibility and testing in the DFSS verify/validate phase. When devices have a longer shelf life, package development should be extended by about 45 days for each year of shelf life.

The package and device are not prequalified for compatibility. A common package-development mistake skips the preliminary evaluation and just dives into package validation. Cutting corners to trim time is short-sighted and usually backfires by extending development schedules and increasing overall validation costs because some part of the package fails. That necessitates retests.

A few common prequalification tests that should be used to detect potential design and manufacturing problems are seal strength and integrity tests on manufactured packages. A seal test, for instance, measures the force needed to open a seal. Such tests point out potential deficiencies in manufacturing and may indicate that the production line needs corrective action. This should be done far in advance of testing package performance, such as for transportation, sterilization, or handling. Prequalification tests should also be the basis for establishing targets for process quality control.

Another test used to prequalify package-device compatibility is dynamic testing associated with transportation and handling. A shaker table reproduces the frequencies and amplitudes that a shipping container is likely to experience, and for a prescribed duration.

Most sterile medical device packages do not typically lose sterility simply sitting on a shelf. Failures often stem from events in manufacturing, during shipping to the sterilization facility, or during distribution. Therefore, proposed packages should always undergo prequalification to isolate potential hazards and determine the package response to each of those hazards.

It is often difficult to determine which shipping configuration to validate. Should the team test just one product in one package? Or six devices in a box? To determine the worst-case scenario, it is necessary to determine the most common shipping configuration before validating a package. In this way, other package configurations of the same or similar products may be covered by one validation.

In the ISO 11607 guidelines, for example, a provision allows validating families of packaged products rather than individual configurations. Before working on a validation, write a protocol. It provides a blueprint for how testing will be done, including its purpose, scope, responsibilities, parameters, production equipment and settings, and acceptance test criteria.

ISO 11607-01 is the foremost guidance document for validating packaging for terminally sterilized medical devices. Packaging must comply with ISO 11607-01 to ensure that the medical device enclosed is kept sterile throughout all the elements and hazards generated by the manufacturing, shipping, and storage environments. The standard has recently been revised to incorporate the provisions of the EN 868-1 standard. As a result, the new ISO 11607-01 consists of two parts: part 1, materials and designs, and part 2, processes.

Medical device manufacturers and package testing professionals should take note of the revisions to the ISO 11607 standard, as the revisions could mean the difference between pass or fail when it comes to package testing and validation, such as random vibration testing, seal peel testing, compression testing, repetitive shock testing, leak testing by dye penetration, bubble leak testing, and drop testing.

Validation qualifies the materials and processes that make a complete package. If one process is not right, the entire system breaks down and the manufacturer risks harm to patients. How many packages must be tested? Finding the right sample size is a daunting task because many factors determine it. For example, what type of test will be done? Quantitative tests provide values, whereas qualitative tests report pass/fail or go/no-go results. Other questions to answer include: What is the sample population? How many samples are available for testing? What are the costs? What are the risks (e.g., confidence intervals, Chapter 3)? Sample sizes are usually too small and produce results that have no statistical significance. Equation (12.1) shows that in using a sample average $\bar{y}$ for an output to estimate the population mean, μ, the error $E|\bar{y} - \mu|$ is less than $Z_{\alpha/2}\sigma/\sqrt{n}$ with confidence $100(1 - \alpha)$.

$$n = \left(\frac{Z_{\alpha/2}\sigma}{E}\right)^2 \tag{12.1}$$

Suppose that a DFSS team wanted the error in estimating the mean seal peal strength of a plastic container to be less than 0.05 lbf, with 95% confidence (i.e., $\alpha = 5\%$ and $\sigma = 0.1$ lbf). With $Z_{\alpha/2} = 1.96$ from the standard normal table, the sample size is given as

$$n = \left[\frac{1.96(0.1)}{0.05}\right]^2 = 15.37$$

which can be rounded up to 16 containers.

A packaging prequalification would have guided package designers to an appropriate material or package. The problem shows up as fractured thermoform trays because the product weight is too great for the impact resistance of the material.

Large or massive devices should use high-impact-resistant plastics such as polycarbonate to reduce the possibility of fracturing during distribution and handling. The design of the thermoform tray is also critical to ensure that it will hold the product firmly so that nothing jettisons through the tray lid.

Pinholes in pouches can be reduced by inserting the pouch into a carton without folding, wrinkling, or creasing the ends. Pinholes may form at creases and folds after sufficient vibration. This effect is exacerbated by folding the package in a complex manner that concentrates stress. The problem is solved simply by using secondary packages (cartons or shelf boxes) large enough to hold the unfolded pouch.

Accelerated aging are often performed at overly elevated temperatures. Manufacturers occasionally accelerate shelf life and expiration-date studies to unrealistic and indefensible limits. This ill-conceived attempt to reduce time and costs is done by raising test temperatures to levels that melt, warp, or produce changes that are uncharacteristic behaviors. Temperatures over 55 °C, for example, are indefensible based on the rationale typically used to justify accelerated-aging protocols.

Accelerated aging is usually performed on packaged medical devices to document expiration dates. Companies can perform real-time aging on products, but the results are often obsolete by the time the test validates a three-year expiration date. The FDA does not require expiration dating for product's that don't have components with defined effective lives, such as batteries. European Directives require that all sterile medical devices must have expiration dates. Therefore, documented evidence must substantiate such claims. Temperature selections for accelerated aging studies should avoid unrealistic failure conditions such as deformation due to melting. This obvious advice is sometimes ignored in the rush to bring products to market.

12.4 DESIGN FOR MANUFACTURE AND DESIGN FOR ASSEMBLY

Design for manufacture (DFM) and design for assembly (DFA) are systematic approaches within the DFX family that the DFSS team can use to analyze carefully each design parameter (DP) that can be defined as a part or subassembly for manual or automated manufacture and assembly and gradually reduce waste. Waste (*muda* in Japanese) may mean any of several things. It may indicate products or features that have no function (do not add value) and those that should have been trimmed using the zigzagging method (Chapter 9) during physical mapping. It may also indicate a proliferation of parts that can be eliminated using the zigzagging method in process mapping. But the most leverage experienced by DFX in the DFSS algorithm, beyond the design axioms, is achieved by attacking the following *muda* sources: (1) assembly directions that need several additional operations, and (2) DPs with unnecessarily tight tolerances.

12.4.1 DFMA Approach

In the DFMA approach (Figure 12.2), significant improvement tends to arise from focusing on simplicity (i.e., reducing the number of stand-alone parts). The Boothroyd–Dewhurst DFA methodology gives the following three criteria against which each part must be examined as it is added to the assembly (Huang, 1996):

1. During operation of the device, does the part move relative to all other parts already assembled?
2. Must the part be a different material, or be isolated from, all other parts already assembled? Only fundamental reasons concerned with material properties are acceptable.

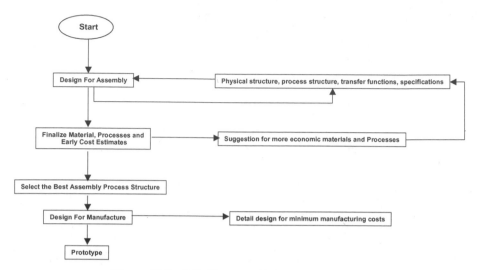

Figure 12.2   DFMA steps. (After Huang, 1996.)

3. Must the part be separate from all other parts already assembled because the necessary assembly or disassembly of other parts would be impossible otherwise?

A "yes" answer to any of these questions indicates that the part must be separate or, using DFA terminology, must be a *critical* part. All parts that are not critical can theoretically be removed or *coupled physically* with other critical parts. Therefore, theoretically, the number of critical parts is the minimum number of separate parts of the design.

Next, the DFSS team estimates the assembly time for the design and establishes its efficiency rating in terms of assembly difficulty. This task can be done when each part is checked for how it will be grasped, oriented, and inserted into the device. Out of this exercise, the device design is rated, and from this rating standard, time is determined for all operations necessary to assemble the part. The DFA time standard is a classification of design features that affect assembly process. The total assembly time can then be assessed, and using medical device industry standard labor rates, the assembly cost and efficiency can be estimated. At this stage, manufacturing costs are not considered, but assembly time and efficiency provide benchmarks for new iterations. After all feasible simplification tasks are introduced, the next step is to analyze the manufacture of individual parts. The objective of DFM within the DFMA is to enable the DFSS team to weigh alternatives, assess manufacturing cost, and make decisions between physical integration (DP synthesis) and increased manufacturing cost. The DFM approach provides experimental data for estimating the cost of many processes. The DFSS team is encouraged to consult with the following studies where deemed appropriate: Dewhurst (1988) for injection molding; Dewhurst and Blum (1989) for die-cast parts; Zenger and Dewhurst (1988) for sheet-metal stamping; and Knight (1991) for powder metal parts.

The DFSS team will create a baseline of the concept or concepts under consideration in the characterize phase and conduct a part-by-part assessment. Once the baseline is completed, the DFMA team will use the output of the DFMA to begin brainstorming new concepts to simplify the device design. The DFSS team will also be using DFMA software tools to evaluate the impact that different design alternatives have on both component and total device cost.

DFMA is an iterative process that allows a DFSS team to review several different concepts based on design mappings (Chapter 9) before selecting the optimal concept and proceeding with the detailed design work. The black belt must ensure that time is allocated in the schedule to accommodate this iterative evaluation process.

The DFSS ICOV calls a characterize phase tollgate review. The initial DFMA analysis and report of the concept(s) must be completed prior to the tollgate review. The DFMA team will then continue to evaluate design changes as the final device concept moves into the optimize phase. The team will also issue an updated report prior to the characterize tollgate review.

A DFMA specialist will be a valuable addition in the characterize phase. The specialist will help the team compare the metrics generated during DFMA analysis to the targets and provide feedback to the team. The specialist will also begin to track the concept's device cost using a commercially available software tool such as the tool depicted in Figure 12.3. Such concurrent costing software can estimate the cost of individual components with 23 different shape-forming processes.

Before starting DFMA analysis on the device design concept under consideration in the characterize phase, the DFSS team should consider a list of items as potential inputs to the analysis, such as manufacturing quality data on an existing baseline device, current manufacturability issues, field reliability issues (field failures), serviceability issues, customer requirements in the QFD, product requirements definition, competitive benchmark analysis, supplier management strategy, lifetime and yearly volume estimates, device cost targets, and previous prototypes results, if applicable. All team members must go through a DFMA overview training session prior to participating in a DFMA analysis. Several analyses are conducted, depending on the ICOV phase of interest.

12.4.2 DFMA in the ICOV DFSS Process

In the DFSS ICOV phases, DFMA can be used as follows:

1. *Identify phase.* The objective is to establish DFMA targets for the device. In this phase, the DFMA activities can include:

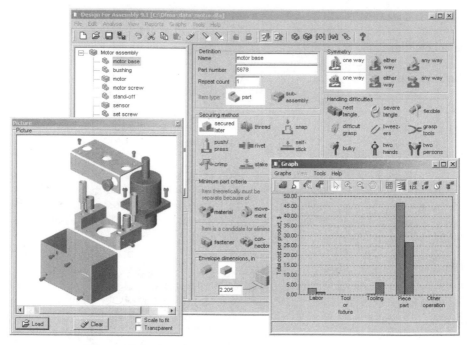

Figure 12.3   Boothroyd–Dewhurst Inc. (BDI) software.

- DFMA of competitors devices (best-in-class)
- DFMA of internal baseline legacy devices
- Using DFMA software to track metrics tracked throughout the DFSS project life cycle: part count, assembly time, number of operations, and DFA index
- Establishing a level of improvement for each metric. Aim high. For example, the average levels of improvement from published DFMA case studies are as follows: part count, over 50%; assembly time, over 50%; and DFA index, double.

2. *Characterize phase.* In this phase the objective for the DFSS team is to conduct a DFMA on the concept or concepts selected. This process provides the biggest benefit at this DFSS phase.

- Create a baseline for the device concept(s) under consideration by using the DFMA software tool of the teams choice and conducting a part-by-part assessment.
- Use the DFMA concurrent costing software tool to evaluate the impact of different design alternatives on both component and product cost.
- This is an iterative process that allows the team to review several concepts before selecting the concept that is optimal from the DFMA perspective.

- DFMA deliverables at the completion of this phase include:
  - A report that includes a list of design recommendations to achieve the DFMA targets.
  - A summary of the DFMA metrics compared to the DFMA targets.
  - If the targets are not met, the results must be reviewed with the team to determine if further analysis is required.

3. *Optimize phase.* In this phase the objective is to conduct DFMA analyses on design changes to evaluate the impact on the DFMA targets. The DFSS team will also continue to look for opportunities to simplify the device design and reduce cost as prototypes and manufacturing equivalent units (MEUs) are being evaluated.

- The DFSS team compares the latest DFA model with the bill of materials (BOM) and assembly process of the MEUs.
- The DFMA specialist in the DFSS team will model any design improvements to determine the impact on the DFMA metrics and cost.
- A DFMA must be conducted on any design modifications identified throughout the optimize phase.
- DFMA deliverables at the completion of this phase include:
  - A report that includes a list of design recommendations to achieve the DFMA targets.
  - A summary of the DFMA metrics that are compared to the targets.
  - If the targets are not met, the results must be reviewed with the DFSS team to determine if further analysis is required.
  - An estimate of the device cost (materials, labor, and tooling).

4. *Verify/validate phase.* In this phase the objective is to complete a final DFMA in preparation for device launch. This is to ensure that the DFA model accurately represents the final design and its configuration, as well as identifying and documenting potential improvement and cost reduction opportunities.

- The team with the DFMA specialist compares the latest DFA model with the final product BOM and assembly process.
- The DFSS team conducts one final postlaunch DFMA review to identify potential improvement or cost-reduction opportunities.
- The final DFA model and associated DFM concurrent costing models will be stored in a database.
- DFMA deliverables at the completion of this phase include:
  - A summary of the DFMA metrics that are compared to the DFMA targets.
  - If DFMA targets are not met, the results must be reviewed with the DFSS team and management.

- The summary will include device cost information as well as a list of potential improvement and cost-reduction opportunities.
- The opportunities identified can feed into future studies.

12.4.3 DFMA Best Practices

As a golden rule, the DFSS team should minimize the number of setups and stages through which a high-level DP (e.g., a part or subassembly) must pass before it becomes a physical entity. This objective is now feasible and affordable due to the significant development in computer numerically controlled (CNC) machines with single-setup machining and multiaxis capabilities. The employment of CNC machines reduces lead times and tooling and setup costs, while responding to customer demands with added flexibility. Single-setup machines are usually equipped with touch-trigger probe measuring part positioning and orientation. By reducing expensive fixtures and setup times, CNC machines gradually become very attractive, with typical savings of over 60% reduction in work in progress. However, the most significant advantages are the high-quality parts produced, improving both the rolled throughput yield (obtained by minimizing the effect of the hidden factories) and the overall DPMO by reducing scrap and rework.

Before embarking on use of the DFA and DFM tools, the team should:

1. Revisit the device physical mapping, the process mapping of the DFSS algorithm, and the marketing strategy. The team should be aware that the DFSS algorithm as a device design strategy is global, whereas the process strategy is usually local, depending on existing manufacturing facilities.

2. Review all processes involved in market analysis, customer attributes, and other requirements (e.g., packaging, maintenance). Where clarification is sought, the team may develop necessary prototypes, models, experiments, and simulation to minimize risks. In doing so, the team should take advantage of available specifications, testing, cost–benefit analysis, and modeling to build the design.

3. Analyze existing manufacturing and assembly functions, operations, and sequence concurrently using simulation tools to examine assembly and subassembly definitions of the device and find the best organization and production methods.

4. Apply the most appropriate rather than the latest technology in the processes identified during process mapping.

5. Follow the axiomatic design (Chapter 9) approach to create "modular" design (i.e., standard physical entities in the form of components, parts, and subassemblies). Modular device entities have many attractive advantages: cost reduction, physical and process mapping configuration ease, facilitation of engineering changes' implementation, more product derivatives, and higher quality and reliability.

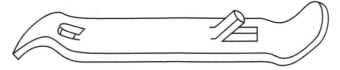

Figure 12.4 Bottle–can opener.

6. Design for the minimum number of parts by using the idea of physical integration, *not* functional coupling (i.e., multi-FR parts with multi-DPs uncoupled in time or space). For example, consider the bottle–can opener shown in Figure 12.4. The FRs are:

- FR1: open beverage bottle
- FR2: open beverage can

The DPs are:

- DP1: beverage opener side
- DP2: can opener side

The design mapping is depicted by

$$\begin{Bmatrix} FR1 \\ FR2 \end{Bmatrix} = \begin{bmatrix} X & 0 \\ 0 & X \end{bmatrix} \begin{Bmatrix} DP1 \\ DP2 \end{Bmatrix}$$

where "X" depicts a relationship between an FR and a DP, and "0" indicates the absense of such a relationship. By definition, the two FRs are independent or uncoupled per Axiom 1 of Chapter 9. A simple device that satisfies the FRs above can be made by stamping sheet metal as shown in Figure 12.4. Note that a single device can be made without a functional coupling and hosted in the same part physically. *Functional coupling should not be confused with physical integration.* In addition, since the complexity of the product is reduced, it is also in line with Axiom 2 of Chapter 9.

7. Choose the appropriate materials for fabrication ease.

8. Apply the layered assembly principles and such factors as parts handling and feeding, orientation, identification, positioning, allowable tolerances, and mating.

9. Use the appropriate DFM and DMA tools. Since DFM and DFA are interlinked, they can be used sequentially according to the road map in Figure 12.2 suggested by Huang (1996), who called the road map the *DFMA approach.*

The DFMA approach usually benefits from poka-yoke techniques, which may be used when components are taking form and manufacturing and assembly issues are considered simultaneously. *Poka-yoke* (mistake-proofing) is a technique for avoiding human error at work, developed by Japanese manufacturing engineer Shigeo Shingo to achieve zero defects. A defect exists in either of two states: It has occurred, calling for defect detection; or it is about to occur, calling for defect prediction. Poka-yoke has three basic functions to use against defects: shutdown, control, and warning. The technique starts by analyzing the process for potential problems; identifying parts by the characteristics of dimension, shape, and weight; and detecting process deviation from nominal procedures and norms.

Example 12.1 (Yang and El-Haik, 2003)   A motor-drive assembly must be designed to sense and control its position on two steel guide rails. The motor is fixed on a rigid base to enable up–down movement over the rails and so support the motor system (Figure 12.5). The motor and a measurement cylindrical sensor are wired to a power supply unit and control unit, respectively. The motor system is fully enclosed and has a removable cover for access to adjust the position sensor when needed. The current design is shown in Figures 12.5 and 12.6.

The motor system is secured to the base by two screws. The sensor is held by a setscrew. To provide suitable friction and to guard against wear, the base is provided with two bushings. The end cover is plate-secured by two end-plate screws, fastened to two standoffs, and screwed into the base. The end plate is fitted with a plastic bushing for connecting wire passage. A box-shaped cover slides over the entire assembly from below the bases. The cover is held in place by four cover screws, two into the base and two into the end cover. Is this a good assembly design?

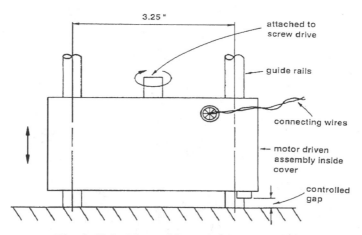

Figure 12.5   Motor-drive assembly front view.

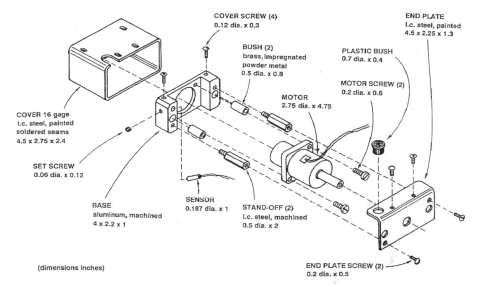

Figure 12.6   Datum design exploded view.

Solution: We need to take the following DFMA steps.

1. Study the current (datum) design and identify all parts and subassemblies. The initial design proposed is formed from 19 elements:

- Two purchased design subassemblies: the motor drive and the sensor
- Eight other parts (e.g., end plate, cover)
- Nine screws

2. Apply the criteria given in Section 12.4.1 to every part to simplify the design and decide on the theoretical possible minimum number of parts.

We need to simplify by achieving the minimum number of parts as follows:

- The motor and the sensor comprise standard purchased subassembly. Thus, no further analysis is required.
- The base is assembled into a fixture, and since there is no other part to assemble to, it is a "critical" part.
- The two bushings don't satisfy the criteria in Section 12.4.1. Theoretically, they can be assembled to the base or can be manufactured of the same material as the end plate and combined with it.
- The setscrew, the four cover screws, and the end-plate screws are theoretically unnecessary. An integral fastening arrangement is possible most of the time.
- The two standoffs can be assembled to the base (do not meet the criteria).
- The end plate is a critical part for accessibility.

If the motor and sensor subassemblies can be snapped or screwed to the base with a snapped-on plastic cover, only four separate items will be needed, resulting in a 79% reduction in parts because only four parts remain as the theoretically possible minimum: motor, sensor, base, and end plate.

3. Revisit all trimmed parts and check any practical, technical, or economic limitations on their removal. For example:

- Some may argue that the two motor screws are needed to secure the motor for higher fastening force.
- Some may argue that the motor screws are needed to hold the sensor because any other alternatives will be uneconomical, due to the low volume.
- Others may argue that the two powder metal bushings may be unnecessary.
  In all cases, it is very difficult to justify the separate standoffs, cover, and the six screws.

4. Estimate the assembly time and costs to account for savings in weighing assembly design alternatives. The DFMA database provides such estimates without detailed drawings. Table 12.2 exhibits the result of the DFMA analysis:

- Total actual assembly time, $T_{assem.actual} = 163$ seconds.
- Total theoretical assembly time, $T_{assem.,theoretical} = 12$ seconds (the theoretical number of parts is four, with an average of 3 seconds assembly time).
- Calculate the datum assembly design, $\eta_{assem.datum}$, efficiency using

TABLE 12.2 DFMA Worksheet for Datum Design

Item	Number	Theoretical Part Count	Assembly Time (s)	Assembly Cost (U.S. cents)
Base	1	1	3.5	2.9
Bushing	2	0	12.3	10.2
Motor subassembly	1	1	9.5	7.9
Motor screw	2	0	21.0	17.5
Sensor subassembly	1	1	8.5	7.1
Setscrew	1	0	10.6	8.8
Standoff	2	0	16.0	13.3
End plate	1	1	8.4	7.0
End-plate screw	2	0	16.6	13.8
Plastic bushing	1	0	3.5	2.9
Thread lead	—	—	5.0	4.2
Reorient	—	—	4.5	3.8
Cover	1	0	9.4	7.9
Cover screw	4	0	34.2	26.0
Total	19	4	160.0	133.0

$$\eta_{\text{assem.,datum}} = \frac{T_{\text{assem.,theoretical}}}{T_{\text{assem.,actual}}} \times 100\%$$

$$= \frac{12}{163} \times 100\%$$

$$= 7.362\% \tag{12.2}$$

SO this is not an assembly-efficient design.

5. Redo step 4 for the optimum design (with the minimum number of parts) after all practical, technical, and economic limitation considerations. Assume that the bushings are integral to the base and that the snap-on plastic cover replaces standoffs, cover, plastic bushing, and six screws, as shown in Figure 12.7. These parts contribute 97.4 seconds in assembly time reduction, which amounts to $0.95 per hour assuming an hourly labor rate of $35 per hour. Other added improvements include using pilot point screws to fix the base, which was redesigned for self-alignment. A worksheet for the optimum design is given in Table 12.3.

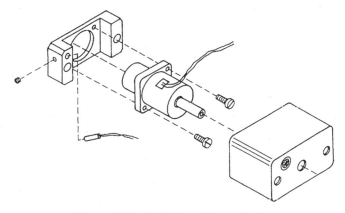

Figure 12.7 DFMA optimum design.

TABLE 12.3 DFMA Worksheet for Optimum Design

Item	Number	Theoretical Part Count	Assembly Time (s)	Assembly Cost (U.S. cents)
Base	1	1	3.5	2.9
Motor subassembly	1	1	4.5	3.8
Motor screw	2	0	12.0	10.0
Sensor subassembly	1	1	8.5	7.1
Setscrew	1	0	8.5	7.1
Thread leads	—	—	5.0	4.2
Plastic cover	1	1	4.0	3.3
Total	7	4	46.0	38.4

- Total actual assembly time, $T_{assem.,actual} = 46$ seconds from the DFMA database.
- Total theoretical assembly time, $T_{assem.,theoretical} = 12$ seconds (the theoretical number of parts is four, with an average of 3 seconds of assembly time).
- Calculate the datum assembly design, $\eta_{assem.,optimum}$, efficiency using

$$\eta_{assem.,optimum} = \frac{T_{assem.,theoretical}}{T_{assem.,actual}} \times 100\%$$

$$= \frac{12}{46} \times 100\%$$

$$= 26.087\% \qquad (12.3)$$

6. Calculate the parts cost savings as shown in Table 12.4. The saving = $35.44 − $21.73 = $13.71 in parts cost, with a new fixed cover cost of $5000.

7. Calculate the total savings from both time (step 4) and parts reduction (step 6):

total savings = savings from assembly time reduction + savings from parts reduction
$$= \$0.95 + \$13.71$$
$$= \$14.66$$

$$(12.4)$$

The break-even volume equals 342 total assemblies.

TABLE 12.4 Cost Differential Worksheet

Proposed Design		Redesign	
Item	Cost[a]	Item	Cost[b]
Base (aluminum)	$12.91	Base (nylon)	$13.43
Bushing (2)	2.40*	Motor screw (2)	0.20*
Motor screw (2)	0.20	Setscrew	0.10*
Setscrew	0.10*	Plastic cover, including tooling	8.00
Standoff (2)	5.19		
End plate	5.89		
End-plate screw (2)	0.20*		
Plastic bush	0.1*		
Cover	8.05		
Cover screw (4)	0.40*		
Total	35.44		21.73

[a]Purchased in quantity; motor and sensor subassemblies purchased not included.
[b]Tooling costs for plastic cover, $5,000.
*Purchased in quantities.

12.5   DESIGN FOR MAINTAINABILITY

The objective of design for maintainability is to assure that a design will perform satisfactorily throughout its intended life with a minimum expenditure of budget and effort. Design for maintainability, design for serviceability, and design for reliability are related because minimizing maintenance and easing service can be achieved by improving reliability. An effective design for maintainability minimizes (1) the downtime for maintenance, (2) user and technician maintenance time, (3) personnel injury resulting from maintenance tasks, (4) cost resulting from maintainability features, and (5) logistics requirements for replacement parts, backup units, and personnel. Maintenance actions can be preventive, corrective, or recycle and overhaul.

Design for maintainability encompasses access and control, displays, fasteners, handles, labels, positioning and mounting, and testing. The DFSS team needs to follow these guidelines:

- Minimize the number of serviceable design parameter modules (DPs) using simple procedures and skills.
- Provide easy access to the serviceable DPs by placing them in serviceable locations. This will also enhance the visual inspection process for failure identification.
- Use common fasteners and attachment methods.
- Design for minimum hand tools.
- Provide safety devices (e.g., guards, covers, switches).
- Design for minimum adjustment and make adjustable DPs accessible.

The DFSS team should devise the criteria for a "repair or discard" decision within the context of life-cycle costing. The major maintainability cost factors to consider include device transportation, shopping and handling, training of maintenance people, repair logistics which encompass the design of service, and production, distribution, and installation of repairable DPs (components and subassemblies).

The *repair procedure* should target:

- Enhancing the field repair capability to react to emergency situations
- Improving current repair facilities to reflect the design changes
- Reducing cost using modularity and standard components
- Decreasing storage space

The *discard procedure* should consider:

- Manufacturing costs
- Simplifying maintenance tasks (e.g., minimum skills, minimum tools, standard attachment methods)

- Work site reliability; train technicians to avoid harming repair equipment
- Repair change adjustment to enable plug-in of new parts rather than field rework

12.6 DESIGN FOR SERVICEABILITY

After the DFSS team finishes DFR and DFMA exercises, the next step is to embark on design for serviceability (DFS), another member of the DFX family. DFS is the ability to diagnose, remove, replace, replenish, or repair any DP (component or subassembly) to original specifications with relative ease. Poor serviceability produces warranty costs, customer dissatisfaction, risk to the end user (patient), and lost sales and market share due to loss loyalty. The DFSS team should check their voice-of-the-customer studies, such as QFD, for serviceability attributes. Ease of serviceability is a performance quality in Kano analysis. The DFSS algorithm strives to have serviceability personnel involved in the early stages, as they are considered a customer segment. Many customers will benefit from DFS both internally and externally as applied in the DFSS algorithm.

The following elements of DFS should be considered by the DFSS team:

1. Customer service attributes
2. Labor time
3. Parts cost
4. Safety
5. Diagnosis
6. Service simplification
7. Repair frequency and occurrence
8. Special tools
9. Failures caused by service procedures

12.6.1 DFS Guidelines

The DFS guidelines are as follows:

1. Reduce service functional requirements (FRs) by minimizing the need for service by tracking devices warranties and developing associated databases. The DFSS team has the opportunity to make their DFS procedure data driven by analyzing the possible failure rates of datum baseline devices (incremental design scenarios) and ranking them using Pareto analysis to address service requirements in prioritized sequence. Use the DFX family to improve reliability. For example, DFMA improves reliability by reducing

the number of parts; Axiom 2 of Chapter 9 helps reduce design stiffness to reduce variation in the FRs, which is a major cause of failures. In addition, axiomatic design helps generate ideas for physical integration for DP consolidation, resulting in fewer separate parts, thus enhancing reliability levels.

2. Identify customer service attributes and appropriate type of service. The type of service required by any customer segment is the determinant of the DFS technique to be used. There are three types: standard operations, scheduled maintenance, and repairs. Standard operations consist of items of normal wear and tear. For standard operations, service ease should be maximized and coupled with mistake-proofing (poka-yoke) techniques. In many industries, the end customer is usually the operator. Scheduled maintenance, if any, is usually recommended in the customer manual. In this category, customers expect less frequency and easier care. Under the pressure of minimum life-cycle cost, many companies are altering scheduled maintenance tasks to standard operations and "do it yourself" procedures. A sound scheduled maintenance procedure should call for better reliability and durability, minimum tools (e.g., a single standard fastener size) and easy removal paths. In repair service, ease of repair is primary. This objective is usually challenged by limited accessibility space and design complexity. Repair service can be greatly enhanced by employing a diagnostics system, repair kits, and modular design practices. Repair issues can take a spectrum of possible causes, ranging from type I and type II errors in diagnostics systems, tools and parts logistics issues, and repair technicality.

3. Practice the DFS approach. If the serviceability requirements have not yet be met, the DFSS team is encouraged to use design mappings by employing the zigzagging method between serviceability FRs and DPs (Chapter 9). Once the team has identified all serviceability mapping, they can move on to consider design alternatives. These alternatives may sometimes not be applicable. In other cases, they may seem to conflict with one another. Nevertheless, the DFSS team should assess whether a six-sigma capable and rounded design is to be established for all requirements, including those related to serviceability. A serviceability set of FRs usually includes proper location, standardization of tools and parts, protection from accelerated failure, ergonomics consideration, and diagnostics functions.

The DFSS team should proceed according to the following steps to devise a sound DFS approach:

1. Review assumptions, serviceability customer CTQs and FRs from the QFD, serviceability types, customer segments, and six sigma targets.

2. Check datum devices and use the data available as a way to predict design performance from a datum's historical database. The team should also benchmark best-in-class competition to exceed customer satisfaction.

3. Identify types of services needed (e.g., standard operation, scheduled maintenance or repair) and map them to appropriate customer segments.

4. Understand all service procedures in the company instructional materials, including steps, sequence, potential problems, and so on.

5. Estimate labor time. Labor time is considered the foundation of serviceability quantification for warranty assessment purposes. Labor time is the sum of repair recognition time, diagnostic time, logistic time, and actual repair time. The team should aim to beat the best-in-class labor time.

6. Minimize all service-problematic areas by reviewing the customer-concern tracking system, determining and eliminating root causes, addressing the problem based on a prioritization scheme (e.g., Pareto analysis of the impact of repair cost), searching for solutions in literature and instructional materials, and predicting future trends.

7. Determine a solution approach. The information extracted from the data gathered will lead to some formulation of a serviceability design strategy. Every separate component or critical part should be addressed for its unique serviceability requirements.

8. Introduce serviceability design parameters (DPs or solution) into the design mappings. These can be categorized based on the answers to the following questions:

a. Orientation
   - Do the parts have easy removal paths?
   - Do the service steps require reorientation?
b. Contamination
   - Can the fluid, if any, be contained prior to or through service?
   - What is the possibility of contaminating parts during service?
c. Access
   - *Assemblability:* Is it possible to group components for ease of service? Check the structure.
     - Is disassembly intuitive?
     - Can asymmetrical components fit one way?
   - *Reachability:* Can the part be reached by hand? by tool? Can the part be removed from the assembly?
   - *Layerability:* Is the part in the assembly layer correlated to frequency of service?
   - *Real estate:* Is it possible to move or size parts for service space?
   - *Efficiency:* Is it necessary to remove parts that obstruct visibility or service?
   - *Diagnostic:* Can the part be accessed for diagnostics without disassembly?

- *Service reliability:* Address potential damage of serviced or removed parts. Have all possibilities for parts minimization using DFMA been exhausted?
  - Consider use of standard parts (e.g., fasteners).

d. Simplicity
  - Customer considerations
    - *Tools:* Design for generic tools.
    - Minimize use of special tools.
    - *Adjustment:* Reduce customer intervention through tuning and adjustment. Use robustness techniques.
    - *Poka-yoke:* Use color codes and very clear instructions.

12.6.2 Application: Pressure Recorder PCB Replacement (see Boothroyd and Dewhurst, 1990; Huang, 1996)

In this approach we study the service disassembly and reassembly processes by identifying all individual steps, including part removal, tool acquisition, pickup and orientation, and insertion. The time standard in this procedure is the result of work by Abbatiello (1995) at the University of Rhode Island. An exploded view is shown in Figure 12.8. The worksheets shown below in the tables were developed to utilize the serviceability time database. The first step of the DFS approach is to complete the disassembly worksheet in Table 12.5. The DFSS team may disassemble the pressure recorder to reach the printed circuit board (PCB), the item requiring service. In the disassembly process, the team will access, row by row, several disassembly locations and record all operations in the disassembly worksheet.

Subassemblies are treated as parts when disassembly is not required for service; otherwise, the disassembly operation recording will continue when removing them. Reference to Abbatiello's (1995) database is referred to in columns 3, 5, and 7. For example, the time of 4.2 seconds in column 4 is the average taken from hours of videotape service work and includes a fraction of time for tool replacement at the end of service. The estimated time for PCB disassembly, T_d, is 104.3 seconds. This time can be converted to labor cost by multiplying by the service labor hourly rate.

The serviceability efficiency, η, is determined by parts necessity for removal or disassembly if they satisfy any of the following:

- The part or subassembly must be removed to isolate the service item(s).
- The part or subassembly removed contains the service item.
- The part or subassembly removed is a functional cover part enclosing the service item. For example, the plastic cover in the pressure recorder does not enclose the PCB, thus is not considered a cover.

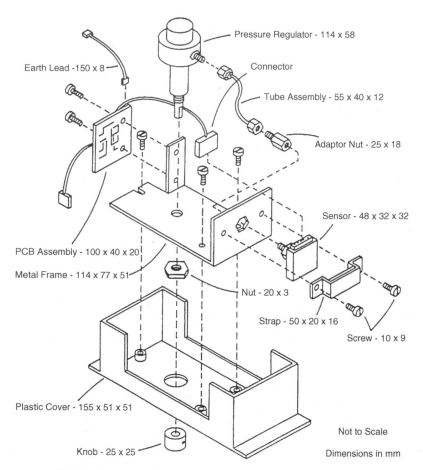

Figure 12.8 Exploded view of pressure recorder assembly.

When a part or subassembly does not satisfy any of the above, it is not considered to be a necessary part for disassembly. The sum in column 11 is the theoretical minimum justifiable and necessary number of disassembly operations, N_m. *In this example, only the removal of PCB is justified; N_m = 1.*

The next step is to fill out the corresponding reassembly worksheet. The reassembly worksheet format is similar to the disassembly worksheet and requires reference to the insertion and fastening database. The reassembly worksheet is shown in Table 12.6.

The DFSS team noted that the total removal time, T_r, equals 130.9 seconds and does not equal the total disassembly time.

Upon completion of both worksheets, the overall service efficiency of the service performed (i.e., replacing the PCB) can be calculated using the following steps:

TABLE 12.5 Disassembly Worksheet: Pressure Recorder

1 ID No.	2 Number of Times Operation Is Repeated	3 Four-Digit Tool Acquisition Code	4 Tool Acquisition Time (s)	5 Four-Digit Item Removal or Operation Code	6 Item Removal or Operation Time (s)	7 Four-Digit Item Set-Aside Code	8 Item Set-Aside Time (s)	9 Operation Time (s) = $4 + 2 \times (6 + 8)$	10^a Operation Cost, (cents) = $9 \times L/36$	11 Number of Service Items and Cover Parts of Functional Connections	Labor Rate ($/h), $L = 30$ Service Task Performed
1	3	5700	4.2	1710	11.3	5500	1.4	42.3	35.25	0	Remove screws
2	1	—	—	5800	4.5	—	—	4.5	3.75	0	Reorientation
3	1	5700	4.2	4100	8	—	—	12.2	10.17	0	Loosen setscrew
4	1	—	—	1500	2.4	5500	1.4	3.8	3.167	0	Remove knob
5	1	—	—	1500	2.4	5500	1.4	3.8	3.167	0	Remove cover
6	1	—	—	5800	4.5	—	—	4.5	3.75	0	Reorientation
7	1	—	—	4401	6.4	—	—	6.4	5.333	0	Unplug screw
8	2	5700	4.2	1700	8	5500	1.4	23	19.17	0	Remove screws
9	1	—	—	1500	2.4	5500	1.1	3.8	3.167	1	Remove PCB
Total								104.3 T_d	86.92 C_d	1 N_m	

[a]Note that the division by 36 in column 10 is to convert dollars to cents and hours to seconds.

1. Calculate the total time of service, T_s, as $T_s = T_d + T_r = 235.2$ seconds.
2. Determine the ideal service time based on the minimum amount of time required for all necessary operations: (1) removal, (2) set-aside, (3) acquisition, and (4) insertion. Several assumptions need to be made:
    a. All parts necessary for the service are placed within easy reach: ideally, with no tools required.
    b. Following DFMA, the *1/3 DFS ideal design* rule of thumb is used, which states that in ideal design for assembly, approximately one in every three parts will need to be unsecured and later resecured by efficient methods such as snap-fit and release fastening.

TABLE 12.6   Disassembly Worksheet: Pressure Recorder

1	2	3	4	5	6	7	8	9	10	Labor Rate ($/h), $L = 30$
ID No.	Number of Times Operation Is Repeated	Four-Digit Tool Acquisition Code	Tool Acquisition Time (s)	Four-Digit Item Acquisition Code	Item Acquisition Time (s)	Four-Digit Item Insertion or Operation Code	Item Insertion or Operation Time (s)	Operation Time (s) = $4 + 2 \times (6 + 8)$	Operation Cost (cents) = $9 \times L/36$	Service Task Performed
1	1	5700	4.2	5601	3.4	001	4.90	12.50	10.42	Add PCB
2	2			5600	1.4	0104	13.80	30.40	25.33	Fasten screws
3	1	5700	4.2			3000	8.60	8.60	7.167	Plug in sensor
4	1					5800	4.50	4.50	3.75	Reorientation
5	1			5600	1.4	0001	6.30	6.30	5.25	Plastic cover
6	1			5600	1.4	0001	6.30	6.30	5.25	Knob
7	1					2700	8.00	8.00	6.667	Fasten setscrew
8	1	5700	4.2			5800	8.70	8.70	7.25	Reorientation
9	3			5600	1.4	0401	45.60	45.60	38	Screw on cover
Total								130.9 T_r	109.1 C_r	

Using these assumptions, the ideal service time for the parts that need no additional removal or insertion can be given by

$$t_{\min} = \frac{3T_{\text{rem.un}} + T_{\text{rem.snap}}}{3} + \frac{2T_{\text{ins.un}} + T_{\text{ins.snap}}}{3} + T_{\text{acq}} + T_{\text{set-aside}} \qquad (12.5)$$

where

$T_{\text{rem.un}}$ = unsecured item removal time (= 2.4 s from the database)
$T_{\text{rem.snap}}$ = snap-fit item removal time (= 3.6 s from the database)
$T_{\text{in.un}}$ = unsecured item insertion time (= 3.8 s from the database)

$T_{\text{ins.un}}$ = snap-fit item insertion time (= 2.2 s from the database)
$T_{\text{set-aside}}$ = item set-aside time (= 1.4 s from the database)
T_{acq} = item acquisition time (= 1.4 s from the database)

Therefore,

$$t_{\min} = \frac{3 \times 2.4 + 3.6}{3} + \frac{2 \times 3.8 + 2.2}{3} + 1.4 + 1.4$$
$$\cong 9\,\text{s} \tag{12.6}$$

and with $N_m = 1$, the time-based efficiency is given by

$$\eta_{\text{time}} = \frac{t_{\min} N_m}{T_s} \times 100\%$$
$$= \frac{9 \times 1}{235.2} \times 100\%$$
$$= 3.8\% \tag{12.7}$$

The efficiency value is very low, leading us to conclude that the service procedure needs to be simplified, possibly using efficient disassembly methods and reconfigure the assembly so that the items needing frequent service are

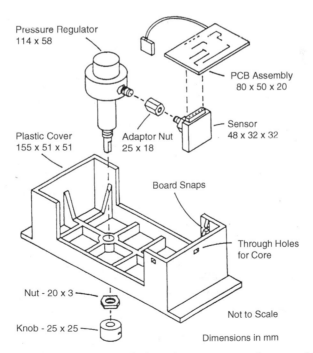

Figure 12.9 Reconfigured view of pressure recorder assembly.

accessed conveniently. In our example, considering PCB as a primary service structure, the assembly is reconfigured so that the board is on the outermost layer (Figure 12.9). Using the same database values, the estimated time for both disassembly and reassembly, T_s, is 16.5 s. Hence, the new efficiency is

$$\eta_{time} = \frac{t_{min}N_m}{T_s} \times 100\%$$

$$= \frac{9 \times 1}{16.5} \times 100\%$$

$$= 54.5\% \tag{12.8}$$

This DFS calculation approach can be extended to multiservice procedures, say $i = 1, 2, \ldots, k$. The overall time-based efficiency is a weighted average of the procedures of interest by the failure frequencies, f_i. This is given by

$$\eta_{overall} = \frac{1}{\sum_{i=1}^{k} f_i} \sum_{i=1}^{k} f_i \eta_i \tag{12.9}$$

12.7   SUMMARY

The DFX family provides a systematic approach to analyzing and improving device design from a spectrum of perspectives. It strengthens teamwork within the concurrent DFSS environment.

The design for manufacturability and assembly (DFMA) approach produces a considerable reduction in parts, resulting in simple and more reliable design with lower assembly and manufacture costs.

Design for reliability (DFR) provides a DFSS team with insights into how and why a proposed design may fail and identifies aspects of a design that may need to be improved. When reliability issues are addressed at early stages of the DFSS algorithm, project cycle time will be reduced.

By Axiom 2 of Chapter 9, a simplified product can be achieved through the sequential application of DFMA followed by design for serviceability (DFS). DFS is the ability to diagnose, remove, replace, replenish, or repair any DP (component or subassembly) to original specifications with relative ease. Poor serviceability produces warranty costs, customer dissatisfaction, and lost sales and market share due to loss of loyalty.

Another DFX family member is design for maintainability, whose objective is to assure that a design will perform satisfactorily throughout its intended life, with a minimum expenditure of money and effort. Design for maintainability, DFS, and DFR are related because minimizing maintenance and easing service can be achieved by improving reliability.

13

DFSS TRANSFER FUNCTION AND SCORECARDS

13.1 INTRODUCTION

In its simplest form, a *transfer function* is a mathematical representation of the relationship between the input and output of system or process. For example, putting a speaker in a room will make the speaker sound different from its performance in a nonenclosed space as a result of the reflections, absorptions, and resonance in the room. This change is the transfer function.

All systems, including medical devices, have a transfer function or a set of transfer functions. Typically the most noticeable change to artificial (human-made) systems is when excited by an energy source. An output response or a design functional requirement is inherent because the system is like a box, an enclosed entity that promotes a reaction to energy excitement. But the transfer function is more than just a change in a system's or process's status; it can also cause major changes in the system's physical embodiment. As designers, DFSS teams usually determine the transfer function(s) of their device through their design activities. They can map the activities and optimize the design output functional requirements and then build the device and its process and take advantage of their knowledge of the transfer function. So exactly what is a transfer function?

A *transfer function* describes the relationship between design parameters or process variables $(x_1, x_2, \ldots, x_n)$ and a functional requirement (y), denoted

Medical Device Design for Six Sigma: A Road Map for Safety and Effectiveness,
By Basem S. El-Haik and Khalid S. Mekki
Copyright © 2008 John Wiley & Sons, Inc.

by the relationship $y = f(x_1, x_2, \ldots, x_n)$. The variable y is the dependent output variable of a process or a system of interest to the customer. In medical device design, the transfer function is used to design and/or monitor a process to detect if it is out of control or if symptoms are developing within the device or its manufacturing processes. Once derived or quantified through design of experiment (DOE; see Chapters 14 and 15), for example, a transfer function $y = f(x_1, x_2, \ldots, x_n)$ can be developed to define the relationship of process variables, which can lead to a plan for controlling the process. The response (y) is an output measure or functional or design requirement, such as yield in a cellular therapy device. The transfer function explains the transformation of the inputs into the output, with x's being design inputs or a process step that is involved in producing the medical device. For example, in a medical device, medicine mixing uniformity for dosage delivery (y) is a function (f) of the mixing cycle volume (x_1), the number of mixing cycles (x_2), the duration of pauses during cycles (x_3), and so on. All of these x's can be defined, measured, and used for optimizing y.

Optimization in a medical device DFSS context means shifting the mean of $y(\mu_y)$ to the target (T_y) and minimizing its variance (σ_y^2). Design transfer functions are tied to design mappings and design hierarchy. These are explained below.

13.2 DESIGN MAPPING

The DFSS project road map (Chapter 9) recognizes three types of mapping as depicted in Figure 13.1:

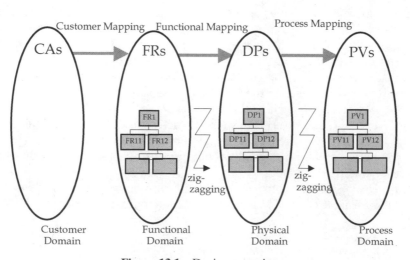

Figure 13.1 Design mappings.

1. Customer mapping (from customer attributes to functional requirements)
2. Functional mapping (from functional requirements to design parameters)
3. Process mapping (from design parameters to process variables)

The medical device DFSS road map of Chapter 7 is focused on providing a solution framework for the design process in order to produce healthy conceptual entities with six sigma quality potential. Mapping from the customer attribute domain to the functional requirement domain (y's) is conducted using quality function deployment (QFD), described in Chapter 8. QFD represents mapping from the raw customer attributes to the functional requirements.

In functional mapping, the following phase, the six sigma conceptual potential of the functional requirements, the y's, is set. This mapping phase presents a systematic approach for establishing capability at the conceptual level in the medical device entity by cascading requirements into a hierarchy while deploying design best practices, such as design principles. The application of design principles, in particular those promoted to axioms, is the team's insurance against repeating already known vulnerabilities. Axiomatic design (Chapter 9) is the prime tool for functional mapping and analysis.

Process mapping is a mapping from the design parameters domain to the process variables domain. Process variables are parameters that can be dialed (adjusted or changed) to deliver design parameters which in turn satisfy a functional requirement. Graphical process mapping, the IDEF [integrated computer-aided manufacturing (ICAM) definition] family,[1] and value stream mapping are several of the techniques used to conceive design process mapping.

In addition to design mappings, Figure 13.1 conveys the concept of design hierarchy, such as systems, subsystems, and components. At a given level of design hierarchy, there exists a set of requirements defined as the minimum set of requirements necessary at that level. Defining acceptable functional requirements may involve several iterations when a limited number of logical questions are employed in the mapping process.

13.2.1 Functional Mapping

Functional mapping is design mapping between functional requirements and design parameters. Functional mapping can be represented graphically or mathematically depicting the input–output or cause-and-effect relationships of functional elements. In its graphical form, block diagrams are used to capture the mapping and comprise nodes connected by arrows depicting such

---

[1]IDEF is a family of mapping techniques developed by the U.S. Air Force (see El-Haik and Roy, 2005).

relationships. A block diagram should capture all design elements within the DFSS project scope and ensure correct flow down to critical parameters. Functional mapping is captured mathematically using mapping matrices, with matrices belonging to the same hierarchical level clustered together. Design hierarchy is built by decomposing design into a number of simpler design matrices that collectively meet the high-level functional requirements identified in the first mapping. The collection of design matrices or blocks forms the conceptual design blueprint and provides a means to track the chain of effects for design changes as they propagate across the device design. The decomposition starts by identifying a minimum set of functional requirements that deliver the device tasks defined by the customer. Both the design principles and the team's creativity guide the decomposition heuristic process of functional definition through logical questions (Chapter 9). Efficient use of design principles can gear the synthesis and analysis design activities to vulnerability-free solutions.

13.2.2 Process Mapping

Process mappings are conceptual representations at different hierarchal levels. These matrices are not stand-alone, and a complete device solution entity for the design project needs to be delivered in some physical form. We call this *embodiment*. The ultimate goal of design mapping is to facilitate design detailing when the relationships are identified in the form of transfer functions or other models. Design mappings, a design analysis step, should be conducted *prior* to design synthesis activities.

A detailed transfer function is useful not only for design optimization but also for further design analysis and synthesis activities. For example, the functional requirement of a given subsystem can be the input signal of another subsystem delivering another requirement, and so on. These relationships create the design hierarchy.

Similar to functional mapping, process mappings can be depicted graphically or mathematically (refer to Chapter 9 for further material). To make the most improvements in any existing process, it is necessary to understand the actual way that the process occurs. In process mapping we need symbols for a process step (Table 13.1), a measurement, a queue, storage, transportation (movement), and a decision.

There are three versions of a process map (Figure 13.2). There is what it was designed to be, which is usually a clean flow based on the process mapping. After embodiment and over time, there is an as-is process map with all the gritty variety that usually occurs because of varying suppliers, customers, operators, and conditions. Take an ATM machine as an example. Does everyone follow the same flow for getting money out? Some may check their balance first and then withdraw, while others may type in the wrong PIN and have to retype it. The last version is the version that we would like it to be, with only value-added steps—clean, intuitive, and works right every time.

TABLE 13.1   Process Mapping Standard Symbols

Symbol	Meaning
☐	Process step or operation (white)
◖	Delay (red)
◯	Quality check, inspection, or measurement (yellow)
▽	Storage (yellow)
◇	Decision (blue)
⇨	Transport or movement of material or transmission of information (yellow)

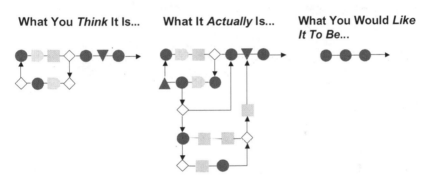

What You *Think* It Is...   **What It *Actually* Is...**   **What You Would *Like* It To Be...**

Figure 13.2   Three versions of a process.

A process map is a pictorial representation showing all of the steps of a process. As a first step, the team should familiarize themselves with the mapping symbols, then walk the process by asking such questions as "What really happens next in the process?", "Does a decision need to be made before the next step?", or "What approvals are required before moving on to the next task?" The team then draws the process using the symbols on a flipchart or overhead transparency. Every process will have a beginning and an end (elongated circles). All processes will have tasks, and most will have decision points (a diamond). Upon completion the team should analyze the map for such items as non-value-added steps, rework loops, duplication, and increased cycle time. A typical high-level process map is shown in Figure 13.3.

A good process map should identify all process steps or operations as well as visible measurement, inspection, rework loops, and decision points. In addition, "swim lanes" are often used when mapping information flow for transactional and business processes. We believe that swim lanes are appropriate

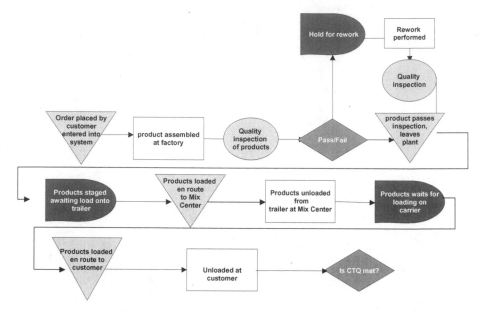

Figure 13.3 High-level process map example.

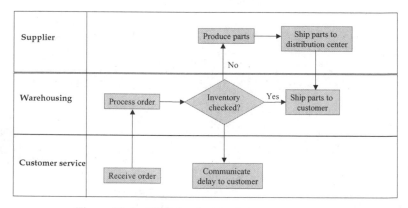

Figure 13.4 High-level swim lanes process map.

for all types of DFSS projects, as they segregate steps by who does them or where they are done and make handoffs visual. The map is arranged on a table where the rows indicate who owns or performs the process step (process owner) and the process flow that changes lanes indicates hand-offs. Hand-off points are where lack of coordination and communication can cause process problems. An example is depicted in Figure 13.4.

Clear distinctions can be made between warehousing and those process steps where customer interactions occur. The swim lane process map example shows a high-level portion of the order receiving process. Another level of detail in each of the process steps will require further mapping if they are within the scope of the project.

Another process mapping technique, *value stream mapping* (VSM), originated in document manufacturing processes that were to be improved using lean manufacturing methods. VMS is equally applicable to discrete event processes. They are most useful with higher-frequency processes even if considering mixed-model processing. In this section we define value stream mapping and its advantages and present the various steps for its construction. Usually, whenever there is a product or service for a customer, there is a value stream. Therefore, value stream mapping is applicable whenever the design team is trying to make waste in a process visible, to eliminate non-value-added steps, actions, and activities. A value-added activity or step is any activity or thing the customer is willing to pay for. Non-value-added activities, those that do not add market form or function or are not necessary should be eliminated, simplified, reduced, or integrated. See El-Haik and Roy (2005) for more details.

13.2.3   Design Mapping Steps

The following synthesis steps can be used in both functional and process mappings. We'll use a functional mapping technique for illustration.

1. Obtain high-level functional requirements using quality function deployment (QFD; see Chapter 8).
2. Define boundaries from the project scope.
3. Conduct the mappings using the techniques from Chapter 9 to the lowest possible level and identify the transfer functions at every level. The lowest level represents very standard design parameters or process variables. For example, in medical device DFSS projects, forms, standards and procedures are at the lowest level.
4. Define the respective hierarchical levels of design mappings.
5. Within a level for each mapping and for each requirement (y), determine the potential mapped-to design parameters and process variables.
6. For compatible analysis, select and use a consistent mapping technique (Chapter 9) for both functional and process mappings.
7. Aggregate the chains of mappings in every hierarchical level into an overall mapping. You will produce something for your project that resembles Figure 13.1.

13.3   DESIGN SCORECARDS AND THE TRANSFER FUNCTION

In a world where data are plentiful and data storage is relatively inexpensive, it is a painful irony that most medical device manufacturers are unable to use those data to make better decisions. These manufacturers are rich in data but poor in knowledge. Hidden within those megabytes of information is useful knowledge about customers, devices, and processes that if uncovered could result in significant cost savings or revenue enhancement. Transfer function models[2] uncover hidden relationships and improve design decision making. DFSS teams can use transfer function models effectively to cleanse, augment, and enhance historical knowledge.

A transfer function is a means of optimization and design detailing and is usually documented in a scorecard. A transfer function should be treated as a living entity within the DFSS road map that passes through its own life-cycle stages. A transfer functions is first identified using functional mapping and then detailed by derivation, modeling, or experimentation. Design transfer functions belonging to the same hierarchical level in the design should be recorded in that hierarchical level scorecard. A scorecard is used to record and optimize the transfer functions. The transfer function is integrated with other DFSS concepts and tools, such as process mapping, DOE, and DFMEA. Functional mapping and process mapping are the premier activities performed in the characterize phase of the DFSS road map (Chapter 7). Both types of design activities, as well as their corresponding techniques, are covered in Chapter 9.

Through several transfer function detailing options, such as DOE, transfer functions can be approximated by an algebraic equation of a polynomial additive model and augmented with some modeling and experimental error. This approximation is valid in any local area or volume of the design space from which it was obtained. In other words, we can infer within the tested space but not predict outside the limits of testing. An error term is usually present to represent the difference between the actual transfer function and the function predicted.

Transfer function additivity is extremely desired in all device design mappings. As the magnitude of the error term is reduced, the transfer function additivity increases, as it implies less interaction.[3] In additive transfer functions, the significance of a design parameter is relatively independent of the effect of other parameters. Medical device solution entities that are designed following the axiomatic design method (Chapter 9) will have additive transfer functions that can be optimized easily, thus reducing the DFSS project cycle time. From an analysis standpoint, this additivity is needed in order to employ statistical analysis techniques such as robust design, DOE, and regression.

---

[2]Usually, *transfer function model* refers to a statistical technique used in forecasting a variable over time. The technique is similar to regression analysis and is often referred to as dynamic regression analysis. Transfer function models are most often used as a relatively simple and effective time-series forecasting technique and is useful forecasting demand and capacity in logistic problems.

[3]Interaction is the cross-product term of a transfer function. In a designed experiment, it occurs when the difference of a functional requirement between levels of one parameter or variable is not the same at all levels of the other factors. See Chapter 14 for more details.

The transfer functions in the functional and process mappings are usually captured in design scorecards, which document and assess DFSS project progress quantitatively, store the learning process, and show all critical elements of a design and their performance. Their benefits include documenting transfer functions and design optimization, predicting final results, enabling communication among all stakeholders in the project, while evaluating how well the device design is supported by production processes.

The set of transfer functions of a given device design are the means for optimizing customer satisfaction. Transfer functions can be derived mathematically, obtained empirically from a DOE, or regressed using historical data. In several cases, no closed mathematical formula can be obtained and the DFSS team must resort to mathematical and/or simulation modeling. In DFSS there should be a transfer function for every functional requirement (y), depicting the functional mapping, and for every design parameter, depicting the process mapping. The transfer functions at a given hierarchy level are recorded in one scorecard.

13.3.1   DFSS Scorecard Development

The scorecard identifies which design parameters contribute most to variation and mean in the response of the transfer function and the optimized design point. Tightening tolerances may be appropriate for the parameters that affect the output most significantly. The team has the freedom to customize the scorecard. During scorecard development, the team should remember that a scorecard has a hierarchical structure that parallels the concerned mapping. There will be a number of scorecards equal to the number of hierarchal levels in the concerned mapping.

The extension of the DFSS methodology from a product to a medical device environment is facilitated by the design scorecard and life-cycle element mapping. Think about a simple database used in a programmable X-therapy device; the process is to build the software code, load it, use it, report it, and update it. The common requirements of a typical design scorecard would be accuracy, completeness, and time requirements for inputting, reporting, and updating steps in this process, as shown in Table 13.2.

13.3.2   Transfer Function Life Cycle

Transfer functions are living entities in the DFSS road map. The life cycle of a transfer function (see Yang and El-Haik, 2003) in the DFSS project passes into the following sequential stages:

1. *Identification:* obtained by mapping between the design domains.

2. *Conceptual treatment:* obtained by fixing, adding, replacing, and deleting some of the independent variables in the codomain to satisfy design principle and axioms (Chapter 9).

TABLE 13.2　Design Scorecard for X-Therapy Device Use

	Quantity	Defects	DPU	RTY	Z_{lt}	Z_{st}
Top level						
Input	100	6	0.06	0.941765	1.569761	3.069761
Report	2	3	1.5	0.22313	−0.76166	0.738336
Maintain	5	6	1.2	0.67032	0.440798	1.940798
Total				0.140858	−1.07647	0.423529
Input level						
Accuracy	100	3	0.03	0.970446	1.887383	3.387383
Completeness	100	1	0.01	0.99005	2.328215	3.828215
Time to input	100	2	0.02	0.980199	2.057868	3.557868
Total	100	6		0.941765	1.569761	3.069761
Report level						
Accuracy	2	1	0.5	0.606531	0.270288	1.770288
Completeness	2	1	0.5	0.606531	0.270288	1.770288
Process time	2	1	0.5	0.606531	0.270288	1.770288
Total	2	3		0.22313	−0.76166	0.738336
Maintain level						
Completeness	5	0	0	1	6	7.5
Accuracy	5	0	0	1	6	7.5
Time to perform	5	2	0.4	0.67032	0.440798	1.940798
Total	5	6		0.67032	0.440798	1.940798

3. *Detailing:* achieved by finding the cause and effect, preferably through a mathematical relationship, between all variables in the mapping domains concerned. Detailing involves validating both the assumed relationship and the sensitivities of all independent parameters and variables [i.e., $y = f(x_1, x_2, \ldots, x_n)$]. Transfer functions can be categorized as (1) empirical, as obtained from testing, or (2) mathematical, in the form of equations, inequalities, and other mathematical relations among design parameters and/or process variables that describe the behavior of the design entity. For some cases it is possible analytically to have equations in closed form. However, in many situations, closed-form solutions are impossible and one can resort to other methods, such as simulation.

4. *Optimization:* obtained by either shifting the mean of the dependent variables or reducing their variation, or both, in the optimize phase of the DFSS road map. This can be achieved by adjusting $(x_1, x_2, \ldots, x_n)$ parameter means and variances. This optimization propagates to the customer domain via the established transfer function in the design mappings, resulting in increased satisfaction.

5. *Validation:* carried out in both mappings.

6. *Maintenance:* obtained by controlling all significant independent variables, after optimization, in-house or outside.

Stages 1 to 6 are experienced in a DFSS project.

7. *Disposal.* stage reached when the design transfer functions are disposed of or reach entitlement in delivering high-level functional requirements when either new customer attributes that can not be satisfied with the current design emerge or when the mean or controlled variance of the requirements are no longer acceptable by the customer. This stage is usually followed by the evolution of new transfer functions to satisfy the needs that have emerged.

8. *Evolution of a new transfer function.* usually follows certain basic patterns of development [according to TRIZ (see Chapter 10)]. Evolutionary trends of the functional performance of a certain design can be plotted over time and have been found to evolve in a manner that resembles an S-curve (Figure 13.5).

The following are enumerations of some possible sources of detailed transfer functions:

1. Direct documented knowledge, such as equations derived from laws of physics (e.g., force = spring constant × displacement). Transfer function variability optimization and statistical inference can be carried out using simulation, generally via the Monte Carlo method or Taylor series expansion. The transfer functions obtained through this source are very dependent on the team's understanding and competency with their design and the discipline of knowledge that it represents.

2. Transfer functions can be obtained by sensitivity analysis to estimate the derivatives, with the prototype process, baseline design, or a credible mathematical model. The sensitivity analysis involves changing one parameter or variable, then requantifying the transfer function (y) to obtain the result, and then comparing the change of both sides to each other. The process is repeated for all independent parameters or variables ($x_1, x_2, \ldots, x_n$).

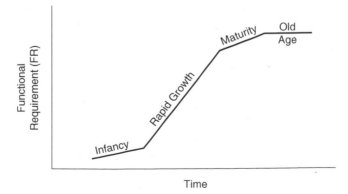

Figure 13.5 S-curve of FR evolution.

3. Design of experiments (DOE) is another source of transfer function detailing. In many perspectives, DOE is another form of sensitivity analysis. DOE analysis runs the inputs throughout their possible experimental ranges, not through incremental area or volume. See Chapters 14 and 15 for more details.

The resulting predictive equation from DOE analysis using statistical packages such as Minitab, for example, is in essence a transfer function. The black belt may take the derivative of the predictive equation to estimate sensitivities. Special DOE techniques such as the response surface method (Yang and El-Haik, 2003), factorial experimentation, and robust design (Chapters 14 and 15) are more appropriate due to the richness of information they yield.

A DOE can be run using physical entities, or mathematically. Additionally, simulation models result from using techniques such as Monte Carlo (Section 13.6) or various computer-aided design and manufacturing products. Mathematical models are descriptive; they provide a representation that is a good and realistic substitute for the real system while retaining characteristics of importance. We simulate the behavior of real systems by conducting virtual experiments on analytical models in lieu of experiments on real systems. Simulation reduces cost and effort and provides a replica of reality for further investigation, including if–then scenarios.

In simulation, the team needs to define design parameters and/or process variables. The simulation model then samples a number of runs from these distributions and forms an output distribution. The statistical parameters of this distribution, such as the mean and variance, are then estimated. Afterward, statistical inference analysis can be used.

4. Regression transfer equations are obtained when the functional requirements are regressed over all input variables or parameters of interest. Multiple regressions, coupled with multivariable analysis of variance (MANOVA) and covariance (MANCOVA), are typically used to estimate parameter (variable) effect. These subjects are beyond the scope of the book.

13.4 TRANSFER FUNCTION MATHEMATICS

In this section we get a view of the role that mathematics plays in describing how design elements change in a transfer function. We graph the types of functions that arise in medical device design with major concentration on polynomials up to quadratic terms. Polynomial transfer functions are continuous and differentiable functions and represent most common components of many useful models. A nonpolynomial function can be approximated by polynomial terms using Taylor series expansion.

In graphing polynomials and other functions, we begin with the assignment of numerical coordinates to points in a plane. These coordinates, called *Cartesian coordinates* in honor of Descartes, a French mathematician, make it possible to graph algebraic equations in two variables (or parameters), lines and curves. Cartesian coordinates also allow calculation of angles and distances and make it possible to write coordinate equations to describe the paths along which objects move and change. Most today are familiar with the notion of x-axis, y-axis, and the point where the coordinates intersect, the origin. Motion from left to right along the x-axis is called motion in the positive x-direction. Along the y-axis, the positive direction is up and the negative direction is down. When plotting data in a Cartesian coordinate plane whose parameters have different units of measures, the units shown on the two coordinate axes may have different interpretations.

If we track the performance of a functional requirement, we can watch their progress on graph paper by plotting points and fitting them with a curve. We extend the curve as new data appear. To what uses can we then put such a curve? We can see what the performance was on any given data point. We can see by the slope of the curve, the rate at which a functional requirement is rising or falling. If we plot other data on the same sheet of paper, we can perhaps see what relation they have to the rise and fall of functional requirements. The curve may also reveal patterns that would be helping us forecast or affect the future with more accuracy than someone who has not graphed the data. In Chapter 14 we introduce plotting one factor effect at a time (commonly known as *mean effect plots*) and the two factor effects (commonly known as *interaction effect plots*), and so on. In addition, graphing helps make a connection between rates of change and slopes of smooth curves. One can imagine the slope as the grade of a roadbed.[4] Consider

$$y = f(x_1) = a_0 + \underbrace{a_1 x_1}_{\text{linear term}} \tag{13.1}$$

It is an equation of linear transfer function where a_0 and a_1 are the y-intercept and slope, respectively. It is a polynomial of the first degree or linear. In this case, the output y, the functional requirement, is called the *dependent variable*, while x, the design parameter, is called the *independent variable*. This relationship can be exemplified by an incremental addition that is replenished at a *constant rate* a_1 with an initial value of a_0. The terms a_0 and $a_1 x_1$ are in units of y. Therefore, the unit of a_1, the slope, is the unit of y per unit of x. This function is graphed in Figure 13.6.

Suppose that there is another design parameter, denoted by x_2, and we are interested in the overall performance of y as a function of the two design parameters. In this case, y can be given as

$$y = f(x_1, x_2) = a_0 + \underbrace{a_1 x_1 + a_2 x_2}_{\text{linear terms}} \tag{13.2}$$

---

[4]Civil engineers calculate the slope of a roadbed by calculating the ratio of the distance it rises or falls to the distance it runs horizontally, calling it the *grade* of the roadbed.

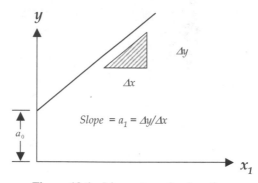

Figure 13.6   Linear transfer function.

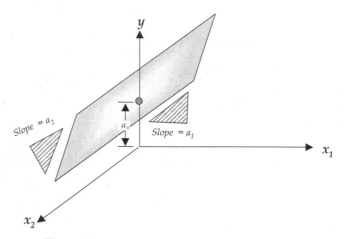

Figure 13.7   Linear transfer function in a plane.

The plot of such a transfer function is given in Figure 13.7. As you may conclude, it is a plane. Note that this transfer function may be enhanced by a cross-product term reflecting the interaction between parameters or factors x_1 and x_2. In Chapter 14 we call this cross-product term *interaction*. This may happen when there is a chemical reaction. Equation (13.2) then becomes

$$y = f(x_1, x_2) = a_0 + \underbrace{a_1 x_1 + a_2 x_2}_{\text{linear terms}} + \underbrace{a_{12} x_1 x_2}_{\text{interaction term}} \tag{13.3}$$

We often encounter transfer functions that change at a *linear rate* rather than a constant rate. That is, the instantaneous rate of change in the design output y relative to a design parameter x_1 is linear similar to (13.1), which means that y is a quadratic function in the independent variables. The functional requirement y in this case is quadratic:

$$y = f(x_1) = a_0 + \underbrace{a_1 x_1}_{\text{linear term}} + \underbrace{a_{11} x_1^2}_{\text{quadratic term}} \qquad (13.4)$$

Quadratic transfer functions are often encountered in customer satisfaction target setting in the context of design mappings (Figure 13.1). In this case, customer satisfaction (y) is highest when an influential independent factor (x) assumes a desired target value. For example, in a restaurant that collects customer feedback, in particular the lunch meal, the highest satisfaction is often encountered when the overall experience took on average of 1 hour. Satisfaction is measured on a 6-point scale from poor (1) to excellent (6). This will allow restaurant management to target employee responsiveness to customers, including friendly table visits as well as prompt delivery. More or less time results in decay in customer satisfaction (y), as depicted in Figure 13.8. Using mathematical treatment, the customer satisfaction is given by

$$y = f(x) = \frac{|y_0 - y_T|}{-x_0^2 + 2x_0 x_T - x_T^2}(x - x_T)^2 + y_T \qquad (13.5)$$

This high-level introduction of linear and quadratic polynomials transfer functions will allow the reader to grasp the forthcoming concepts in the book. Both represent building blocks of most often encountered medical device transfer functions. Other forms are listed below. The reader can extend such forms to three (introducing x_3), four (by introducing x_4), and so on, independent factors (variables or parameters):

$$y = f(x_1, x_2) = a_0 + \underbrace{a_1 x_1 + a_2 x_2}_{\text{linear terms}} + \underbrace{a_{12} x_1 x_2}_{\text{interaction term}} + \underbrace{a_{11} x_1^2 + a_{22} x_2^2}_{\text{quadratic terms}} \qquad (13.6)$$

$$y = f(x_1, x_2, x_3) = a_0 + \underbrace{a_1 x_1 + a_2 x_2 + a_3 x_3}_{\text{linear terms}}$$

$$+ \underbrace{a_{12} x_1 x_2 + a_{13} x_1 x_3 + a_{23} x_2 x_3}_{\text{interaction terms}} + \underbrace{a_{11} x_1^2 + a_{22} x_2^2 + a_{33} x_3^2}_{\text{quadratic terms}} \qquad (13.7)$$

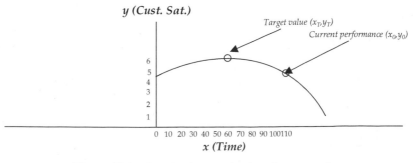

Figure 13.8 Quadratic transfer function example.

When empirical methods are used to obtain a transfer function, the result is an approximation, and not exact because of the inclusion of experimental error as well as the effect of unaccounted for design parameters, process variables, and noise factors. An error term will represent the difference between the actual and empirical transfer functions. The notation $\hat{y}$ is used to reference a transfer function obtained empirically.

13.5 TRANSFER FUNCTION AND OPTIMIZATION

To be valid, a transfer function that includes random parameters or variables, which have probabilistic uncertainty, must incorporate the parameter or variable uncertainty. Transfer function is design DNA. The evaluation of transfer functions that contain random parameters or variables (independent variables) by point estimates alone does not include the uncertainty and therefore does not offer complete representation.

Without clear justifications for preferring one value in the entire uncertainty domain, point estimates are not credible. Ignoring variability (uncertainty) may result in misleading conclusions. Therefore, transfer functions detailing should take into consideration all possible sources of uncertainty, including uncontrollable factors (noise factors; refer to Chapter 15) to gain DFSS optimization credibility.

Optimization in the context of medical device DFSS of a requirement, say y, is carried in two steps: first, minimizing its variance (σ_y^2), and second, shifting the mean (μ_y) to the target (T_y). This two-step optimization implies design robustness and when coupled with a six sigma target means a six sigma design. In conducting optimization, design transfer functions are the workforce. Some of the transfer functions are readily available from existing knowledge. Others will require perhaps some intellectual or monetary capital to obtain.

A key philosophy of DFSS project mapping is that during the optimization phase, *inexpensive parameters* can be identified and studied, and can be combined in a way that will result in performance that is insensitive to uncontrolled, yet adversely influential factors (noise factors). The team's task is to determine for each design parameter the combined best settings (parameter targets), which have been judged by the design team to have the potential to improve a medical device the most. By varying the parameter target levels in the transfer function (design point), a region of nonlinearity can be identified. This area of nonlinearity is the most optimized setting for the parameter under study. Consider two settings or means of a design parameter (x), setting 1 (x^*) and setting 2 (x^{**}) that have the same variance and probability density function (statistical distribution), as depicted in Figure 13.9. Consider, also, the given curve of a hypothetical transfer function, which is in this case a nonlinear function in the design parameter (x). It is obvious that setting 1 produces less variation in the functional requirement (y) than setting 2 by capitalizing on

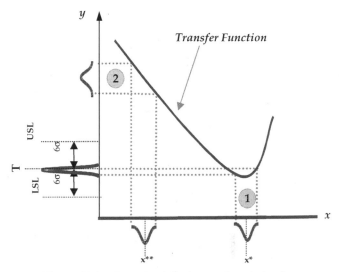

Figure 13.9 Transfer function and optimization.

nonlinearity.[5] Setting 1 (x^*) will also produce a lower quality loss, a concept that is entertained in Chapter 15. In other words, the design produced by setting 1 (x^*) is more robust (optimized) than that produced by setting 2. Setting 1 (x^*) robustness is evident in the amount of variation transferred through the transfer function to the y response in Figure 13.9.[6] When the distance between the specification limits is six times the standard deviation ($6\sigma_y$), a six-sigma-level optimized y is achieved. When all design functional requirements are released at this level, a six-sigma design is obtained.

The black belt and the rest of the DFSS team need to detail the transfer functions in the context of the DFSS algorithm if they want to optimize, validate, and predict the exact performance of their project scope in the intended environment. However, the team should be cautious about the predictability of some of the transfer functions, due to the stochastic effects of noise factors in the intended environment that are particularly hard to predict. The team should explore all knowledge to obtain the transfer functions desired. For example, stack-up based on tolerances may contain descriptions of functionality that is based on a lumped-mass model and geometry. Transfer functions that are obtained by means other than direct documented knowledge are approximate, and for purposes of the DFSS road map are valid until proven wrong or are disposed of, due to the evolution of other concepts that have been adopted.

---

[5]Leveraging interactions between the noise factors and the design parameters comprise another popular empirical parameter design approach.
[6]Also, the flatter quadratic quality loss function in Figure 13.2.

13.6   MONTE CARLO SIMULATION

When we use the word *simulation*, we refer to any analytical method meant to replicate a real-life process, especially when another transfer function is too mathematically complex or too difficult to reproduce. Without the aid of simulation, a developed model will generally reveal a single outcome, the most likely or average scenario. Analysis uses simulation to automatically analyze the effect of varying inputs on outputs of the modeled process. One type of spreadsheet simulation is Monte Carlo simulation,[7] which randomly generates values for variables continuously to simulate a process.

The random behavior in gambling games is similar to how Monte Carlo simulation selects variable values at random to simulate a model. When a dice is rolled, you know that a 1, 2, 3, 4, 5, or 6 will come up, but you don't know which for any particular trial. It's the same with design parameters and process variables, which have a known range of values but an uncertain value for any particular time or event.

For each parameter or variable (one that has a range of possible values), the DFSS team defines the possible values with a probability distribution. The type of distribution you select is based on the conditions surrounding that variable. Distribution types include normal, uniform, exponential, triangular, and so on (see Chapter 3). To add this sort of function to an Excel spreadsheet, you would need to know the equation that represents this distribution. In commercially available packages such as Crystal Ball, these equations are calculated for you automatically. They can even fit a distribution to any historical data available.

A simulation calculates multiple scenarios of a model by repeatedly sampling values from the probability distributions for the device parameters and using those values for the advancement of transactions in the process. Simulations can consist of, hundreds or even thousands of trials in just a few seconds. During a single Monte Carlo trial, a simulation model selects a value randomly from the defined possibilities (the range and shape of the distribution) for each process variable and then recalculates the spreadsheet.

Monte Carlo simulation is a popular simulation method to evaluate the uncertainty of a functional requirement (y). It involves some sampling from the independent parameter or variable probability distributions to provide their values. A random number generator is used to obtain the parameter value based on the probability density function. When all independent parameters or variables are quantified, the functional requirement is quantified to have its numerical result. This process is repeated for a desired number of iterations. A histogram of the results is then built from the answer and can be used for statistical inference. The black belt needs to:

[7]Monte Carlo simulation was named for Monte Carlo, Monaco, where the primary attraction is gambling. Gambling implies the use of chance and probability similar to the simulation mechanism of employing randomness. Games of chance such as roulette wheels, dice, and slot machines exhibit random behavior.

- Determine the applicable distribution of y
- Estimate the parameters of that distribution
- Use the distribution for optimization and inference. For example, assuming y normality, we can use the following upper z-value:

$$z_y = \frac{\text{USL} - \mu_y}{\sigma_y}$$

to calculate the defects per million.

The drawbacks of this method include the following:

- Simulation time may be an issue, in particular, for some complex mathematical forms of transfer functions and a large number of iterations.
- Identifying the proper probability distribution functions for the independent parameters and variables may be difficult, due to lack of data or an understanding of the underlying physics.
- Randomness of the random number generator may be an issue.

Tables of ready-to-use random numbers are available to be used, especially in Monte Carlo simulations, where random sampling is used to estimate certain requirements. Also, most simulation software packages have the capability of automatic random number generation. The detail of sampling from probability distributions is not within the scope of this chapter [see, e.g., El-Haik and Alaomar (2006)].

Monte Carlo simulation models are time-independent (static) models that deal with a fixed-state process. In such spreadsheet-like models, certain variable values are changed by random generation, and a certain measure or more are evaluated through such changes without considering the timing and dynamics of such changes, a prime disadvantage that is handled by discrete event simulation models. In discrete event simulation, the time dimension is live.

13.7 SUMMARY

Design can be defined by a series of mappings between four domains. The DFSS project road map recognizes three types of mapping:

1. Customer mapping (from customer attributes to functional requirements)
2. Functional mapping (from functional requirements to design parameters)
3. Process mapping (from design parameters to process variables)

Transfer functions are a mathematical relationship relating a design response, usually a functional requirement, with design parameters and/or process variables. Transfer functions are a DFSS optimization vehicle. They facilitate the DFSS optimization of outputs related to the medical device entity of interest by defining the true relationship between input and output variables. Optimization in this context means minimizing the requirement variability and shifting its mean to some target value desired by customer. Design scorecards are used to document the transfer function as well as the optimization calculations.

14

FUNDAMENTALS OF EXPERIMENTAL DESIGN

14.1 INTRODUCTION

Design of experiments (DOE) is a method used to obtain a transfer function (Chapter 13). DOE and robust parameter design (Chapter 15) are the two most popular methods used to obtain transfer functions empirically.

In the mid-1920s, the British statistician Ronald Fisher put the finishing touches on a method for making breakthrough discoveries. Some 70 years later, Fisher's method, now known as design of experiments, has become a powerful tool for engineers, researchers, and six-sigma parishioners. Fisher developed DOE as a research design tool to improve farm yields in the early 1930s. Fisher was a geneticist working on improving crop yields in England using supervised field trials, fertilizers, and seed varieties as experimental factors. In his study, Fisher encountered such issues as uncontrollable variation in the soil from plot to plot and the limited number of plots available for any given trial. Fisher solved these issues by the arrangement of fertilizers or seed varieties in the field. This action minimized the effects of soil variation in the analysis of the plot yields. Fisher also developed the correct method for analyzing designed experiments called *analysis of variance* (ANOVA). This analysis method breaks up the total variation in the data into components from different sources. His analysis of variance delivers surprisingly precise results when applied to a well-structured matrix, including small sizes. Today, these components are called *signals* and *noise* with estimated effects calculated

Medical Device Design for Six Sigma: A Road Map for Safety and Effectiveness,
By Basem S. El-Haik and Khalid S. Mekki
Copyright © 2008 John Wiley & Sons, Inc.

as the sum of squares and the signal-to-noise ratio. There is a signal component for each controlled source (factor) in the experiment and a noise component representing variations not attributable to any of the controlled variations. ANOVA using the signal-to-noise ratio provides precise allocations of the effects of the factors and interactions. The ANOVA solutions developed for these problems work just as well in today's six sigma environment as they did in twentieth-century agriculture.

DOE provides a powerful tool within the DFSS road map to accomplish break-through improvements in product, service, or process efficiency and effectiveness by optimizing its fulfillment of the critical-to characteristics (CTs), functional requirements (FRs), and design parameters (DPs). In each case we create a response variable (y) and vary the factors that can cause a change in the performance of the response y. We can have $CT = f(FRs)$ or $CT = f(DPs)$ or $FR = f(DPs)$ or $DP = f(PVs)$. It is important to note that most problem-solving experimentation occurs in the relationships between DPs and PVs (process mapping); if these do not yield breakthrough performance, the design team should visit the FRs and look at options. The most proper utilization of a DOE is in the optimize phase within the road map of Figure 7.1. Optimization in a DOE sense implies finding the proper settings of significant factors that enable the DFSS team to shift the mean and to reduce variation in their design requirements or responses. DOE has been available for decades, but its penetration in industry have been limited. Besides ignorance and lack of proper training, implementation had been resisted by the discipline required as well as the use of statistical techniques. Scientists managers, and medical device designers usually fear the use of statistics. Six sigma belts play a big role in helping their teams and satellite members overcome such emotional barriers.

Traditionally, the approach to experimentation in a process, for example, required changing only one factor at a time (OFAT). Soon it was found that the OFAT approach is incapable of detecting *interactions*[1] among the factors, which is a more probable and possible event than most professionals think. Therefore, DOE is also called *statistically designed experiment*. The purpose of the experiment and data analysis is to establish and detail the transfer functions[2] between outputs (e.g., design parameters) and experimental factors (e. g., process variables and noise factors) in a mapping, generally using a P-diagram, as illustrated in Figure 14.1. A transfer function is a means of optimization and design detailing and is usually documented in the scorecard. A transfer function is treated as a living entity within the DFSS methodology that passes through its own life-cycle stages. A transfer function is first identified using the proper mapping method (Chapter 9) and then detailed by derivation, modeling, or experimentation. The prime uses of the transfer function

---

[1]Interaction could be two-level, three-level, and so on. In a two-level interaction, a change in the response (output) of factor A occurs when factor B changes.
[2]Recall that DOE is a transfer function detailing method, as presented in Chapter 13.

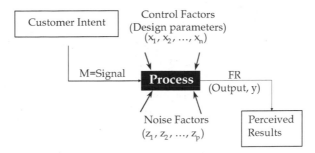

Figure 14.1 P-diagram.

are optimization and validation. Design transfer functions belonging to the same hierarchical level in the design structures (system or subsystem or component) should be recorded in that hierarchical-level scorecard (Chapter 13). A scorecard is used to record and optimize the transfer functions. The transfer function concept is integrated with other DFSS concepts and tools such as mapping or robust design P-diagrams[3] (Figure 14.1) within the rigor of design scorecards (Yang and El-Haik, 2003).

In Fischer's experiments, the output or response variable (y) was usually the yield of a certain farm crop. Controllable factors, $x = (x_1, x_2, \ldots, x_n)$, were usually the farm variables, such as the amount of various fertilizers applied, watering pattern, and selection of seeds. Uncontrollable factors, $z = (z_1, z_2, \ldots, z_p)$, could be soil types, weather patterns, and so on (see Figure 14.1). In early agricultural experiments, the experimenter would like to find the cause-and-effect relationship between the yield and controllable factors. That is, the experimenter would like to know how different types of fertilizers, their application quantities, the watering pattern, and types of seeds would influence the yield of the crop.

Today, DOE implementation has expanded to all industries. For example, the two sides of medical packaging are achieved by a heated platen tool used to seal them together thermally. Failure of a seal during sterilization or handling would result in loss of sterility and thus affect patient safety. The process variables during the sealing operation are platen temperature, with the range 100 to 150°C; pressure applied, with the range 30 to 110 psi; and dwell time, with the range 0.5 to 2.3 s. Each of these variables must be controlled within the correct limits to achieve acceptable seal quality. DOE is the most efficient method of determining these limits for process validation.[4] The range investigated for each factor is chosen based on knowledge of the system. The design team should be able to assess the acceptable processing window on form, fill,

---

[3]See Appendix 11A for robust design–based FMEA that uses the P-diagram.
[4]Process validation usually includes installation qualification, for the equipment; operational Qualification, which demonstrates that the equipment consistently operates to specification under normal conditions; and performance qualification, which is used when the process is challenged to produces devices within specification when operated under challenged conditions.

and seal equipment. Using their knowledge and experience, 10 temperatures, three pressure levels, and five dwell times were investigated, resulting in 150 separate runs. Using a DOE approach it was possible to complete the trial with only limited runs using a fractional factorial array, a classical DOE approach.

Besides the classical DOE school, Taguchi methods provide another route for quality optimization strategy that builds robustness into design entity during the DFSS optimization phase. The Taguchi method is a combination of sound engineering design principles and Taguchi's version of DOE, called an *orthogonal array experiment*. In this chapter we introduce both schools of DOE for transfer function detailing (Chapter 13). Other aspects of DOE methods within DFSS are described by Yang and El-Haik (2003).

DOE is a general form of hypothesis testing (Chapter 3), a method of inferential statistics that tests the viability of a hypothesis about a certain population parameter in the light of experimental data.

14.2 CLASSICAL DESIGN OF EXPERIMENT

In a DOE, we deliberately change experimental factors (those that we can control) and observe their effects on the output responses, the design requirements. Experimental runs are conducted randomly to prevent trends and to allow the factorial effects to reveal their true, unbiased significance. Randomness is a very important aspect of classical DOE, where data collection and result interpretation both depend on this assumption. The data obtained in the experiment are used to fit empirical models relating an output y to the experimental factors, the x's.

Mathematically, we are trying to find the following transfer function relationship:

$$y = f(x_1, x_2, \ldots, x_n) + \varepsilon \qquad (14.1)$$

where ε (lowercase Greek epsilon) represents experimental error or experimental variation. The existence of ε means that there may not be an exact functional relationship between y and $(x_1, x_2, \ldots, x_n)$. This is because the uncontrollable factors $(z_1, z_2, \ldots, z_p)$ will influence the requirement y but are not accounted for in (14.1) and there are experimental and measurement errors in the experiment in both y and $(x_1, x_2, \ldots, x_n)$. A DOE study within a DFSS study road map will follow a multiple-step methodology as described below.

14.2.1 Study Definition

DOE is used in research as well as in product and service optimization settings, although sometimes for very different objectives. The primary purpose in scientific research is usually to show the statistical significance of an effect that a particular factor exerts on the dependent variable of interest (a design requirement denoted as y). In an optimization DOE, the primary objective is usually to extract the maximum amount of *unbiased* information regarding the factors affecting a medical device from as few observations as possible (to minimize cost). While in the research application, DOE techniques are used to uncover the interactive nature of application that is manifested in higher-order interactions of factors (those involving three or more factors). In a robust design variability experiment (Chapter 15), interaction effects are often regarded as a nuisance, as they only complicate the process of identifying significant factors revealed in the main effects.

In either case, this is not trivial. The DFSS team needs to decide on the objective of the DOE study or studies within the DFSS project road map. Do they want to reduce defects? Is it to improve current device performance? What is the study scope within the mapping (Chapter 9)? Do they work on process, or a subprocess? Is one DOE sufficient?

To develop an overall DOE, we suggest the following steps:

1. Define the problem and set the objectives.
2. Select the responses.
3. Select the factors and levels.
4. Identify the noise variables.
5. Select the design strategy.
6. Plan the experiment:
   a. Resources
   b. Supplies
   c. Schedule
   d. Sample size
   e. Risk assessment

Defining the Problem and Setting the Objectives The following process should be followed:

1. Understand the current state of the DFSS project by reviewing and developing an understanding of the technical domains that are active in the medical device or devices being optimized. A review of the physical laws, process and system behaviors, and underlying assumptions is appropriate at this stage.

2. Develop a shared vision for optimizing device functional decomposition or mappings. The team is advised to conduct a step-by-step review of the DOE methodology to understand and reinforce the importance of each strategic activity associated with experimentation and to facilitate consensus on the criteria for completion of each activity.

3. Appreciate what elements of experimental plan development will require the greatest time commitment. The team will also need to discuss the potential impact associated with compromise of the key DOE principles, if any.

4. Plan time allocation. The team needs to develop a work plan that includes timing for several individual DOE sequences if required.

5. Plan time for measurement system(s) verification.

6. Develop a P-diagram for preliminary experimentation to determine the most important sources of variation, including the noise factors.

7. Plan for selection of experimental factors and logistical considerations for building test samples and other elements.

8. Allocate funds to perform the DOE plan. Estimate costs and seek resource approval to conduct the DOE test plan. Budget for multiple optimization experiments.

9. Add something about risk considerations. What effect will experimental conditions have on safety, yield, scrap, and rework? Will they affect the customer, or will they be contained internally? What will happen with the experimental units'? Will they be scrapped or usable?

Selecting the Response   The purpose of describing a medical device in terms of its inputs and outputs is to structure development of the DOE strategy. The description provided by design mapping provides an effective summary as to what level of optimization is taking place, what measurement approach the DOE optimization will be based on, and what major sources of variation influence the medical device. The following actions are suggested:

1. Definition of the DOE responses should be revisited by developing a characterization of boundary conditions and describing the system delivering them in terms of its inputs and outputs using a P-diagram. The description is also a characterization of the basic function of the system, which has been identified in Chapter 9 using the mapping (decomposition or requirement cascade) techniques of the team's choice. The response can be generalized as a measurement characteristic related to the mappings of a device map (e.g., a functional requirement or design parameter). It may be helpful to list various measurement characteristics, which can be viewed as alternative measurement approaches.

2. After study definition, the team needs to select what requirements will be optimized. Here, we explore the case of a single requirement (y). In selecting a response variable, the DFSS team should select the left-hand side of a defined transfer function as depicted in the project design mappings. DOE will be used to detail their design and to provide other useful information about the design under study. It is desirable for the y to be a continuous variable characteristic of the device (e.g., concentration versus color visual judgment). This will make data analysis much easier and more meaningful, and a variable that can be measured easily and accurately.

Choosing Factors, Levels, and Ranges In general, every step used in a device allows for the adjustment of various factors that affect its resulting quality. Experimentation allows a design team to adjust the settings in a systematic manner and to learn which factors have the greatest impact on the resulting functional requirement or design parameter. Using this information, the settings can be improved constantly until optimum quality is obtained.

Factors can be classified as control or noise. *Control factors* are design parameters or process variables which are freely specified by the design team through receiving their knowledge of the concept design and the technology that is being developed for the purpose of device optimization.

There are two types of factors, continuous and discrete. A *continuous factor* can be expressed over a defined real number interval with one continuous motion of the pencil: for example, weight, speed, and price are continuous factors. A *discrete factor* is also called a *categorical variable* or *attribute variable*. For example, types of marketing strategy, types of delivery methods (face to face or via a third party), and types of operating system are discrete factors. Historical information and brainstorming by the team will facilitate a P-diagram listing of potential factors belonging to the categories (response, control, and noise[5]) and aid in structuring the development of a DOE strategy.

A key aspect of DFSS philosophy is that during the design stage, inexpensive parameters can be identified and studied and can be combined in a way that will result in performance that is insensitive to uncontrollable sources of variation. The team's task is to determine the combined best settings (parameter targets) for each of the control parameters that have been judged by the design team to have potential to improve the output(s) of interest. Factors will be selected in a manner that will enable target values to be varied during experimentation with no major impact on medical device cost. The greater the number of potential control factors that are identified, the greater the opportunity for optimization of the functional output in the presence of noise factors.

Identifying the Noise Factors *Noise factors* cause a functional requirement (response y) to deviate from the intended performance or target desired by the customer. Noise factors can be classified into external sources (use and environment), unit-to-unit sources (production and supplier variation), and deterioration sources (wear-out, or the general effects of use over time). A concept used to account for noise factors, advanced by Taguchi within his robustness methodology, is explored in Chapter 15. For a classical DOE setting, the subject of this chapter, it is important to have the design team

---

[5]Robust design classification includes another category not mentioned here: the signal factor. A *signal* is a parameter controlled by the customer/user of the device (or by the output from another device) to express the intended value of response that needs to be produced (Chapter 15).

conduct such a categorization of input factors (both control and noise) and document such a classification in the P-diagram. Selected factors of both categories deemed experimentation candidates by the team are considered as factorial variables in the same array of DOE testing. The idea is to look for interaction between the two categories in order to reduce variation in functional requirements (DOE responses).

In a DOE study, each experimental factor will be changed at least once; that is, each factor will have at least two settings. Otherwise, that factor will not be a variable but a fixed factor in the experiment. The various settings of a factor in the experiment are called *levels*. For a continuous factor, those levels often correspond to different numerical values. For example, thermally heated packaging process for a medical device levels could 205°F, 225°F, and 245°F. For continuous factors, the range of variable is also important; if the range of a variable is too small, we may miss lots of useful information. If the range is too large, the extreme values might give infeasible experimental runs or defective or unusable output. For a discrete variable, the number of levels is often equal to the number of useful choices. For example, in a marketing DOE, if the color of a device is a factor, the number of levels will depend on how many preferred choices there are and which levels the team wants to test in this experiment (e.g., transparent versus colored). The choice of the number of levels in an experiment depends on time and cost considerations. The more levels we have in experimental factors, the more information we get from the experiment, but there will be more experimental runs, leading to higher cost and a longer time to conclusion.

Selecting the Design Strategy   The choice of DOE objectives (recall step 1 of this section) has a profound effect on the decision whether to conduct a research, optimization, or screening DOE. In science and research, the primary focus is on experimental designs with up to perhaps five factors, and more emphasis is focused on the significance of interactions. However, experimentation in industry is broader in implementation, with many factors whose interaction effects cannot be evaluated. The primary focus of the discussion is placed on the derivation of unbiased main effect (and perhaps, two-way) estimates with a minimum number of observations.

Although DOE is used primarily for optimization in the DFSS road map, there are many situations where the knowledge is not profound, and the team may resort to exploring factor relations via a *screening DOE*. In this type of DOE, the objective is to segregate the vital few significant factors while withholding factors known to have little effect. It is not uncommon that very many different factors may potentially be important. Special designs (e.g., Plackett–Burman designs, Taguchi orthogonal arrays) have been developed to screen such large numbers of factors in efficiently, that is, with the least number of observations necessary. For example, you can design and analyze an experiment with n factors and only $n + 1$ runs in which you will be able to estimate the main effects for each factor, and thus can quickly identify which effects are important and most likely to yield improvements in the medical device under study.

A *confirmation DOE* is used to prove the significance of what is found in a screening DOE. In most cases, the confirmation type is used to detail design transfer functions as well as optimization. When a transfer surface is desired rather than a transfer function (Chapter 13), a special optimization technique called *response surface methodology* is generally used to find the optimum design in the design space. In these cases, a *verification DOE* should be performed to confirm the predictability of the transfer function or surface for all responses of interest and that the medical device remains optimum or robust under use conditions.

The purpose of DOE strategy is to coordinate data collection plan into a comprehensive experimentation and all knowledge about the device under development. The plan should be designed to maximize research and development efficiency through use of a sound testing array, functional requirements (responses), and other statistical data analysis.

The DFSS team is encouraged to explore experimentally as many factors as is feasible, to investigate the functional performance potential of the design being adopted from the characterize phase of the DFSS project map. Transferability of the improved functional performance to the customer environment will be maximized as a result of the use of a sound optimization strategy during data collection.

Data from the optimization experiment will be used to generate an analytical model which will aid in improving the design sigma level in the DOE response selected. The validity of this model and the resulting conclusions will be influenced by the experimental and statistical assumptions made by the team. For example, what assumptions can be made regarding the existence of interactions among factor main effects? What assumptions can be made (if any) regarding the underlying distribution of the experimental data? What assumptions can be made regarding the effect of nuisance factors on the variance of the response?

Develop the Measurement Strategy   The objective of developing a measurement strategy is to identify a validated measurement system or systems in order to observe the output of the medical device that is being developed or improved. The measurement strategy is the foundation of any experimentation effort. In optimization DOE, the team should revisit the objective and express (in quantifiable terms) the level of functional performance that is to be expected from the DOE. An opportunity statement for optimized performance translated in terms of improvement will help rationalize cost versus quality trade-offs, should they arise. Note that binary variables (pass/fail) or any discrete (attribute) data are symptoms of poor functional choices and are not experimentally efficient for optimization.

The team needs to validate that the measurement approach has a high strength of association to changing input conditions for the device under design. The way to determine and quantify this association is by using a correlation analysis. The design requirement (y) is measured over a range of input parameter values. The input variable can be any important design parameter, and the analysis can be repeated for additional parameters in an effort to determine the degree of correlation. In this context, measurement repeatability improves with increasing positive correlation. Interpretation of the quality of a measurement system can be accomplished by applying confidence intervals to a plot of y data calculated using data statistics. When statements about the data are bounded by confidence intervals, a much clearer picture can be derived which influences conclusions about what the data are saying. The ability to make precise statements from the data increases with increasing sample sizes. A black belt can calculate the appropriate sample size for a desired confidence region using the statistical methods reviewed in Chapter 3. The following formula can be used to approximate the number of replications[6] (n) that are needed to bring the confidence interval half-width (h_w) down to a certain specified error amount at a certain significance level (α):

$$n = \left(\frac{Z_{\alpha/2}s}{h_w} \right)^2 \tag{14.2}$$

where s is the sample standard deviation.

In analyzing a measurement system, the team needs to assure its repeatability and reproducibility. The team should analyze and verify that the repeatability error of the measurement system is orders of magnitude smaller than the tolerance of interest for the specimens to be measured. Otherwise, it will become difficult to measure the actual effect of design parameter changes during experimentation because the effect on the system response will be masked by excessive measurement error. Taking repeated samples and using the average for a response could reduce the effect of measurement error.

Experimental Design Selection   A number of considerations enter into the various types of designs. In the most general terms, the goal is always to allow the design team to evaluate in an unbiased (or least biased) way the consequences of changing the levels of a particular factor, that is, regardless of how other factors were set. In more technical terms, the team attempts to generate designs where main effects are *unconfounded* among themselves and in some cases, even unconfounded with the interaction of factors.

Experimental methods are finding increasing use in the health care industry to optimize devices, processes, and services. Specifically, the goal of these methods is to identify optimum settings for the various factors that affect an entity of interest. The general representation of the number of experiments

---

[6]To *replicate* is to run each combination of factor levels in the design more than once. This allows estimation of the "pure error" in the experiment.

is l^k, where l is the number of levels of decision variables and k is the number of factors. Using only two levels of each control factor (*low, high*) often results in 2^k factorial designs. The easiest experimental method is to change one design factor while other factors are kept fixed. Factorial design therefore looks at the combined effect of multiple factors on system performance.

Fractional and full factorial DOE are the two types of factorial design. The major classes of designs that are typically used in experimentation are:

- $2k$ full factorial
- 2^{k-p} (two-level, multifactor) designs, screening designs for a large numbers of factors
- 3^{k-p} (three-level, multifactor) designs (mixed designs with two- and three-level factors are also supported)
- Central composite (or response surface) designs
- Latin square designs
- Taguchi robust design analysis[7] (Chapter 15)
- Mixture designs and special procedures for constructing experiments in constrained experimental regions

The type of experimental design selected will depend on the number of factors, the number of levels in each factor, and the total number of experimental runs that can be afforded. In this chapter we consider primarily full factorial designs (2^k type) and fractional factorial designs (2^{k-p} type) on the classical DOE side. If the number of factors and levels are given, full factorial experiment will need more experimental runs, thus be more costly, but it also provides more information about the design under study. The fractional factorial will need fewer runs and thus be less costly, but it will also provide less information about the design (discussed in subsequent sections).

Conduct the Experiment Classical DOE of random effects uses runs (observation) that are created either by running trials of factor combinations or by using representative analytical modeling to simulate the DOE combinations desired. The experimental samples should be as representative of production intent as reasonable (as close to production pedigree as possible).

The sample set utilization described here suggests how many samples are required. The test sample combinations are defined by DOE methods to preserve orthogonality, where the factors are independent of each other and are prepared accordingly. Experimental conditions should be clearly labeled for identification, with consideration for imposed noise factors. A data collection form will help to organize data collection during experimentation. In addition,

---

[7]Interestingly, many of these experimental techniques have made their way from other industries into the health care area, and successful implementations have been reported.

it is important to record and identify the specific experimental combination for each sample. This information can be used to re-create the actual conditions and to regenerate the data if necessary. The team should also record the actual run order to assist in the re-creation of conditions if it should become necessary later in the analysis. To verify the level and precise combination of factor conditions during each experimental trial, a record needs to be collected of the actual conditions for each experimental sample at the time the response data are recorded. When running an experiment, we must complete the following steps:

1. Check the performance of measurement devices.
2. Check that all planned runs are feasible.
3. Watch out for possible drifts and shifts during the run.
4. Avoid unplanned changes (e.g., swap operators halfway through).
5. Allow time (and backup material) for unexpected events.
6. Get all parties involved to buy-in.
7. Preserve all the raw data.
8. Record everything that happens.
9. After the experiment has been completed, reset all factors to their original state.

Analysis of DOE Raw Data There are several statistical methods of analyzing designs with random effects. The ANOVA technique discusses numerous options for estimating variance components for random effects and for performing approximate hypothesis tests using F-tests based on synthesized error terms. Statistical methods will be used. A large portion of this chapter is dedicated to how to analyze the data from a statistically designed experiment. From an analysis of experimental data, we are able to identify the significant main and interactions effects, the arguments of the transfer function or transfer surface. Not all the factors are the same in terms of their effects on the output. When the DFSS team changes the level of a factor, if its impact on the response is relatively small compared with inherited experimental variation due to uncontrollable noise factors and experimental error, this factor might be insignificant. If a factor has a large impact on both the response mean and the variance, it might be significant. Sometimes, two or more factors may have interactions; in this case, their effects on the output will be complex. However, it is also possible that none of the experimental factors are found to be significant, in which case the experiment is inconclusive in finding influential factors, yet leaves us with a knowledge of factors that are not significant. This situation may indicate that we may have missed important factors in the experiment. DOE data analysis can identify significant and insignificant factors by using ANOVA; that is, the DFSS team will be able to rank the relative importance of factor effects and their interactions using ANOVA with a numerical score.

As a typical output, DOE data analysis provides an empirical mathematical transfer function relating the output (y) to experimental factors. The form of transfer function could be linear or polynomial with significant interactions. DOE data analysis can also provide graphical representations of the mathematical relationship between experimental factors and output, in the form of main effect charts and interaction charts.

Additionally, if there were an ideal direction of goodness for the output, for example, if y were customer satisfaction, the direction of goodness for y would be the higher, the better. By using the mathematical transfer function model, DOE data analysis identifies the best setting of experimental factors to achieve the best possible result for the output.

An advantage of using DOE for optimization includes the ability to use statistical software to develop the transfer function to make predictions about any combination of the factors in between and slightly beyond the various levels, and to generate types of informative two- and three-dimensional plots. In addition, the design team needs to be aware of the fact that DOEs do not compare results directly against a control or standard. They evaluate all effects and interactions and determine if there are statistically significant differences among them. Statistical confidence intervals can be calculated for each response optimized. A large effect might result, but if the statistical error for that measurement is high, the effect will not be believed. In other words, we get a large change in output but cannot be certain that it was due to anything that we did.

Conclusions and Recommendations   Once the data analysis has been completed, the DFSS team can draw practical conclusions about the study. If the data analysis provides enough information, we might be able to make recommendations for some changes in the design to improve its robustness and performance. Sometimes the data analysis cannot provide enough information and additional experiments may need to be run. When the experimental analysis is complete, one must verify whether or not the conclusions are good. These are the validation or confirmation runs. The interpretation and conclusions from an experiment may include a "best" setting to use to meet the goals of the experiment. Even if this setting has been included in the experiment, you should run it again as part of the confirmation runs to make sure that nothing has changed and that the response values are close to their predicted values. Typically, it is very desirable to have a stable performance. Therefore, one should run more than one test at the best or optimum factorial settings. A minimum of three runs should be conducted. If the time between actually running the experiments and conducting the confirmation runs is more than the average time span between the experimental runs, the DFSS team must be careful to ensure that nothing else has changed since the original data collection. If the confirmation runs don't produce the results expected, the team needs to verify that they have the correct settings for the confirmation runs, revisit the transfer function model to verify the best settings from the analysis, and verify that they had the correct predicted value for the confirmation runs. Otherwise, the transfer function model may not predict very well in the defined design space. Nevertheless, the team still learns from the experiment and should use the information gained to design another follow-up or substitute experiment.

14.3 FACTORIAL EXPERIMENT

In the DFSS project road map (Chapter 7), an experimental design is usually checked for optimization (i.e., to produce a credible transfer function or surface plot). This usually means determining how an output of a medical device responds to a change in some factor. In addition, a DOE is conducted following the DFSS optimization phase to validate or confirm the transfer function obtained. In either case, careful planning (Section 14.2) at the outset of the DOE will save a great deal of resources.

If the response (y) under consideration is dependent on one factor, the DOE strategy is simple: Conduct an experiment by varying the factor and measure the corresponding response at these values. A transfer function is obtained by fitting a line or a curve to the experimental observations. In a classical DOE, the best factor levels are used to obtain a certain level of information, the predictive equation or the transfer function. The proper choice of experimental conditions increases the information obtained from the experiment. The recognition and measurement of interactions is of real value in the study of devices where interaction is common. A DOE can also be used to reduce the resources needed in experimenting by eliminating redundant observations, ending up with approximately the same amount of information from fewer experimental runs.

Most experiments involve two or more experimental factors. In this case, factorial designs are the most frequently used. By a factorial design, we mean that all combinations of factor levels will be tested in the experiment. For example, if we have two factors in the experiment, factors A and B, each having multiple levels (A has a levels and B has b levels), then in a factorial experiment, we are going to test all ab combinations. In each combination, we may duplicate the experiment several times, say, n times. Then there are n replicates in the experiment. If $n = 1$, the experiment is called a *single replicate*. Therefore, for two factors, the total number of experimental observations (runs) is equal to abn. For example, in an experiment of two factors, factors A and B, with each factor at two levels, the number of runs equals $2 \times 2 \times n = 4n$. In general, a two-factor factorial experiment has the arrangement shown in Table 14.1. Each cell of Table 14.1 corresponds to a distinct factor-level combination, known as a *treatment* in DOE terminology.

TABLE 14.1 General Arrangement for a Two-factor factorial Design

Factor	Factor B			
A	1	2	...	b
1	Y_{111}	Y_{121}	...	Y_{1b1}
	Y_{112}	Y_{122}	...	Y_{1b2}
2	Y_{211}	Y_{221}	...	Y_{2b1}
	Y_{212}	Y_{222}	...	Y_{2b2}
...	:	:	:	:
a	Y_{a11}	Y_{a21}	...	Y_{ab1}
	Y_{a12}	Y_{a22}	...	Y_{ab2}

14.3.1 Mathematical Transfer Function

If we denote A as x_1 and B as x_2, one possible mathematical transfer function model is

$$y = f_1(x_1) + f_2(x_2) + f_{12}(x_1, x_2) + \varepsilon \qquad (14.3)$$

Here $f_1(x_1)$ is the main effect of A, $f_2(x_2)$ is the main effect of B, and $f_{12}(x_1, x_2)$ is the interaction of A and B.

14.3.2 Interaction Between Factors

An interaction between factors occurs when the change in response from the one level to another level of one factor is not the same as the change in response at the same two levels of a second factor (i.e., the effect of one factor is dependent on a second factor). Interaction plots are used to compare the relative strength of the effects across factors.

If there is no interaction, a transfer function with two parameters can be written as

$$y = f_1(x_1) + f_2(x_2) + \varepsilon \qquad (14.4)$$

where $f_1(x_1)$ is a function of x_1 alone, and $f_1(x_2)$ is a function of x_2 alone, we call the model an *additive model* (Chapter 13). However, if the interaction effect is not equal to zero, we do not have an additive transfer function model. Figure 14.2 depicts several interaction plot scenarios. In case (a), the response is constant at the three levels of factor A but differs for the two levels of factor B. Thus, there is no main effect of factor A, but a factor B main effect is present. In case (b), the mean responses differ at the levels of factor A, but the means are almost equal at the levels of factor B. In cases (c) and (d) both factors affect the response (y). In case (c), the mean response difference between the factor B levels varies with the factor A levels. The effect on response depends on factor B, and therefore the two factors interact. In case

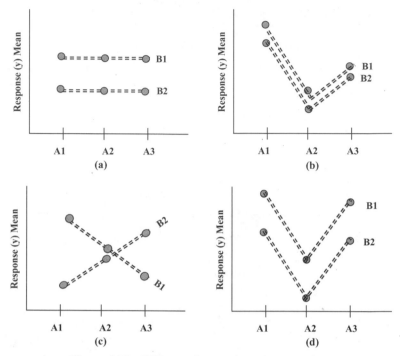

Figure 14.2   Different interaction plot scenarios.

(d), the effect of factor A on the response (*y*) is independent of factor B; that is, the two factors do not interact.

The greater the departure of the lines from the parallel state, the higher the degree of interaction. Interaction can be synergistic or nonsynergistic. In the former the effect of taking both factors together is more than the added effects of taking them separately; and vice versa for the nonsynergistic case. In both, the corresponding interaction plots are not parallel. Lack of interaction can be depicted by parallel lines in an interaction plot.

Let's look at an example. In reference to the Auto 3D device case study (Chapter 20), during the design of the disposable subsystem, the product development team wanted to understand the impact on flow rate when changing to the diluent's concentration under different sterilization dose and environmental conditioning factors. Figure 14.3 shows the interaction relationship between the diluent concentration, sterilization dose, and environmental conditioning. The plot shows a strong interaction between diluent concentration and both sterilization dose and environmental conditioning but, as expected, no interaction between environmental conditioning and sterilization dose.

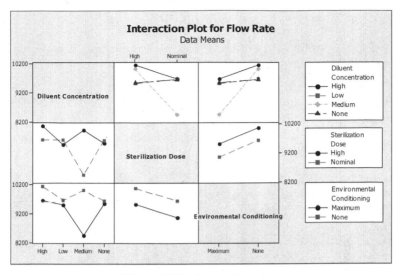

Figure 14.3 Interaction plot.

14.4 ANALYSIS OF VARIANCE

Analysis of variance[8] (ANOVA) is used to investigate and model the relationship between a response variable (y) and one or more independent factors. In effect, ANOVA extends the two-sample t-test for testing the equality of two population means to a more general null hypothesis of comparing the equality of more than two means versus them not all being equal. ANOVA includes procedures for fitting ANOVA models to data collected from a number of different designs and graphical analysis for testing an equal-variance assumption, confidence interval plots, and graphs of main effects and interactions.

For a set of experimental data, the data probably varies due to changing of experimental factors, while some of the variation might be caused by unknown or unaccounted for factors, experimental measurement errors, or variation within the controlled factors themselves.

Several assumptions need to be satisfied for ANOVA to be credible:

1. The probability distributions of the response (y) for each factor level combination (treatment) is normal.
2. The response (y) variance is constant for all treatments.
3. The samples of experimental units selected for the treatments must be random and independent.

[8]ANOVA differs from regression in two ways: The independent variables are qualitative (categorical), and no assumption is made about the nature of the relationship (i.e., the model does not include coefficients for variables).

The ANOVA method produces the following:

1. A decomposition of the total variation of the experimental data to its possible sources (main effect, interaction, or experimental error)
2. A quantification of the variation due to each source
3. Calculation of significance [i.e., which main effects and interactions have significant effects on response (y) data variation]
4. Transfer function when the factors are continuous variables (noncategorical in nature)

ANOVA Steps in a Two-Factor Completely Randomized Experiment (Yang and El-Haik, 2003)

Step 1 Decompose the total variation in the DOE response (y) data to its sources (treatment sources: factor A, factor B, factor A × factor B interaction, and error). The first step in ANOVA is a sum of squares calculation which produces variation decomposition. The following mathematical equations are needed:

$$\bar{y}_{i..} = \frac{\sum_{j=1}^{b} \sum_{k=1}^{n} y_{ijk}}{bn} \text{ (row average)} \tag{14.5}$$

$$\bar{y}_{.j.} = \frac{\sum_{i=1}^{a} \sum_{k=1}^{n} y_{jik}}{an} \text{ (column average)} \tag{14.6}$$

$$\bar{y}_{ij.} = \frac{\sum_{k=1}^{n} y_{ijk}}{n} \text{ (treatment or cell average)} \tag{14.7}$$

$$\bar{y}_{...} = \frac{\sum_{i=1}^{a} \sum_{j=1}^{b} \sum_{k=1}^{n} y_{ijk}}{abn} \text{ (overall average)} \tag{14.8}$$

It can be shown that

$$\underbrace{\sum_{i=1}^{a} \sum_{j=1}^{b} \sum_{k=1}^{n} (y_{ijk} - \bar{y}_{...})^2}_{SS_T} = \underbrace{bn \sum_{i=1}^{a} (\bar{y}_{i..} - \bar{y}_{...})^2}_{SS_A} + \underbrace{an \sum_{j=1}^{b} (\bar{y}_{.j.} - \bar{y}_{...})^2}_{SS_B}$$

$$+ \underbrace{n \sum_{i=1}^{a} \sum_{j=1}^{b} (\bar{y}_{ij.} - \bar{y}_{i..} - \bar{y}_{.j.} + \bar{y}_{...})^2}_{SS_{AB}} + \underbrace{\sum_{i=1}^{a} \sum_{j=1}^{b} \sum_{k=1}^{n} (y_{ijk} - \bar{y}_{ij.})^2}_{SSE}$$

$$\tag{14.9}$$

or simply,

$$SS_T = SS_A + SS_B + SS_{AB} + SSE \qquad (14.10)$$

SS_T denotes the total sum of squares, which is a measure for the total variation in the whole data set; SS_A is the sum of squares due to factor A, which is a measure of total variation caused by main effect of A; SS_B is the sum of squares due to factor B, which is a measure of total variation caused by main effect of B; SS_{AB} is the sum of squares due to factor A and B interaction (denoted as AB) as a measure of variation caused by interaction; and SSE is the sum of squares due to error, which is the measure of total variation due to error, all shown here together with their degrees of freedom:

$$
\text{total sum of squares, } SS_T \atop DF = abn-1
\ =
\begin{cases}
\text{factor A sum of squares (SS}_A) \\
DF = a-1 \\
+ \\
\text{factor B sum of squares (SS}_B) \\
DF = b-1 \\
+ \\
\text{interaction AB sum of squares (SS}_{AB}) \\
DF = (a-1)(b-1) \\
+ \\
\text{error sum of squares (SSE)} \\
DF = ab(n-1)
\end{cases}
$$

Step 2   Test the null hypothesis toward the significance of the factor A mean effect and factor B mean effect as well as their interaction. The vehicle of test is the mean square calculations. The *mean square* of a source of variation is calculated by dividing the source of variation sum of squares by its degrees of freedom.

The actual amount of variability in the response data depends on the data size. A convenient way of expressing this dependence is to say that the sum of squares has degrees of freedom (df) equal to its corresponding variability source data size reduced by one. Based on statistics, the number of degrees of freedom associated with each sum of squares is as given in Table 14.2.

TABLE 14.2   Degrees of Freedom for a Two-Factor Factorial Design

Effect	Degrees of Freedom
A	$a-1$
B	$b-1$
AB interaction	$(a-1)(b-1)$
Error	$ab(n-1)$
Total	$abn-1$

Test for main effect of factor A:
H_0: no difference among the mean levels of factor A ($\mu_{A1} = \mu_{A2} = \ldots = \mu_{Aa}$)
H_a: at least two factor A mean levels differ

Test for main effect of factor B:
H_0: no difference among the mean levels of factor B ($\mu_{B1} = \mu_{B2} = \ldots = \mu_{Ba}$)
H_a: at least two factor B mean levels differ

Test for main effect of factor A × factor B interaction:
H_0: factors A and B do not interact in the response mean
H_a: factors A and B interact in the response mean

Step 3 Compare the *F*-test of the mean square of the experimental treatment sources to the error to test the null hypothesis that the treatment means are equal.

- If the test results in nonrejection of the null hypothesis, refine the experiment by increasing the number of replicates (n) or by adding other factors if the response is unrelated to the two factors.

In the *F*-test, the term F_0 will be compared with $F_{critical}$, defining the null hypothesis rejection region values with the appropriate degrees of freedom. If F_0 is larger than the critical value, the corresponding effect is statistically significant. Several statistical software packages, such as Minitab, can be used to analyze DOE data conveniently; spreadsheet packages such as Excel can also be used.

In ANOVA, a sum of squares is divided by its corresponding degrees of freedom to produce the mean square, which is used in the *F*-test to see if the corresponding effect is statistically significant. An ANOVA is often summarized in a table similar to Table 14.3.

TABLE 14.3 ANOVA Table

Source of Variation	Sum of Squares	Degree of Freedom	Mean Square	F_0
A	SS_A	$a - 1$	$MS_A = \dfrac{SS_A}{a-1}$	$F_0 = \dfrac{MS_A}{MSE}$
B	SS_B	$b - 1$	$MS_B = \dfrac{SS_B}{b-1}$	$F_0 = \dfrac{MS_B}{MSE}$
AB	SS_{AB}	$(a-1)(b-1)$	$MS_{AB} = \dfrac{SS_{AB}}{(a-1)(b-1)}$	$F_0 = \dfrac{MS_{AB}}{MSE}$
Error	SSE	$ab(n-1)$		
Total	SS_T	$abn - 1$		

Test for main effect of factor A:

Test Statistic: $F_{0,a-1,ab(n-1)} = MS_A/MS_E$ with a numerator Df of $a - 1$ and a denominator df of $ab(n - 1)$.

H_0 hypothesis rejection region: $F_{0,a-1,ab(n-1)} \geq F_{\alpha,a-1,ab(n-1)}$ with a numerator Df of $a - 1$ and a denominator df of $ab(n - 1)$.

Test for main effect of factor B:

Test statistic: $F_{0,b-1,ab(n-1)} = MS_B/MSE$ with a numerator Df of $b - 1$ and a denominator df of $ab(n - 1)$.

H_0 hypothesis rejection region: $F_{0,b-1,ab(n-1)} \geq F_{\alpha,b-1,ab(n-1)}$ with a numerator df of $b - 1$ and a denominator df of $ab(n - 1)$.

Test for main effect of factor A × factor B interaction:

Test statistic: $F_{0,(a-1)(b-1),ab(n-1)} = MS_{AB}/MS_E$ with a numerator df of $(a - 1)(b - 1)$ and a denominator df of $ab(n - 1)$.

H_0 hypothesis rejection region: $F_{0,(a-1)(b-1),ab(n-1)} \geq F_{\alpha,(a-1)(b-1),ab(n-1)}$ with a numerator df of $(a - 1)(b - 1)$ and denominator df of $ab(n - 1)$.

The interaction null hypothesis is tested first by computing the F-test of the mean square for interaction with the mean square for error. If the test results in nonrejection of the null hypothesis, proceed to test the main effects of the factors. If the test results in rejection of the null hypothesis, we conclude that the two factors interact in the mean response (y). If the test of interaction is significant, a multiple comparison method such as Tukey's grouping procedure can be used to compare any or all pairs of the treatment means.

Next, test the two null hypotheses that the mean response is the same at each level of factors A and B by computing the F-test of the mean square for each factor main effect to the mean square for error. If one or both tests result in rejection of the null hypothesis, we conclude that the factor affects the mean response (y). If both tests result in nonrejection, an apparent contradiction has occurred. Although the treatment means apparently differ, the interaction and main effect tests have not supported that result. Further experimentation is advised. If the test for one or both main effects is significant, a multiple comparison such as Tukey's grouping procedure is used to compare the pairs of the means corresponding to the levels of the significant factor(s).

The results and data analysis methods discussed above can be extended to the general case where there are a levels of factor A, b levels of factor B, c levels of factor C, and so on, arranged in a factorial experiment. There will be $abc \ldots n$ total trials if there are n replicates. Clearly, the number of trials needed to run the experiment will increase very fast with the increase in number of factors and number of levels. In practical application, we rarely use a general full factorial experiment for more than two factors. Two-level factorial experiments are the most popular experimental methods.

In the ANOVA table given in Table 14.4, there are three effects: factor A, cycle volume; factor B, push velocity; and factor C, temperature. The larger

TABLE 14.4   ANOVA Table

Source of Variation	Sum of Squares	Degrees of Freedom	Mean Square	F	p-Value
Factor A: cycle volume	6780.67	3	2260.22	217.12	0.005
Factor B: push velocity	32.00	1	32.00	3.07	0.222
Factor C: temperature	2303.51	1	2303.51	221.28	0.004
Error	20.82	2	10.41		
Total	9137.00	7			

the sum of squares of a treatment effect, the more variation is caused by that effect, and the more important the effect is. In this example, the sum of squares for cycle volume is 6780.67 $(mm^3)^2$, the sum of squares for push velocity is 32.00 $(mm/s)^2$, and the sum of squares for temperature is 2303.51 $(°F)^2$. From the ANOVA table, the F-test is a better measure of relative importance and the p-value can be used to determine if a factor effect is statistically significant.

Note that the most commonly used criterion is to compare the p-value at the 5% significance level. If the p-value is less than 5%, the effect is significant. In this example the F-test value for cycle volume is 217.12 and the p-value is 0.5%, which indicates statistical significance; in addition, the F-test value for push velocity is 3.07 and the p-value is 22.2%, which indicates statistical insignificance; nevertheless, the F-test value for temperature is 221.28 and the p-value is 0.4%, which also indicates statistical significance.

Overall, the results of the ANOVA table show that both cycle volume and temperature have a significant impact on the response variable, whereas the push velocity has no impact on the same response variable.

14.5 2^K FULL FACTORIAL DESIGNS

In many cases, it is sufficient to consider the factors affecting a device at two levels. For example, the patient for a device may be male or female; adult or a child, and so on. The black belt would like to determine whether any of these changes affect the results of a system. The most intuitive approach to studying those factors would be to vary the factors of interest in a full factorial design, that is, to try all possible combinations of levels. Such experiment is called 2^k, which is an experiment with k factors each with two levels; that is, the number of treatment combinations in a two-level full factorial of k factors is $2 \times 2 \dots 2 = 2^k$. If there are n replicates at each treatment combination, the total number of experimental trials is $2^k n$. Because there are only two levels for each factor, we call them the low and high levels. For example, if a factor is "age," with two levels, "child" and "adult," then "child" is the low level and "adult" is the high level.

TABLE 14.5 2^2 Experimental Design

Run Number	$A(X_1)$	$A(X_2)$
1	−1	−1
2	+1	−1
3	−1	+1
4	+1	+1

Two-level factorial designs are the most popular because it is a full factorial design with the least number of runs, an ideal situation for screening experiments. The two-level factorial designs are the basis of the fractional factorial designs that are discussed next.

The number of necessary runs in a full 2^k experiment will increase geometrically. For example, if the black belt wants to study seven factors, the necessary number of runs in the experiment would be $2^7 = 128$. To study 10 factors, he or she would need $2^{10} = 1024$ runs in the experiment. Because each run may require time-consuming and costly setting and resetting of the medical device, it is often not feasible to require that many different runs for the experiment. In these conditions, fractional factorials are used that sacrifice interaction effects so that main effects may still be computed correctly.

The standard layout for a two-level design uses a binary notation with +1 and −1 notation denoting the high and low levels, respectively, for each factor. For example, Table 14.5 describes an experiment in which four trials (or runs) were conducted, with each factor set to high or low during a run according to whether the matrix had a +1 or −1 set for the factor during that trial. The substitution of +1 and −1 for the factor levels is called *coding*. This aids in the interpretation of the coefficients and helps mathematically to fit a transfer function experimental model. Also note in Table 14.5 use of the functional argument of X_1 and X_2, which denotes the coding of a hypothetical factor A and factor B, respectively.

14.5.1   Design Layout

If the experiment had more than two factors, there would be additional columns in the layout matrix corresponding to the extra factors (i.e., a column per factor). In a full 2^k factorial design, the number of distinct experimental runs, $N = 2^k$. For example, if $k = 4$, then $N = 2^4 = 16$; if $k = 5$, then $N = 2^5 = 32$; and so on.

Table 14.6 gives a standard layout for a 2^4 factorial experiment. The run number is sequenced by standard order, which is featured by the sequence −1 +1 −1 +1 . . . for factor A, −1 −1 +1 +1 for factor B, −1 −1 −1 −1 and +1 +1 +1 +1 for factor c, and so on. In general, for a 2^k experiment, the first column starts with −1 and alternates in sign for all 2^k runs; the second column starts with −1 repeated twice and then alternates with 2 in a row of the opposite sign

TABLE 14.6   Experimental Layout for a 2^4 Design

Run No.	A	B	C	D	1	2	...	n	Response Total[a]
	Factor				Replicate				
1	−1	−1	−1	−1					(1)
2	1	−1	−1	−1					a
3	−1	1	−1	−1					b
4	1	1	−1	−1					ab
5	−1	−1	1	−1					c
6	1	−1	1	−1					ac
7	−1	1	1	−1					bc
8	1	1	1	−1					abc
9	−1	−1	−1	1					d
10	1	−1	−1	1					ad
11	−1	1	−1	1					bd
12	1	1	−1	1					abd
13	−1	−1	1	1					cd
14	1	−1	1	1					acd
15	−1	1	1	1					bcd
16	1	1	1	1					abcd

[a]Computed by adding the replicate row in a given run.

until all 2^k places are filled; the third column starts with −1 repeated four times, then four repeats of +1's and so on; the ith column starts with 2^{i-1} repeats of −1 followed by 2^{i-1} repeats of +1; and so on. This is known as *Yates' standard order*.

Every run (simultaneously experimenting combination of factorial levels) can also be represented by the symbols in the last column of the table, where the symbol depends on the corresponding levels of each factor.

14.5.2   Data Analysis

For a 2^k full factorial experiment, the numerical calculations for ANOVA, main effect chart, interaction chart, and mathematical transfer function model become easier, compared with a general full factorial experiment. Here we give a step-by-step procedure for the entire data analysis.

14.5.3   DOE Application

Many disposable parts in the medical device applications use injection molding parts. Shrinkage, y, is often a major problem, and often a molded die for parts is built larger than nominal size to allow for part shrinkage. In the following experimental situation a new die is being produced, and it is important to find the injection molding parameters that minimize mold shrinkage. In the following experiment the response values are deviations from nominal.

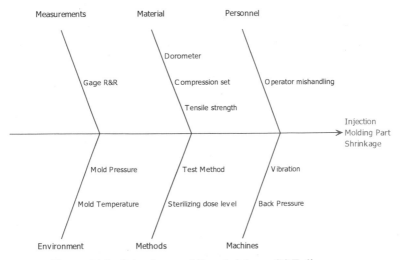

Figure 14.4   Injection molding shrinkage C&E diagram.

TABLE 14.7   DOE Factors and Levels

Factor Name	Measurement Unit	Low Level	High Level
A: injection velocity	in./sec	10 (−1)	25 (1)
B: mold temperature	°F	212 (−1)	302 (1)
C: mold pressure	psi	450 (−1)	1000 (1)

The design and development team created a cause-and-effect diagram (see Appendix 4A) to list all possible factors (controllable and uncontrollable), which has potential effects on mold shrinkage. Figure 14.4 show an injection molding shrinkage cause-and-effect diagram. The factors mold temperature, mold pressure, and injection velocity were selected to be included in a preliminary screening experiment from which the factors for a more complete analysis could be determined. Table 14.7 lists the screening factors and their associated levels. The response of the experiment is measured as the difference from a nominal value of a critical-to-quality dimension, which here we call *shrinkage*.

Step 1: Preparation   First develop an analysis matrix for data collection. For example, in a 2^3 factorial experiment, the analysis matrix is shown in Table 14.8. Interaction columns are obtained by multiplying the corresponding columns of factors involved. Interaction columns are not shown in Table 14.8, for formatting reasons.

Step 2: Compute Contrasts

$$\text{Contrast}_A = -(1) + a - b + ab - c + ac - bc + abc = 5.59294$$

$$\text{Contrast}_B = -(1) - a + b + ab - c - ac + bc + abc = 6.11858$$

TABLE 14.8 Screening Factors and Response

Run	A: Injection Velocity	B: Mold Temperature	C: Mold Pressure	Shrinkage (in × 1000) Rep. 1	Rep. 2	Total
1	−1	−1	−1	3.88233	3.94833	(1) = 7.83066
2	1	−1	−1	3.83211	3.94708	a = 7.77919
3	−1	1	−1	4.06448	4.09293	b = 8.15741
4	1	1	−1	4.97790	5.09239	ab = 10.07029
5	−1	−1	1	3.80594	3.92012	c = 7.72606
6	1	−1	1	3.77069	3.95922	ac = 7.72991
7	−1	1	1	3.78831	3.82620	bc = 7.61451
8	1	1	1	5.60662	5.73557	abc = 11.34219

$$\text{Contrast}_C = -(1) - a - b - ab + c + ac + bc + abc = 0.57512$$

$$\text{Contrast}_{AB} = (1) - a - b + ab + c - ac - bc + abc = 5.68818$$

$$\text{Contrast}_{AC} = (1) - a + b - ab - c + ac - bc + abc = 1.87012$$

$$\text{Contrast}_{BC} = (1) + a - b - ab - c - ac + bc + abc = 0.88287$$

$$\text{Contrast}_{ABC} = (1) + a + b - ab + c - ac - bc + abc = 1.75948$$

Step 3: Compute Effects Effects are calculated using the Minitab, alias structure:

Alias Structure I =
Injection Velocity
Mold Temperature
Mold Pressure
Injection Velocity * Mold Temperature
Injection Velocity * Mold Pressure
Mold Temperature * Mold Pressure
Injection Velocity * Mold Temperature * Mold Pressure

The factorial effects are:

Injection Velocity = 0.69033

Mold Temperature = 0.84861

Mold Pressure = 0.06060
Injection Velocity × Mold Temperature = 0.62724

Injection Velocity × Mold Pressure = 0.24505

Mold Temperature × Mold Pressure = 0.12407

Injection Velocity × Mold Temperature × Mold Pressure = 0.20622

A normal probability plot and a Pareto chart for factor effects are shown in Figures 14.5 and 14.6. From these we can conclude that injection velocity,

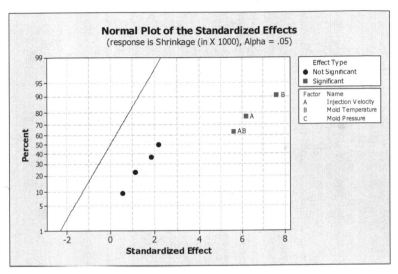

Figure 14.5 Normal probability plot of factor effects.

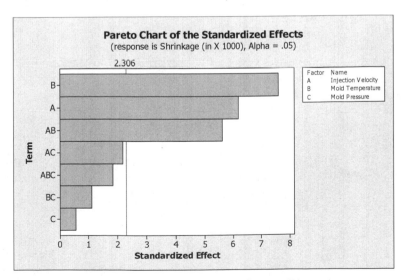

Figure 14.6 Pareto chart of factor effects.

TABLE 14.9 ANOVA Table of the DOE Model

Source of Variation	Sum of Squares	Degrees of Freedom	Mean Square	F-Test	p-Value
Main effects	4.8015	3	1.60050	32.29	0.000
Two-way interactions	1.8755	3	0.62516	12.61	0.002
Three-way interactions	0.1701	1	0.17011	3.43	0.101
Residual error	0.3966	8	0.04957		
Total	7.2436	15			

TABLE 14.10 Effects and Coefficients Table of the DOE Model

Term	Effect	Coefficient	p-Value
Constant	—	4.27003	0.000
Injection velocity	0.69033	0.34517	0.000
Mold temperature	0.84861	0.42431	0.000
Mold pressure	0.06060	0.03030	0.601
Injection velocity × mold temperature	0.62724	0.31362	0.000
Injection velocity × mold pressure	0.24505	0.12252	0.059
Mold temperature × mold pressure	0.12407	0.06204	0.297
Injection velocity × mold temperature × mold pressure	0.20622	0.10311	0.101

mold temperature, and the interaction between injection velocity and mold temperature stand out as significant effects.

Step 4: Compute the Sum of Squares See Table 14.9.

Step 5: Complete the ANOVA Table ANOVA for the shrinkage response shows that significant main effects and two-way interactions exist in the screening DOE model, as shown in Table 14.9. Further flow-down in the ANOVA for each of the main effects and their associated interactions is shown in Table 14.10. The analysis of variance depicts the same conclusion as that of the normal probability plot along with the Pareto chart of effects.

Step 6: Plot Main Effects and Interaction Charts for All Significant Effects See Figures 14.7 and 14.8.

Step 7: Validate ANOVA assumes that the data collected are normally and independently distributed with the same variance in each treatment combination or factor level. These assumptions can be evaluated by the residuals defined as $e_{ijl} = y_{ijl} - \bar{y}_{ij}$. That is, the residual is just the difference between the observations and the corresponding treatment combination (cell) averages (Hines and Montgomery, 1990).

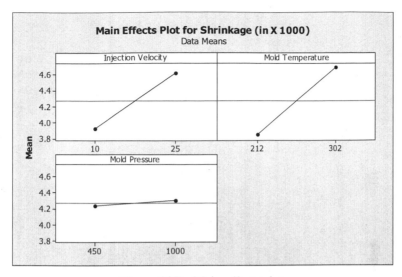

Figure 14.7 Main effects plot.

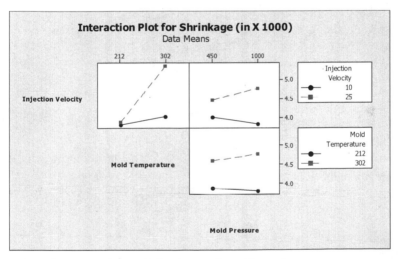

Figure 14.8 Interaction effects plot.

Plotting the residuals on normal probability paper, looking for a straight-line fit, can check the normality assumption. To check the assumption of equal variance at each factor level, we plot the residual against the factor levels and compare the spread in the residuals. It is also useful to plot the residuals against fitted values or treatment combination averages. The variability in the residuals should not in any way depend on the value of cell averages. When a pattern appears in those plots, indicating nonnormality, it suggests the need for transformation, that is, analyzing the data in a different metric

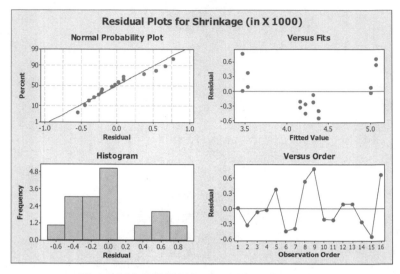

Figure 14.9　ANOVA assumption diagnostics.

or dimension. In some problems the dependency of residuals scatter in fitted values is very important. We would like to select the level that improves y in the direction of goodness; however, this level may also cause more variation in y from observation to observation.

Plotting the residuals against the time or run order in which the DOE was performed can check the independence assumption. A pattern in this plot such as a sequence of positive and negative residuals may indicate that the observations are not independent. This indicates that the time or run order is important, or factors that change over time are important and have not been included in the DOE.

Figure 14.9 presents the residual analysis. The normal probability plot of these residuals does not appear to deviate from normality. The graph of residuals versus fitted values does not reveal any unusual pattern. See Appendix 14A for comments on DOE graphical analysis.

Step 8: Establish Transfer Function Model　Similar to regression, ANOVA involves statistical analysis of the relationship between a response and one or more factors. It is not surprising to formulate ANOVA as a regression analysis. We can establish a regression transfer function model for the DOE data. Here are the rules:

1. Only significant effects are included in the model. If A and AB are significant, all factorial effects that include B are in (e.g., without B, we cannot have AB).
2. We use the mathematical variable x_1 to express A, x_2 for B, x_3 for C, and so on. The mathematical variables x_1x_2 represent AB interaction; x_1x_3, AC interaction; $x_1x_2x_3$, ABC interaction; and so on.

With y = shrinkage response, X_1 = injection velocity, X_2 = mold temperature, and X_3 = mold pressure, and from Table 14.10, we can define the response transfer function as follows:

$$\text{shrinkage (in multiples of 1000)} = y$$
$$\cong 4.27003 + 0.34517x_1 + 0.42431x_2 + 0.31362x_1x_2$$

Step 9: Determine Optimal Settings Depending on the objective of the problem, we can determine the optimum setting of the factor levels by examining the main effects and interactions plots. If there is no interaction, the optimal setting can be determined by looking at one factor at a time. If there are interactions, we have to look at the interaction plot first. For this example, since we want to minimize shrinkage, we will set the injection velocity at 10 in./sec and the mold temperature at 212°F. Other nonsignificant factors can be set based on other criteria, such as economy or ease of operation.

Note that these optimal settings are based on mean or central tendency ANOVA analysis. A similar study can be conducted on the variability of the requirement, which is not presented here. According to the Six Sigma Professionals, Inc.[9] training material the two analyses need to be contrasted against each other to decide on the final optimal setting.

14.5.4 The 2^3 Design

A two-level full factorial design of three factors is classified as a 2^3 design. This design has eight runs. Graphically, we can represent the 2^3 design by the cube shown in Figure 14.10. The arrows show the direction of increase of the factors. The numbers 1 through 8 at the corners of the design box refer to the standard order of the runs. In general, cube plots can be used to show the

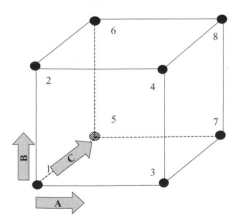

Figure 14.10 A 2^3 full factorial design with factors A, B, and C.

[9]www.SixSigmaPI.com.

relationships among two to eight factors for two-level factorial or Plackett–Burman designs.

As the number of control factors increase, full factorial design may lead to running huge numbers of trials even when using only two levels of each factor. This is particularly critical when running multiple replications at each factor–level combination. For example, experimenting with 10 control factors, each with two levels, requires $2^{10} = 1024$ experiments. Running only five replications at this factorial design will result in 5120 runs, which requires significant time and computations. Hence, strategies of factor screening and developing fractional factorial design are often used to cope with a large number of control factors.

14.5.5 The 2^3 Design with Center Points

Center points are usually added as in Figure 14.11 to validate the assumption in a 2^k factorial design concerning the linearity of factorial effects. In a 2^k factorial design this assumption can be satisfied approximately rather than being exact. The addition of center points of n_C replicates to a factorial design is the team's insurance against unknown curvature (nonlinearity) while providing an error estimate without affecting the factorial effects estimation.

In a 2^k design, center points are represented by $(0, 0, 0, \ldots, 0)$, indicating the design center as in Figure 14.12. For k quantitative factors, let $\bar{y}_F$ be the average of the 2^k factorial points and let $\bar{y}_C$ be the average of the n_C center points. When the difference $\bar{y}_F - \bar{y}_C$ is large, the center points lie far from the planes passing through the factorial points and curvature exists. A single

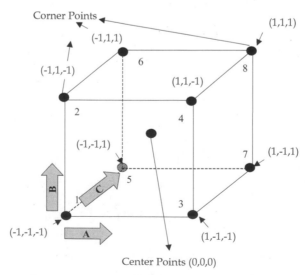

Figure 14.11 A 2^3 full factorial design with factors A, B, and C and center points.

degree of freedom is usually given for the sum of squares of nonlinearity or curvature that can be calculated using

$$SS_{\text{curvature}} = \frac{n_F n_C (\bar{y}_F - \bar{y}_C)}{n_F n_C} \tag{14.11}$$

with $n_C - 1$ degrees of freedom and n_F is the number of factorial design points. For a 2^3 design, $n_F = 8$. When center points are added to the 2^3 design, it produces a potential transfer function with quadratic terms such as

$$y = f(x_1, x_2, x_3) = a_0 + \underbrace{a_1 x_1 + a_2 x_2 + a_3 x_3}_{\text{linear terms}}$$

$$+ \underbrace{a_{12} x_1 x_2 + a_{13} x_1 x_3 + a_{23} x_2 x_3}_{\text{interaction terms}} + \underbrace{a_{11} x_1^2 + a_{22} x_2^2 + a_{33} x_3^2}_{\text{quadratic terms}} + \varepsilon \tag{14.12}$$

where ε is the error term.

Each of the coefficients a_{11}, a_{22}, and a_{33} can be tested for curvature significance using the hypothesis $H_0 = a_{11} + a_{22} + a_{33} = 0$ versus H_a: at least one quadratic term coefficient $\neq 0$.

14.6 FRACTIONAL FACTORIAL DESIGNS

As the number of factors k increases, the number of runs specified for a full factorial can quickly become very large. For example, when $k = 6$, $2^6 = 64$. However, in this six factor experiment, there are six main effects: say, A, B, C, D, E, F, 15 two-factor interactions; AB,AC,AD,AE,AF,BC, BD,BE, BF, CD, CE,CF, DE,DF,EF, 20 three-factor interactions; ABC,ABD, . . . , 15 four-factor interactions; ABCD, . . . , 6 five-factor interactions; one six-factor interaction.

Fractional factorial design is a good solution for experimental design with limited resources (see Yang and El-Haik, 2003, Chap. 127). Fractional factorial design procedure usually starts by selecting a subset of combinations to test. The subset is selected by focusing on the main effects of control factors and some interactions of interest. The subset size represents 2^{k-p} of the 2^k possible factorial designs. Determining the p subset, which can be 1, 2, 3, and so on, depends on the level of confounding in 2^{k-p} fractional factorial designs, where one effect is confounded with another if the two effects are determined using the same formula. Factor screening provides a smaller treatment subset by screening out factors with little or no impact on performance using methods such as Plackett–Burman designs, supersaturated design, group-screening designs, and frequency-domain methods.

In general, practitioners have found that in an optimization experiment, higher-order interaction effects that involve three factors or more are rarely found to be significant. Usually, some main effects and two-factor interactions are significant. However, in a 2^6 experiment, out of 63 main effects and interactions, 42 of them are higher-order interactions; only 21 of them are main effects and two-factor interactions. As k gets larger, the overwhelming proportion of effects in the full factorials will be higher-order interactions. Since those effects are most likely to be insignificant, a lot of experimental resources are wasted in full factorial design. That is, as the number of factors k increases, most of data obtained in the full factorial are used to estimate higher-order interactions, which are most likely to be insignificant.

Fractional factorial experiments are designed to reduce greatly the number of runs and to use the information from the experimental data wisely. Fractional experiments require only a fraction of the runs of a full factorial; for two-level experiments, it uses only $\frac{1}{2}, \frac{1}{4}, \frac{1}{8}, \ldots$ of runs from a full factorial. Fractional factorial experiments are designed to estimate only the main effects and two-level interactions, not to estimate three-factor and other higher-order interactions.

14.6.1 The 2^{3-1} Design

Detailed accounts of how to design 2^{k-p} experiments can be found, for example, in Box et al. (1978), Montgomery (1991), or Gunst et al. (1989), to name only a few of the many textbooks on this subject. In general, it will use successively highest-order interactions to generate new factors.

Consider a two-level full factorial design for three factors: namely, the 2^3 design. Suppose that the experimenters cannot afford to run all eight-treatment combinations; however, they can afford four runs. If a subset of four runs (i.e., $p = 1$) is selected from the full factorial, it is a 2^{3-1} design. Now let us look at Table 14.11, where the original analysis matrix of a 2^3 design is divided into two portions. In this table we simply rearrange the rows such that the highest interaction, ABC's contrast coefficients, are all +1's in the first four

TABLE 14.11   A 2^{3-1} Design

Treatment Combination	Factorial Effects							
	I	A	B	C	AB	AC	BC	ABC
A	+1	+1	−1	−1	−1	−1	+1	+1
B	+1	−1	+1	−1	−1	+1	−1	+1
C	+1	−1	−1	+1	+1	−1	−1	+1
abc	+1	+1	+1	+1	+1	+1	+1	+1
Ab	+1	+1	+1	−1	+1	−1	−1	−1
Ac	+1	+1	−1	+1	−1	+1	−1	−1
Bc	+1	−1	+1	+1	−1	−1	+1	−1
(1)	+1	−1	−1	−1	+1	+1	+1	−1

rows, all −1's in the second four rows. The second column in this table is called *identity column* or *I column*, because it is a column with all +1's. If we select the first four runs as our experimental design, it is called a *fractional factorial design* with the defining relation I = ABC, where ABC is called the *generator*.

In Table 14.11 we can find that since the entire contrast coefficient for ABC are +1's, we will not be able to estimate the effect of ABC at all. For other main effects and interactions, the first four runs have an equal number of +1's and −1's, so we can calculate the effects of them. However, we can find that the contrast coefficients of factor A are identical to those of BC interaction, and the contrast coefficients of factor B are exactly the same as those of AC, as well as C and AB. Since the effects are computed based on the contrast coefficient, there is no way we can distinguish the effect of A and BC, B and AC, and C and AB. For example, when we estimate the effect of A, we are really estimating the combined effect of A and BC. This mixup of main effects and interactions is called an *alias* or *confounding*. All alias relationships can be found from the defining relation I = ABC. If we simply multiply A at both sides of the equation, we get AI = AABC. Since multiplying identical columns will give an I column, the equation above becomes A = BC. Similarly, we can get B = AC and C = AB. The first half fraction based on I = ABC is called the *principal fraction*. If we use the second half of Table 14.11, the defining relationship will be I = −ABC. Because all ABC coefficients are equal to −1's, we can easily determine that A = −BC, B = −AC, and C = −AB. Therefore, A is aliased with −BC, B is aliased with −AC, and C is aliased with −AB. We will lose the information about the highest-order interaction effect completely, and we will lose partially some information about lower-order interactions.

14.6.2 Half-Fractional 2^k Design

The half-fractional 2^k design is also called a 2^{k-1} design, because it has $N = 2^{k-1}$ runs. We can use the definition relationship to lay out the experiment; here we give the procedure to lay out a 2^{k-1} design, and illustrate that with an example.

1. Compute $N = 2^{k-1}$, determine the number of runs. For example, for $k = 4$, $N = 2k^{-1} = 2^3 = 8$.

2. Create a table with N runs, and lay out the first k − 1 factors in standard order (Table 14.12). For example, for $k = 4$, the factors are A, B, C, and D, and the first $k − 1 = 3$ factors are A, B, and C. We will lay out the first three columns with A, B, and C in standard order.

3. Use a defining relation to create the last column. In the example above, if we use I = ABCD as the defining relation, then D = ABC, we then can get the D column by multiplying the coefficients of the A, B, and C columns in

TABLE 14.12   A 2^{3-1} Standard Order Table

Run	Factor				Replicate				Response Total[a]
	A	B	C	D	1	2	...	n	
1	−1	−1	−1	−1					(1)
2	1	−1	−1	−1					a
3	−1	1	−1	−1					b
4	1	1	−1	−1					ab
5	−1	−1	1	−1					c
6	1	−1	1	−1					ac
7	−1	1	1	−1					bc
8	1	1	1	−1					abc

[a]Computed by adding the replicate row in a given run.

each row. In the example above, I = ABCD, we can derive the following alias relationships:

$$A = BCD, B = ACD, C = ABD, D = ABC \qquad AB = CD, AC = BD, AD = BC$$

Unlike a 2^{3-1} design, the main effects are not aliased with two-factor interactions, but two-factor interactions are aliased with each other. If we assume that three-factor interactions are not significant, main effects can be estimated free of aliases. Although both 2^{3-1} and 2^{4-1} are half-fractional factorial designs, 2^{4-1} has less confounding than 2^{3-1}. This is because their *resolutions* are different.

14.6.3   Design Resolution

A 2^{k-p} design means that we study overall k factors; however, p of those factors were generated from the interactions of a full 2^{k-p} factorial design. As a result, the design does not give full resolution; that is, there are certain interaction effects that are confounded with other effects. In general, a design of resolution R is one where no main effects are confounded with any other interaction of order less than $R - 1$. In a resolution III ($R = $ III) design, no main effects are confounded with any other interaction of order less than $R - I = III - I = II$. Thus, main effects in this design are confounded with two-way interactions, and consequently, all higher-order interactions are equally confounded.

The resolution is defined as the length of the shortest "word" in a defining relation. For example, the defining relation of a 2^{3-1} design is I = ABC; there are three letters in the defining relation (word), so it is a resolution III design. The defining relation of a 2^{4-1} design is I = ABCD; there are four letters in the defining relation, so it is a resolution IV design. Resolution describes the degree to which estimated main effects are aliased (or confounded) with estimated two-level interactions, three-level interactions, and so on. Higher-resolution designs have less severe confounding but require more runs.

A resolution IV design is "better" than a resolution III design because we have a less severe confounding pattern in the resolution IV design than in the resolution III situation; higher-order interactions are less likely than low-order interactions to be significant. A higher-resolution design for the same number of factors will, however, require more runs. In two-level fractional factorial experiments, the following three resolutions are used most frequently.

- *Resolution III designs.* Main effects are confounded (aliased) with two-factor interactions.
- *Resolution IV designs.* No main effects are aliased with two-factor interactions, but two-factor interactions are aliased with each other.
- *Resolution V designs.* No main effect or two-factor interaction is aliased with any other main effect or two-factor interaction, but two-factor interactions are aliased with three-factor interactions.

14.6.4 One-Fourth Fractional 2^k Design

When the number of factors, k, gets larger, 2^{k-1} designs will also require many runs. Then a smaller fraction of factorial design is needed. A one-fourth fraction of factorial design is also called a 2^{k-2} design. For a 2^{k-1} design, there is one defining relationship; each defining relationship is able to reduce the number of runs by half. For a 2^{k-2} design, two defining relationships are needed. If one P and one Q represent the generators chosen, I = P and I = Q are called *generating relations* for the design. Also, because I = P and I = Q, then I = PQ. I = P = Q = PQ is called the *complete defining relation*.

Consider a 2^{6-2} design. In this design, there are six factors: say, A, B, C, D, E, and F. For a 2^{6-1} design, the generator would be I = ABCDEF and we would have a resolution VI design. For a 2^{6-2} design, if we choose P and Q to have five letters, for example, P = ABCDE, Q = ACDEF, then PQ = BF, from I = P = Q = PQ, the complete defining relation, I = ABCDE = ACDEF=BF, we will only have resolution II! In this case even the main effects are confounded, so clearly it is not a good design. If we choose P and Q to be four letters (e.g., P = ABCE, Q = BCDF), then PQ = ADEF and I = ABCE = BCDF = ADEF. This is a resolution IV design. Clearly, it is also the highest resolution that a 2^{6-2} design can achieve. Now we can develop a procedure to lay out a 2^{k-2} design, and we illustrate that with an example.

1. *Compute* N = 2^{k-2} *and determine the number of runs.* For example, for k = 6, N = 2k^{-2} = 2^4 = 16.

2. *Create a table with* N *runs, and lay out the first* k − 2 *factors in standard order* (Table 14.13). For example, for $k = 6$, the factors are A, B, C, D, E, and F. The first $k − 2 = 4$ factors are A, B, C, and D. We will lay out the first four columns with A, B, C, and D in standard order.

TABLE 14.13   A 2^{6-2} Design Standard Order

| | | | Factor | | | |
Run	A	B	C	D	E = ABC	F = BCD
1	−1	−1	−1	−1	−1	−1
2	1	−1	−1	−1	1	−1
3	−1	1	−1	−1	1	1
4	1	1	−1	−1	−1	1
5	−1	−1	1	−1	1	1
6	1	−1	1	−1	−1	1
7	−1	1	1	−1	−1	−1
8	1	1	1	−1	1	−1
9	−1	−1	−1	1	−1	1
10	1	−1	−1	1	1	1
11	−1	1	−1	1	1	−1
12	1	1	−1	1	−1	−1
13	−1	−1	1	1	1	−1
14	1	−1	1	1	−1	−1
15	−1	1	1	1	−1	1
16	1	1	1	1	1	1

3. *Use the defining relation to create the last two columns.* In example above, if we use I = ABCE as the defining relation, then E = ABC, I = BCDF, and F = BCD.

A 2^k fractional factorial design having 2^{k-p} runs is called a $1/2^p$ fraction of a 2^k design or a 2^{k-p} fractional factorial design. These designs need p independent generators. The selection of those generators should make the resulting design have the highest possible resolution. Montgomery (1997) lists many good 2^{k-p} fractional factorial designs.

2^{k-p} designs are the "engine" of DOE because they can analyze many factors simultaneously with relative efficiency in few experimental runs. The experiment design is also straightforward because each factor has only two settings. The simplicity of these designs is a major flaw. That is, the underlying use of two-level factors is the belief that mathematical relationship between response and factors are basically linear in nature. This is often not the case, and many variables are related to the response in nonlinear aspects. Another problem of fractional designs is the implicit assumption that higher-order interactions do not matter; but sometimes they do. In this case it is nearly impossible for a fractional factorial experiment to detect higher-order interaction effects.

The richness of information versus cost of two-level designs is depicted in Figure 14.12, in which "RSM" represents the response surface methodology.[10]

---

[10]See Yang and El-Haik (2003) for response surface methodology within a product DFSS context.

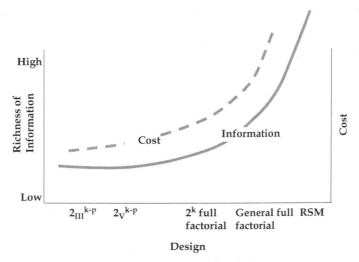

Figure 14.12 Richness of information versus the cost of two-level designs.

The curves in the figure are chosen to indicate the conceptual nonlinearity of both cost and information richness (in terms of design transfer function) and not to convey exact mathematical equations. Clearly, there is trade-off between what you want to achieve and what you are able to pay. It is a value proposition.

14.7 OTHER FACTORIAL DESIGNS

14.7.1 Three-Level Factorial Design

These designs are used when factors need to have more than two levels. For example, if the black belt suspects that the effect of the factors on the dependent variable of interest is not simply linear, the black belt needs at least three levels in order to test for the linear and quadratic effects and interactions for those factors. The notation 3^k is used. It means that k factors are considered, each at three levels. This formulation is more suitable with factors that are categorical in nature, with more than two categories.

The general method of generating fractional factorial design at three levels (3^{k-p} designs) is very similar to that described in the context of 2^{k-p} designs. Specifically, one starts with a full factorial design and then uses the interactions of the full design to construct new factors by making their factor levels identical to those for the respective interaction terms (i.e., by making the new factors aliases of the respective interactions).

The three levels are (usually) referred to as low, intermediate, and high levels. These levels are expressed numerically as 0, 1, and 2. One could have considered the digits −1, 0, and +1, but this may be confused with respect to the two-level designs since 0 is reserved for center points. Therefore, the 0, 1, 2 scheme is usually recommended. The reason that the three-level designs were proposed is to model possible curvature in the transfer function and to handle the case of nominal factors at three levels. A third level for a continuous factor facilitates investigation of a quadratic relationship between the response and each of the factors. Unfortunately, the three-level design is prohibitive in terms of the number of runs, and thus in terms of cost and effort.

14.7.2 Box–Behnken Designs

In the case of 2^{k-p} designs, Plackett and Burman (1946) developed highly fractionalized designs to screen the maximum number of (main) effects in the least number of experimental runs. The equivalent in the case of 3^{k-p} designs are the Box–Behnken designs (Box and Draper, 1987). These designs do not have simple design generators (they are constructed by combining two-level factorial designs with incomplete block designs) and have complex confounding of interaction. However, the designs are economical and therefore particularly useful when it is expensive to perform the necessary experimental runs. The analysis of these types of designs proceeds basically in the same way as was described in the context of 2^{k-p} designs. However, for each effect we can now test for linear and quadratic (i.e., nonlinear) effects. Nonlinearity often occurs when a medical device performs near its optimum.

14.8 SUMMARY

Design of experiments (DOE) is a structured method for determining the transfer function relationship between factors affecting a device and the output of that device (y). In essence, it is a methodology for conducting and analyzing controlled tests to evaluate the effect of factors that control the value of a variable or a group of responses. DOE refers to experimental methods used to quantify indeterminate measurements of factors and interactions between factors statistically through observance of forced changes made methodically as directed by systematic tables.

There are two main bodies of knowledge in DOE: experimental design and experimental data analysis. Two types of experimental design strategy are discussed in this chapter: full factorial and fractional factorial. Full factorial design is used to obtain more information when affordable since the size of experiment will grow exponentially with the number of experiment factors and levels. Fractional factorial design obtains less information from the experiment, but its experiment size will grow much more slowly than that of full factorial. In addition, we can adjust the resolution of fractional factorial design so that it can obtain needed information while retaining a manageable experimental size. Therefore, fractional factorial design becomes the workhorse of

DOE. DOE design is critical in creating orthogonal designs, those in which the factors are independent of each other.

The main DOE data analysis tools include ANOVA, empirical transfer function model building, and main effects and interactions charts. ANOVA is able to identify the set of significant factors and interactions and rank the relative importance of each effect and interaction in terms of their effect on design output. Empirical transfer function models, main effect plots, and interaction plots show the empirical relationship between design output and design factors. They can also be used to identify optimal factor-level settings and the corresponding optimal design performance levels.

APPENDIX 14A

14A.1   Diagnostic Plots of Residuals

Before accepting particular ANOVA results or a transfer function that includes a particular number of effects, the DFSS black belt should always examine the distribution of residual values. These are computed as the difference between the predicted values (as predicted by the current model) and the observed values. He or she can compute the histogram for these residual values as well as probability plots or generate them from a statistical package such as Mintab. Parameter estimates and ANOVA tables are based on the assumption that the residuals are normally distributed. The histogram provides one way to visually check whether this assumption holds.

The normal probability plot is another common tool used to assess how closely a set of observed values (residuals in this case) follows a theoretical distribution. In this plot the actual residual values are plotted along the horizontal x-axis; the vertical y-axis shows the expected normal values for the respective values after they were rank-ordered. If all values fall onto a straight line, we can be satisfied that the residuals follow the normal distribution.

14A.2   Pareto Chart of Effects

The Pareto chart of effects is often an effective tool for communicating the results of an experiment, in particular to laypeople. In this graph, the ANOVA effect estimates are sorted from the largest absolute value to the smallest absolute value. A column represents the magnitude of each effect, and often, a line going across the columns indicates how large an effect has to be statistically significant.

14A.3   Square and Cube Plots

Square and cube plots are often used to summarize values predicted for the response variable given the respective high and low settings of the factors. The square plot will show the values predicted for two factors at a time. The cube plot will show the values predicted for three factors at a time.

14A.4 Interaction Plots

A general graph for showing the means is the standard interaction plot, where points connected by lines indicate the means. This plot is particularly useful when there are significant interaction effects in the analysis.

15

ROBUST PARAMETER DESIGN FOR MEDICAL DEVICES

15.1 INTRODUCTION

In the context of this book, the terms *quality* and *robustness* can be used interchangeably. *Robustness* is defined as a design attribute that represents reduction of the variation of the functional requirements (FRs), design parameters (DPs) or process variables (PVs) of a device and having them on target as defined by the customer (Taguchi, 1986; Taguchi and Wu, 1986; Phadke, 1989; Taguchi et al., 1989, 1999).

Variability reduction has been the subject of robust design (Taguchi, 1986) through methods such as parameter design and tolerance design. The principal idea of robust design is that statistical testing of a product or process should be carried out at the developmental stage, also referred to as the off-line stage. To make the medical device robust against the effects of variation sources in the production and use environments, the design entity is viewed from the point of view of quality and cost (Taguchi, 1986; Taguchi and Wu, 1986; Taguchi et al., 1989, 1999; Nair, 1992).

Quality is measured by quantifying statistical variability through measures such as standard deviation or mean square error. The main performance criterion is to achieve the DPs (e.g., target on average), while simultaneously minimizing variability around this target. Robustness means that a medical device performs its intended functions under all operating conditions (different causes of variations) throughout its intended life. The undesirable and

Medical Device Design for Six Sigma: A Road Map for Safety and Effectiveness,
By Basem S. El-Haik and Khalid S. Mekki
Copyright © 2008 John Wiley & Sons, Inc.

uncontrollable factors that cause a DP under consideration to deviate from target value, called *noise factors* affect quality adversely, and ignoring them will result in a medical device not optimized for conditions of use and possibly failure. Eliminating noise factors may be expensive. Instead, the DFSS team seeks to reduce the effect of the noise factors on DP performance by choosing design parameters and their settings, which are insensitive to the noise.

In DFSS, robust design is a disciplined methodology that seeks to find the best expression of a medical device design. *Best* is defined carefully to mean that the design is the lowest-cost solution to the specification, which itself is based on identified customer needs. Taguchi has included design quality as one more dimension of product cost. High-quality devices minimize these costs by performing, consistently, at targets specified by the customer. Taguchi's philosophy of robust design is aimed at reducing the loss due to variation of performance from the target value based on a portfolio of concepts and measures such as quality loss function, signal-to-noise ratio, optimization, and experimental design. *Quality loss* is the loss experienced by customers and society and is a function of how far performance deviates from target. The quality loss function relates quality to cost and is considered a better evaluation system than the traditional binary treatment of quality (i.e. within/outside specifications). The quality loss function of a functional requirement, a design parameter, or a process variable [generically denoted as response (y)] has two components: mean (μ_y) deviation from targeted performance value (T_y) and variance (σ_y^2). It can be approximated by a quadratic polynomial of the response of interest.

15.2 ROBUST DESIGN FUNDAMENTALS

In Taguchi's philosophy, robust design consists of three phases (Figure 15.1). It begins with the *concept design phase*, followed by the *parameter design* and *tolerance design phases*. Unfortunately, the concept phase has not received the attention it deserves in the quality engineering community: hence the focus on it in this book.

The goal of parameter design is to minimize the quality loss expected by selecting design parameter settings. The tools used are quality loss function, design of experiment, statistics, and optimization. Parameter design optimization is carried out in two sequential steps: variability, then minimization of σ_y^2 and mean (μ_y) adjustment to target (T_y). The first step is conducted using the

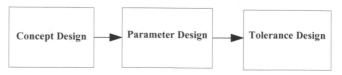

Figure 15.1 Taguchi's robust design.

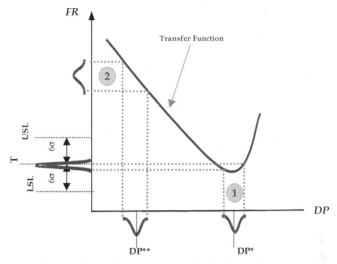

Figure 15.2 Robustness optimization definition.

mapping parameters or variables (x's) (in the context of Figure 9.1) that affect variability, while the second step is accomplished via the design parameters, which affect the mean but do not influence variability adversely. The objective is to carry out both steps at low cost by exploring the opportunities in the design space.

15.2.1 Robust Design and DFSS

Consider two settings or means of a design parameter (DP)—setting 1 (DP*) and setting 2 (DP**)—having the same variance and probability density function (statistical distribution) as depicted in Figure 15.2. Consider also the given curve of a hypothetical transfer function (A mathematical form of the design mapping, see Chapter 13), which is in this case a nonlinear function in the design parameter, DP. It is obvious that setting 1 produces less variation in the functional requirement (FR) than setting 2 by capitalizing on nonlinearity.[1] This also implies lower information content and thus a lower degree of complexity based on axiom 2 of Chapter 9. Setting 1 (DP*) will also produce a lower quality loss, similar to the scenario on the right of Figure 15.3. In other words, the design produced by setting 1 (DP*) is more robust than that produced by setting 2. Setting 1 (DP*) robustness is evident in the amount of variation transferred through the transfer function to the FR response of Figure 15.2 and the flatter quadratic quality loss function in Figure 15.3. When the distance between the specification limits is six times the standard deviation

---

[1]In addition to nonlinearity, leveraging interactions between the noise factors and the design parameters are another popular empirical parameter design approach.

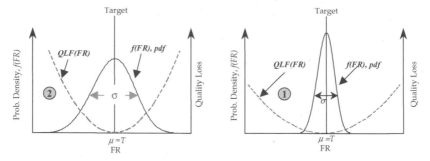

Figure 15.3   Quality loss function scenarios of Figure 15.2.

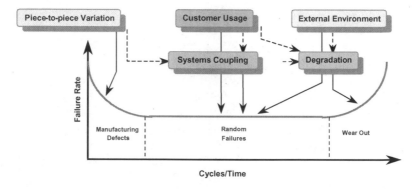

Figure 15.4   Effect of noise factors during the medical device life cycle. (See Fowlkes and Creveling, 1995.)

($6\sigma_{FR}$), a six sigma-level optimized FR is achieved. When all design FRs are released at this level, a six sigma design is obtained.

The important contribution of robust design is the systematic inclusion into experimental design of noise variables: variables over which the designer has little or no control. A distinction is also made between internal noise, such as component wear, material variability, and environmental noise, which the designer cannot control (e.g., humidity, temperature). Robust design's objective is to suppress, as far as possible, the effect of noise by exploring the levels of the factors to determine their potential for making a medical device insensitive to these sources of variation in the respective responses of interest (e.g., the FRs).

The noise factors affect the FRs at different segments in the life cycle. As a result, they can cause dramatic reduction in product reliability as indicated by the failure rate. The bathtub curve in Figure 15.4 implies that robustness can be defined as reliability over time. Reliability is defined as the probability that the design will perform as intended: deliver the FRs to satisfy the customer attributes (Figure 9.1) throughout a specified time period when operated under stated conditions. One reason for early life failures is manu-facturing variability. The unit-to-unit noise causes failure in the field when the product is subjected to external noise. The random failure rate of the DPs that characterizes most of the product life is the performance of design subject to external noise. Notice that the coupling vulnerability contributes to the unreli-ability of the design in customer hands. Deterioration noise is active at the end of product life. Therefore, a product is said to be robust (and therefore reliable) when it is insensitive to the effect of noise factors even though the sources themselves have not been eliminated (Fowlkes and Creveling, 1995).

Parameter design is the most used phase in the robust design method. The objective is to design a solution entity by making the functional requirement insensitive to the variation. This is accomplished by selecting the optimal levels of design parameters based on testing and using an optimization crite-rion. Parameter design optimization criteria include both quality loss function and signal-to-noise ratio (SN). The optimum levels of the x's or the design parameters are the levels that maximize SN and are determined in an experi-mental setup from a pool of economical alternatives. These alternatives assume the testing levels in search for the optimum.

15.3 ROBUST DESIGN CONCEPTS

Several robust design concepts are presented below as they apply to medical device and product development in general.

15.3.1 Concept 1: Output Classification

An output response of a product or a process can be classified as static or dynamic from a robustness perspective. A *static* entity has a fixed target value. The parameter design phase in the case of the static solution entity is to bring the response mean (μ_y) to the target (T_y). On the other hand, the *dynamic* response expresses a variable target, depending on customer intent. In this case the optimization phase is carried over a range of useful customer applica-tions called the *signal factor*. This factor can be used to set y to an intended value; for example, we may want to minimize or eliminate bacterial infection or contamination or maximize sterilization delivered by certain devices.

Parameter design optimization requires the classification of output responses (depending on the mapping of infestation in the context of Figure 9.1) as *smaller-the-better* (e.g., minimize contamination), *larger-the-better* (e.g., increase sterilization effectiveness), *nominal-the-best* (where keeping the device on a single performance objective is the main concern: e.g., meeting cell collection yield), and *dynamic* (where energy-related functional perfor-mance over a prescribed dynamic range of use is the perspective: e.g., medica-tion delivery flow rate as prescribed by a caregiver).

When robustness cannot be assured by parameter design, we resort to the tolerance design phase. Tolerance design is the last phase of robust design. The practice is to upgrade or tighten tolerances of some design parameters so that quality loss can be reduced. However, the tightened tolerance practice will usually add cost in the process to control the tolerance. El-Haik (2005) formulated the problem of finding the optimum design parameter tolerance that minimizes both quality loss and tolerance control costs (Chapter 16).

The important contribution of robust design is the systematic inclusion into experimental design of noise variables, those variables over which the designer has no or little control. A distinction is also made between internal noise, such as material variability, and environmental noise, which the design team cannot control. Robust design's objective is to suppress, as far as possible, the effect of noise by exploring the levels of the factors to determine their potential for making the medical device insensitive to these sources of variation.

15.3.2   Concept 2: Quality Loss Function

Traditional inspection schemes represent the heart of online quality control. Inspection schemes depend on the binary characterization of design parameters (i.e., being within the specification limits or outside the specification limits). A process is called *conforming* if all the design parameters inspected are within their respective specification limits; otherwise, it is *nonconforming*. This binary representation of the acceptance criteria for a design parameter, for example, is not realistic since it characterizes, equally, entities that are marginally off on either specification limits and entities that are marginally within these limits. In addition, this characterization does not discriminate between entities off marginally and those off significantly. The point here is that it is not realistic to assume that as we move away from the nominal specification in a device, the quality loss is zero as long as you stay within the set tolerance limits. Rather, if the device functional requirement is not exactly on target, loss will result, for example, in terms of customer satisfaction. Moreover, this loss is probably not a linear function of the deviation from nominal specifications, but rather, a quadratic function similar to what is shown in Figure 15.3. Taguchi proposed a continuous and better representation than this dichotomous characterization, the quality loss function (Taguchi and Wu, 1980). The loss function provides a better estimate of the monetary loss incurred by production and customers as an output response (y) deviates from its targeted performance value (T_y). The determination of T_y implies the nominal-the-best and dynamic classifications.

A quality loss function can be interpreted as a means to translate variation and target adjustment to a monetary value. It allows design teams to perform a detailed optimization of cost by relating technical terminology to economical measures. In its quadratic form, a quality loss is determined by first finding the functional limits,[2] $T_y \pm \Delta_y$, of the concerned response. The functional limits are the points at which the process would fail (i.e., produce unacceptable performance in approximately half of customer applications). In a sense, these represent performance levels that are equivalent to average customer tolerance. Kapur (1988) continued with this line of thinking and illustrated the derivation of specification limits using Taguchi's quality loss function. A quality loss is incurred due to the deviation from the intended targeted performance (T_y) of the response (y or FR), caused by the noise factors. Let L denote the quality loss function, taking the numerical value of the FR and the targeted value as arguments. By Taylor series[3] at FR = T, and with some assumptions about the significant of the expansion terms, we have

$$L(\mathrm{FR}, T) \cong K(\mathrm{FR} - T_{\mathrm{FR}})^2 \qquad (15.1)$$

Let FR $\in [T_y - \Delta_y, T_y + \Delta_y]$, where T_y is the target value and Δy is the functional deviation from the target (see Figure 15.2). Let A_Δ be the quality loss incurred due to the symmetrical deviation, (Δy); then by substituting in equation (15.5) and solving for K, we obtain

$$K = \frac{A_\Delta}{(\Delta y)^2} \qquad (15.2)$$

In the Taguchi tolerance design method, the quality loss coefficient K can be determined on the basis of losses in monetary terms by falling outside *customer tolerance limits* (*design range*) instead of the specification limits generally used in process capability studies (e.g., *producer limits*). The specification limits are most often associated with the design parameters. Customer tolerance limits are used to estimate the loss from the customer perspective, or the quality loss to society, as proposed by Taguchi. Usually, customer tolerance is wider than manufacturer tolerance. In this chapter we side with the terminology of design range limits and note any deviation from this practice where applicable.

Let $f(y)$ be the probability density function (pdf) of y; then via the expectation operator, E, we have

$$E[L(y, T)] = K[\sigma_y^2 + (\mu_y - T_y)^2] \qquad (15.3)$$

(see Figure 15.5). Equation (15.3) is fundamental. Quality loss has two ingredients: loss incurred due to variability (σ_y^2) and loss incurred due to mean deviation from target, $(\mu_y - T_y)^2$. The latter term is generally minimized by

---

[2]Functional limits or customer tolerance in robust design terminology is synonymous with design range in axiomatic design approach terminology (see Chapter 9).

[3]The assumption here that L is a higher-order continuous function such that derivatives exist and that it is symmetrical around $y = T$.

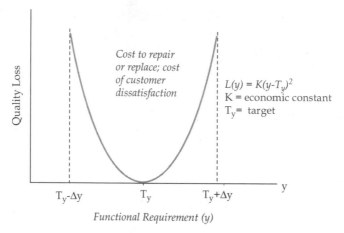

Figure 15.5   Quality loss function.

adjustment of the mean of the critical few *design parameters*, the affecting *x*'s.

The derivation in (15.3) suits the nominal-is-best classification. Other quality loss function mathematical forms may be found in El-Haik and Roy (2005). The following forms of loss function are borrowed from that paper.

1. *Larger-the-better loss function.* For functions such as "increase yield" (*y* = yield), we would like a very large target: ideally, $T_y \to \infty$. The requirement (output *y*) is bounded by the lower functional specifications limit y_l. The loss function is then given by

$$L(y, T_y) = \frac{K}{y^2} \qquad \text{where } y \geq y_l \tag{15.4}$$

Let μ_y be the average *y* numerical value of the medical device range (i.e., the average around which performance delivery is expected). Then, by Taylor series expansion around $y = \mu_y$, we have

$$E[L(y, T_y)] = K\left(\frac{1}{\mu_y^2} + \frac{3}{\mu_y^4}\sigma_y^2\right) \tag{15.5}$$

2. *Smaller-the-better loss function.* Functions such as "reduce audible noise" would like to have zero as their target value. The loss function in this category and its expected values are given.

$$L(y, T) = Ky^2 \tag{15.6}$$

and

$$E[L(y, T)] = K(\sigma_y^2 + \mu_y^2) \tag{15.7}$$

In the development above as well as in the next sections, the average loss can be estimated from a parameter design or even a tolerance design experiment by substituting the experiment variance S^2 and average $\bar{y}$ as estimates for σ_y^2 and μ_y into the equations above.

Recall the two-settings example in Figure 15.2. It was obvious that setting 1 is more robust [i.e., produces less variation in the functional requirement (y)] than setting 2 by capitalizing on nonlinearity as well as lower quality loss, similar to the scenario on the right of Figure 15.3. Setting 1 (DP*) robustness is even more evident in the flatter quadratic quality loss function.

Since quality loss is a quadratic function of the deviation from a nominal value, the goal of the DFSS project should be to minimize the squared deviations or variance of a requirement around nominal (ideal) specifications rather than the number of units within specification limits (as is done in traditional SPC procedures).

Several books have been published on these methods: for example, Ross (1988) and Phadke (1989), and within the context of product DFSS, Yang and El-Haik (2003), to name a few, and it is recommended that the reader refer to those books for further specialized discussions. Introductory overviews of Taguchi's ideas about quality and quality improvement may also be found in Kacker (1985).

15.3.3 Concept 3: Signal, Noise, and Control Factors

A medical device that is designed with six sigma quality should always respond in exactly the same manner to the signals provided by the customer. When you press the ON button of the remote control for your TV set, you expect the set to switch on. In a DFSS-designed TV set, the starting process would always proceed in exactly the same manner; for example, after 3 seconds of pressing the remote, the set comes to life. If, in response to the same signal (pressing the ON button) there is random variability in this process, the quality is less than ideal. For example, due to such uncontrollable factors as speaker conditions, weather conditions, battery voltage level, and set wear, the set may sometimes start only after 20 seconds, and finally, not at all. We want to minimize the variability in output response due to noise factors while maximizing response to signal factors.

Noise factors are those factors that are not under the control of the design team. In this example, those factors include speaker conditions, weather conditions, battery voltage level, and set wear. Signal factors are those factors that are set or controlled by the customer (end user) to make use of the intended functions of a device.

The goal of a medical device DFSS project is to find the best experimental settings (in the absence of an off-the-shelf transfer function) of factors under the team's control that are involved in the design, in order to minimize quality loss; thus, the factors in the experiment represent control factors. Signal, noise and control factors (design parameters) are usually summarized in a P-diagram similar to Figure 14.1.

15.3.4 Concept 4: Signal-to-Noise Ratios

A conclusion of previous sections is that quality can be quantified in terms of the respective device's response to noise and signal factors. The ideal medical device would only respond to customer signals and would be unaffected by random noise factors. Therefore, the goal of the DFSS project can be stated as attempting to maximize the signal-to-noise (SN) ratio for the device. The SN ratios described in the following paragraphs have been proposed by Taguchi (1987).

1. *Smaller-is-better.* In cases where the DFSS team wants to minimize the occurrence of undesirable device responses, the following SN ratio would computed:

$$SN = -10 \log_{10}\left(\frac{1}{N} \sum_{n=1}^{N} y_i^2 \right) \tag{15.8}$$

The constant, N, represents the number of observations (that have y_i as their response) measured in an experiment or in a sample. Experiments are conducted and the y measurements are collected. For example, bacteria killed in a sterilization process could be measured as the y variable and analyzed via the SN ratio. Note that this ratio is an expression of the assumed quadratic nature of the loss function.

2. *Nominal-the-best.* Here, the DFSS team has a fixed signal value (nominal value), and the variance around this value can be considered the result of noise factors:

$$SN = -10 \log_{10} \frac{\mu^2}{\sigma^2} \tag{15.9}$$

This signal-to-noise ratio could be used whenever ideal quality is equated with a particular nominal value. For example, the time delay with respect to a target commitment in a cell extraction process could be measured as the y variable and analyzed via this SN ratio. The effect of the signal factors is zero, since the target date is the only intended or desired state of the process.

3. *Larger-is-better.* Examples of this type of medical device requirement are therapy device yield and purity. The following SN ratio should be used:

$$SN = -10 \log_{10}\left(\frac{1}{N} \sum_{n=1}^{N} \frac{1}{y_i^2} \right) \tag{15.10}$$

4. *Fraction defective.* This SN ratio is useful for minimizing a requirement's defects (i.e., values outside the specification limits) or minimizing the percent of software error states:

$$SN = 10\log_{10}\frac{p}{1-p} \tag{15.11}$$

where p is the proportion defective.

15.3.5 Concept 5: Orthogonal Arrays

The orthogonal array aspect of Taguchi robust design methods is the one most similar to traditional DOE technique. Taguchi has developed a system of tabulated designs (arrays) that allow for the maximum number of main effects to be estimated in an unbiased (orthogonal) manner, with a minimum number of runs in the experiment. Latin square designs, 2^{k-p} designs (Plackett–Burman designs, in particular), and Box–Behnken designs are also aimed at accomplishing this goal. In fact, many of the standard orthogonal arrays tabulated by Taguchi are identical to fractional two-level factorials, Plackett–Burman designs, Box–Behnken designs, Latin squares, Greco-Latin squares, and others.

Orthogonal arrays provide an approach to efficient design of experiments that improves our understanding of the relationship between device design parameters and process variables (control factors) and the desired output performance (functional requirements). This efficient design of experiments is based on a fractional factorial experiment which allows an experiment to be conducted with only a fraction of the possible experimental combinations of factorial values. Orthogonal arrays are used to aid in the design of an experiment. An orthogonal array will specify the test cases that should be used to conduct the experiment. Frequently, two orthogonal arrays are used: a control factor array and a noise factor array, the latter used to conduct the experiment in the presence of difficult-to-control variation so as to develop a robust device.

In Taguchi's experimental design system, all experimental layouts will be derived from about 18 standard orthogonal arrays. Let's look at the simplest orthogonal array, the L$_4$ array, shown in Table 15.1. The values inside the

TABLE 15.1   L$_4$(2^3) Orthogonal Array

	Column		
Expt. No.	1	2	3
1	1	1	1
2	1	2	2
3	2	1	2
4	2	2	1

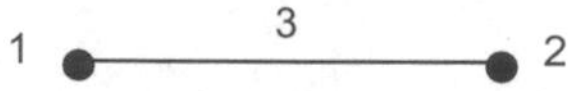

1 ●————3————● 2

Figure 15.6   Linear graph for L_4.

array, 1 and 2, represent two different levels of a factor. Using "−1" for substitute "1" and "+1" for "2," Table 15.1 becomes Table 15.2. Clearly, this is a 2^{3-1} fractional factorial design, with defining relation I (see Chapter 14) = −ABC, where column 2 of L_4 is equivalent to the A column of the 2^{3-1} design, column 1 is equivalent to the B column of the 2^{3-1} design, and column 3 is equivalent to column C of the 2^{3-1} design, with C = −AB.

In each of Taguchi's orthogonal arrays there are corresponding linear graph(s). Linear graphs are used to illustrate the interaction relationships in the array; for example, the linear graph for the L_4 array is given in Figure 15.6. The numbers 1 and 2 represent columns 1 and 2 of the L_4 array; 3 is above the line segment connecting 1 and 2, which means that the interaction of columns 1 and 2 is confounded with column 3, which is perfectly consistent with C = −AB in the 2^{3-1} fractional factorial design.

For larger orthogonal arrays, not only there are both linear graphs and interaction tables to explain interaction relationships among columns. For example, the L_8 array in Table 15.3 has the linear graph shown in Figure 15.7 and the interaction table shown in Table 15.4.

TABLE 15.2 L_4 Using −1 and +1 Notation

	Column		
Expt. No.	1	2	3
1	−1	−1	−1
2	−1	1	1
3	1	−1	1
4	1	1	−1

TABLE 15.3 $L_8(2^7)$ Orthogonal Array

	Column						
Expt. No.	1	2	3	4	5	6	7
1	1	1	1	1	1	1	1
2	1	1	1	2	2	2	2
3	1	2	2	1	1	2	2
4	1	2	2	2	2	1	1
5	2	1	2	1	2	1	2
6	2	1	2	2	1	2	1
7	2	2	1	1	2	2	1
8	2	2	1	2	1	1	2

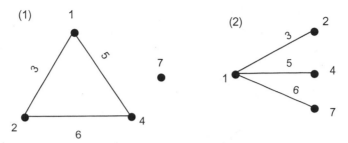

Figure 15.7 Linear graphs for L_8.

TABLE 15.4 Interaction Table for L_8

Column	Column						
	1	2	3	4	5	6	7
1	(1)	3	2	5	4	7	6
2		(2)	1	6	7	4	5
3			(3)	7	6	5	4
4				(4)	1	2	3
5					(5)	3	2
6						(6)	1
7							(7)

This approach to designing and conducting an experiment to determine the effect of design factors (parameters or variables) and noise factors on a performance characteristic is represented in Figure 15.8.

The factors of concern are identified in an *inner array* or *control factor array*, which specifies the factorial levels. The *outer array* or *noise factor array* specifies the noise factor or the range of variation the device will be exposed to in its life cycle. This experimental setup allows identification of the control factors values or levels that will produce the best performing, most reliable, or most satisfactory device over the expected range of noise factors.

15.3.6 Concept 6: Parameter Design Analysis

After the experiments are conducted and the SN ratio is determined for each run, a mean SN ratio value is calculated for each factor level. These data are analyzed statistically using ANOVA techniques as described in Chapter 14. Very simply, a control factor with a large difference in the SN ratio from one factor setting to another indicates that the factor is a significant contributor to achievement of the performance response. Little difference in the SN ratio from one factor setting to another indicates that the factor is insignificant with

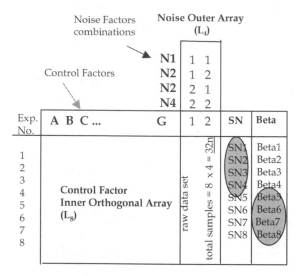

Figure 15.8 Parameter design orthogonal array experiment.

respect to the response. With the understanding desired from experiments and subsequent analysis, the design team can:

1. Identify control factor levels that maximize output response in the direction of goodness and minimize the effect of noise, thereby achieving a more robust design.

2. Perform two-step robustness optimization[4]:

   a. *Robustness optimization step 1:* Choose factor levels to reduce variability by improving the SN ratio. The level for each control factor with the highest SN ratio is selected as the parameter's best target value. All of these best levels will be selected to produce the robust design levels or optimum levels of design combination. A response table similar to Figure 15.9 that summarizes SN gain is generally used. Control factor effects are calculated by averaging SN ratios corresponding to the individual control factor levels, as depicted by the orthogonal array diagram. In this example, the robust design levels are as follows: factor A at level 2, factor C at level 1, and factor D at level 2, or simply A2C1D2. Identify control factor levels that have no significant effect on the functional response mean or variation. In these cases, tolerances can be relaxed and cost reduced. This is the case for factor B of Figure 15.9.

---

[4]Robustness two-step optimization can be viewed as a two-response optimization of the functional requirement (y). Step 1 targets optimizing the variation (σ_y), and step 2 targets shifting the mean (μ_y) to target T_y. For more than two functional requirements, the optimization problem is called *multiresponse optimization*.

Control Factors	A	B	C	D
Level 1	0.62	1.82	(3.15)	0.10
Level 2	(3.14)	1.50	0.12	(2.17)
Gain (meas. in dB)	2.52	0.32	3.03	2.07

Figure 15.9 Signal-to-noise ratio response table example.

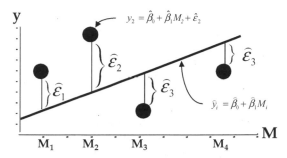

Figure 15.10 Best-fit line of a dynamic robust design DOE.

   b. *Robustness optimization step 2:* Select factor levels to adjust mean performance. This is better suited for dynamic characteristic robustness formulation with sensitivity defined as beta (β). In a robust design, the individual β values are calculated using the same data from each experimental run, as in Figure 15.6. The purpose of determining the beta values is to characterize the ability of control factors to change the average value of the functional requirement (y) across a specified dynamic signal range, as in Figure 15.10. The resulting beta performance of a functional requirement (y) is illustrated by the slope of a best-fit line in the form of $y = \beta_0 + \beta_1 M$, where β_1 is the slope and β_0 is the intercept of the functional requirement data, which are compared to the slope of an ideal function line. A best-fit line is obtained by minimizing the squared sum of error (ε) terms (Figure 15.10).

   In dynamic systems, a control factor's importance in decreasing sensitivity is determined by comparing the gain in SN ratio from level to level for each factor, comparing the relative performance gains between each control factor, and selecting those that produce the largest gains. That is, the same analysis and selection process is used to determine control factors which can best be used to adjust the mean functional requirement. These factors may be the same ones that have been chosen on the basis of SN improvement, or they may be factors that do not affect optimization of the SN ratio.

   Most analyses of robust design experiments amount to a standard ANOVA of the respective SN ratios, ignoring two-way or higher-order interactions. However, when estimating error variances, one customarily pools together main effects of negligible size. It should be noted at this point that, of course, all of the designs discussed in Chapter 14 (e.g., 2^k, 2^{k-p}, 3^{k-p}) can be used to analyze SN ratios that you computed. In fact, the many additional diagnostic plots and other options available for those designs (e.g., estimation of quadratic components) may prove very useful when analyzing design variability (SN ratios). As a visual summary, an SN ratio plot is usually displayed using the experiment average SN ratio by factor levels. In this plot, the optimum settings (the largest SN ratio) for each factor can easily be identified.

For prediction purposes, the DFSS team can compute the SN ratio expected given optimum settings of factors (ignoring factors that were pooled into the error term). The SN ratios predicted can then be used in a verification experiment in which the design team actually sets the process accordingly and compares the resulting SN ratio observed with the ratio predicted by the experiment. If major deviations occur, one must conclude that the simple main effects model is not appropriate. In those cases, Taguchi (1987) recommends transforming the dependent variable to accomplish additivity of factors, that is, to make the main effects model fit. Phadke (1989, Chap. 6) also discusses in detail, methods for achieving additivity of factors.

15.4   APPLICATION: DYNAMIC FORMULATION

The medical device heat sealer (MDHS) shown in Figure 15.11 is a system that utilizes a heating element (press bar) which fuses the material (plastic bag) to generate a seal. During research and development of the MDHS, and as a result of a screening designed experiment, it became obvious that a good

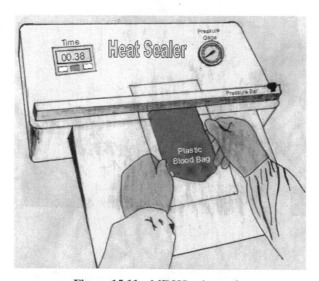

Figure 15.11   MDHS schematic.

seal is a result of three significant design parameters (control factors): factor A, dwell time; factor B, press bar pressure; and factor C, press bar temperature.

The product development team noticed a variation in seal strength when plastic bags were sealed at different temperature and humidity levels. Room temperature and humidity are uncontrollable factors (noise factors) and a good seal must be robust against those noise factors.

A dynamic formulation Taguchi experiment was conducted to define an appropriate level for each of the three control factors that make the system robust in the presence of temperature and humidity noise factors. Figure 15.12 shows the MDHS P-diagram, which indicates the signal, control factors, noise factors, the ideal function, and error states. This diagram lists all the experimental factors required for optimization, with an experiment output defined as seal strength (y) measured using a destructive peel test. The input signal (M) is the plastic bag thickness. The linear ideal function is formulated as $y = \beta M$ in Figure 15.12. A target value, together with upper and lower specification limits, was defined for the seal strength. Table 15.5 lists the control factors (inner array) and noise factors (outer array). In addition, the table lists the input signal levels.

An L_8 Taguchi orthogonal array (see in Figure 15.8 and Table 15.3) is used, with control factors A, B, and C listed in columns 1, 2, and 4, respectively, to avoid any interaction confounding effects (see Figure 15.7 for L_8 linear graph settings). Experimental output was measured by setting up conditions (different combinations for control factors and noise factors at different signals) for each experimental run.

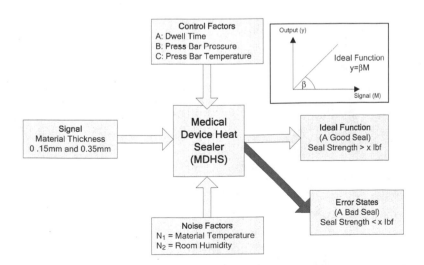

Figure 15.12 Medical device heat sealer P-diagram.

TABLE 15.5 Medical Device Heat Sealer Experiment Parameters

	Low Level	High Level	Units
Control factors			
A: dwell time	0.75	1.25	seconds
B: press bar pressure	85	100	psi
C: press bar temperature	176 (80)	212 (100)	°F (°C)
Signal input, *M*			
Bag sheet thickness	0.15	0.35	mm
	Best Case	Worst Case	
Noise factors			
N_1: material room temperature	86 (30)	40 (4)	°F (°C)
N_2: material room humidity	5	90	%RH

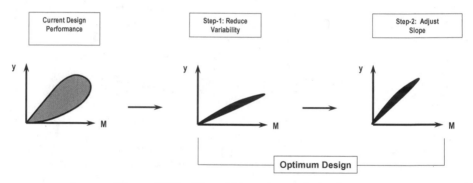

Figure 15.13 Taguchi two-step optimization.

In this experiment, the DFSS team was interested in optimizing the seal strength by identifying the nominal value of each control factor in the presence of noise factors. A surrogate noise approach was followed as compound best and worst case noise factors were chosen under each experimental run. Minitab was used to analyze the experimental results. The experimental output seal strength (*y*) direction of goodness is to maximize the sensitivity of the ideal function (i.e., maximize the seal strength for all thicknesses tested after minimizing the variability envelope around the function, as depicted in Figure 15.13). This is usually done in two steps:

1. The team wants to reduce function variability.
2. The team adjusts the slope (β) to the desired level. In this case, the team wants β to be maximized.

The sensitivity, slope β, and SN ratio were calculated for each run and stored in Table 15.6. The seal strength SN ratio main effects plot for the experiment control factors is shown in Figure 15.14 and values are provided

TABLE 15.6 MDHS Experiment Minitab Results

Run No.	A: Press Bar Pressure	B: Dwell Time	C: Press Bar Temperature	Signal	SN Ratio	Sensitivity (Ibf/mm)
1	1	1	1	0.15	−20.06	8.14
2	1	1	1	0.35	−22.07	8.95
3	1	1	2	0.15	−15.39	33.51
4	1	1	2	0.35	−16.93	36.86
5	1	2	1	0.15	−24.68	4.49
6	1	2	1	0.35	−27.15	4.94
7	1	2	2	0.15	−23.47	21.14
8	1	2	2	0.35	−25.81	23.26
9	2	1	1	0.15	−23.47	21.14
10	2	1	1	0.35	−25.81	23.26
11	2	1	2	0.15	−17.82	27.26
12	2	1	2	0.35	−19.60	29.98
13	2	2	1	0.15	−29.83	7.62
14	2	2	1	0.35	−32.82	8.39
15	2	2	2	0.15	−23.55	21.08
16	2	2	2	0.35	−25.91	23.19

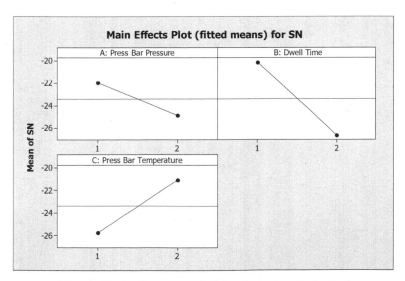

Figure 15.14 Seal strength SN ratio main effects plot.

in Table 15.7. The sensitivity main effects plot for the experiment control factors is shown in Figure 15.15 and values are provided in Table 15.8.

For the ANOVA, the team plots the residuals on normal probability paper, looking for a straight-line fit to check the normality assumption. To check the assumption of equal variance at each factor level, the team plots the residual against the factorial levels and compares the spread in the residuals. It is also

TABLE 15.7   Seal Strength SN Ratio Minitab ANOVA Results

Source of Variation	Sum of Squares	Degrees of Freedom	Mean Square	F	p-Value
A: Press bar pressure	33.8	1	33.8	10.8	0.006
B: Dwell time	169.3	1	169.3	54.11	0.000
C: Press bar temperature	87.4	1	87.4	27.94	0.000
Error	37.5	12	3.1		
Total	328.1	15			

TABLE 15.8   Seal Strength Sensitivity Minitab ANOVA Results

Source of Variation	Sum of Squares	Degrees of Freedom	Mean Square	F	p-Value
A: Press bar pressure	26.56	1	26.56	1.38	0.263
B: Dwell time	351.38	1	351.38	18.25	0.001
C: Press bar temperature	1045.67	1	1045.67	54.30	0.000
Error	231.11	12	19.26		
Total	1654.72	15			

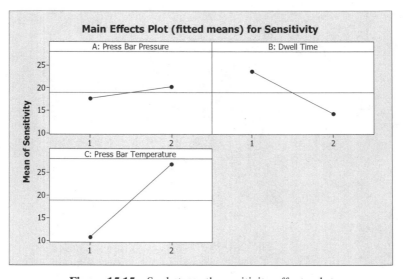

Figure 15.15   Seal strength sensitivity effects plot.

useful to plot the residuals against fitted values or treatment combination averages. The variability in the residuals should not in any way depend on the averages. When a pattern appears in those plots indicating nonnormality, it suggests the need for transformation: that is, analyzing the data in a different metric or dimension. In some problems the dependency of residual scatter in fitted values is very important.

Plotting the residuals against the time or run order can check the independence assumption. A pattern in this plot, such as a sequence of positive and negative residuals, may indicate that the observations are not independent. This indicates that the time or run order is important, or factors that change over time are important and have not been included in the DOE.

Figures 15.16 and 15.17 present the residual analysis of the heat sealer seal strength SN ratio and sensitivity. The normal probability plot of these

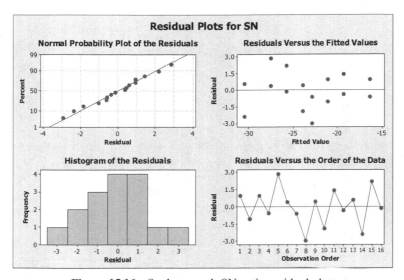

Figure 15.16 Seal strength SN ratio residual plot.

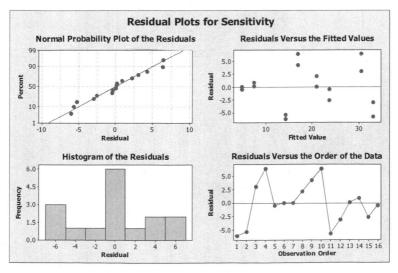

Figure 15.17 Seal strength sensitivity residual plot.

residuals does not appear to deviate from normality. The graph of residuals versus fitted values does not reveal any unusual pattern.

The SN ratio analysis indicates that there is a group of factors that are statistically significant from a variability perspective (i.e., have a large delta gain in Table 15.9). The rule of thumb is that any SN gain that is less than 1 decibel (dB) is considered not significant. The rank of each factor and the delta gains are also depicted graphically in Figure 15.14. All control factors are significant, with factor B the most significant, with a gain of 6.5 dB (i.e., flipping between this factor's levels will give us a better than reduction in variability). From an SN ratio perspective, the recommended factorial levels are:

A: dwell time at level A1 = 0.75 s
B: press bar pressure at level B1 = 85 psi
C: press bar temperature at level C2 = 176°F or 80°C or, in short, the combination A1B1C2.

The sensitivity (β) analysis indicates that there is a group of factors that are statistically significant in terms of the mean (i.e., have a large delta gain in Table 15.10). The rank of each factor and the delta gains are also depicted graphically in Figure 15.15. All control factors are significant, with factor C the most significant, with a gain of 16.17 lbf/mm (i.e., flipping between this factor's levels will give us a better than 90% reduction in variability). From a sensitivity perspective, the recommended factorial levels are:

A: dwell time at level A1 = 1.25 s
B: press bar pressure at level B1 = 85 psi
C: press bar temperature at level C2 = 176°F or 80°C or, in short, the combination A2B1C2.

TABLE 15.9   Response Table for SN Ratios

Level	Factor A	Factor B	Factor C
1	−21.94	−20.15	−25.74
2	−24.85	−26.65	−21.06
Delta	2.91	6.5	4.6
Rank	3	1	2

TABLE 15.10   Response Table for Sensitivity β

Level	Factor A	Factor B	Factor C
1	17.66	23.64	10.87
2	20.24	14.26	27.04
Delta	2.58	9.38	16.17
Rank	3	2	1

The DFSS team noticed that the two analyses conflict at the factor A optimum level. In this example, they favored SN gain over sensitivity gain (i.e., selecting A1 over A2). That is, the optimum combination is A1B1C2.

The seal strength optimum SN ratio transfer function predicted is given in (15.12) and is evaluated for the optimum combination A1B1C2:

$$SN_y\big|_{predicted,optimum} = -23.395 + \sum_{i=1}^{3}\left(\overline{factor_i} + 23.395\right)$$
$$= -16.36\,dB \tag{15.12}$$

where $\overline{factor_i}$ is the average SN ratio value at the significant factorial level in the optimum combination.

The seal strength optimum sensitivity transfer function predicted is given in (15.13) and is evaluated for the optimum combination A1B1C2:

$$\beta\big|_{predicted,optimum} = 18.95 + \sum_{i=1}^{3}\left(\overline{factor_i} - 18.95\right)$$
$$= 30.44\,1bf/mm \tag{15.13}$$

where $\overline{factor_i}$ is the average sensitivity at the significant factorial level.

The current design SN performance is given as

$$SN_y\big|_{predicted,current} = -23.395 + \sum_{i=1}^{3}\left(\overline{facor_i} + 23.395\right)$$
$$= -21.04\,dB \tag{15.14}$$

$$\beta\big|_{predicted,current} = 18.95 + \sum_{t=1}^{3}\left(\overline{factor_i} - 18.95\right)$$
$$= 14.27\,1bf/mm \tag{15.15}$$

The current design SN ratio is −21.04 dB and the β is 14.27 1bf. The SN delta gain (ΔSN) predicted = −16.36 + 21.04 = 4.68 dB. The sensitivity (β) delta gain (Δβ) predicted = 16.17 1bf/mm.

Next, the robustness of this parameter optimization can be verified experimentally. This requires prediction and confirmation runs for both the optimum and the current design combinations. Each treatment combination was predicted, and then two runs at these combinations were measured using the same experimental setup. These confirmation runs were performed at both levels of noise. The results of these confirmation runs, including mean and SN ratio, are shown in Table 15.11.

The confirmed SN ratio = 4.35 dB and the confirmed β = 15.04 1bf/mm. In other words, the team predicted a gain of 4.68 dB, but they were able to

TABLE 15.11 Confirmation Run Results

Design	β	SN Ratio
Optimum	29.82	−15.96
Current	14.78	−20.31

confirm 4.35 dB. This amounts to a 60% reduction in variability. They also predicted a sensitivity gain of 16.17 lbf/mm, but they were only able to confirm 15.04 lbf/mm. The confirmation runs gave very good results.

15.5 SUMMARY

To summarize briefly, when using robustness methods, a DFSS team first needs to determine the design or control factors that can be controlled. These are the factors in the experiment for which the team will try different levels. Next, they decide to select an appropriate orthogonal array for the experiment. Next, they need to decide on how to measure the design requirement of interest. Most SN ratios require that multiple measurements be taken in each run of the experiment; so that the variability around the nominal value cannot otherwise be assessed. Finally, they conduct the experiment and identify the factors that most strongly affect the chosen signal-to-noise ratio, and they reset the process parameters accordingly.

16

MEDICAL DEVICE TOLERANCE DESIGN

16.1 INTRODUCTION

In this chapter we deal with the problem of how, and when, to specify tightened tolerances for a medical device so that quality and performance are enhanced. Every device (or its manufacturing processes) has a number—perhaps a large number—of design parameters (or process variables). We explain here how to identify the critical parameters and variables to target when tolerances have to be tightened.

It is a natural impulse to believe that the quality and performance of any device can easily be improved by merely tightening up on some or all of its tolerance requirements (see www.itl.nist.gov/div898/handbook/pri/section5/pri56.htm). By this we mean that if a specified parameter is, say, machining to $\pm 2 \, \mu m$, we naturally believe that we can obtain better performance by specifying machining to $\pm 1 \, \mu m$. This can become expensive, however, and is often not a guarantee of much better performance. One has merely to witness the high initial and maintenance costs of such tight-tolerance-level parameters in a medical device to realize that tolerance design—the selection of critical tolerances and the respecification of those critical tolerances—is not a task to be undertaken without careful thought. In fact, it is recommended that only after extensive robust parameter design studies have been completed should tolerance design be carried out as a last resort to improve the quality and productivity of a device.

Medical Device Design for Six Sigma: A Road Map for Safety and Effectiveness,
By Basem S. El-Haik and Khalid S. Mekki
Copyright © 2008 John Wiley & Sons, Inc.

In the medical device DFSS road map (Chapter 7), the objective of tolerance design is to gain optimization beyond that gained through parameter optimization and transfer function detailing to achieve a six-sigma-capable design. In this step, the DFSS team determines allowable deviations in design parameters and process variables, tightening tolerances and upgrading only where necessary to meet the functional requirements. Where possible, tolerances may also be loosened. In tolerance design, the purpose is to assign tolerances to a device based on overall tolerable variation in the functional requirements, the relative influence of different sources of variation on the whole, and the cost–benefit trade-offs.

Tolerance design can be conducted analytically based on the validated transfer function obtained, or empirically, via testing. In either case, the inputs of this step are twofold: The team should have a good understanding of the product and process requirements; and their translation into product and process specifications using quality function deployment (QFD) (Chapter8).

The going-in position in the DFSS algorithm is to use tolerances that are as wide as possible for cost considerations, then optimize the function of the design and process through a combination of suitable design parameters. Following this, it is necessary to identify those customer-related functional requirements that are not met through parameter design optimization methods. Tightening tolerances and upgrading materials and other parameters will usually be required to meet six sigma functional requirements targets. Systematic application of DFSS principles and tools such as QFD allows the identification of customer-sensitive requirements and the development for these characteristics of target values to meet customer expectations. It is vital that these characteristics be traced down to lowest-level mappings and that appropriate targets and ranges be developed. By definition, *tolerance* is the permissible deviation from a specified value or a standard.

For a medical device, customers (clinics, doctors, hospitals, and patients) often have explicit or implicit requirements and allowable requirement variation ranges, called *customer tolerance*. In the next stage, customer requirements and tolerances will be mapped into design functional requirements and functional tolerances. For a design to deliver its functional requirements to satisfy functional tolerances, it is required that the design parameters be set to the right nominal values and their variations be within design parameter tolerances. For design development, the last stage is to develop manufacturing process variable set points and tolerances.

16.2 TOLERANCE DESIGN AND DFSS

In the DFSS process, functional requirement tolerance development is the first important step. It translates ambiguous, mostly verbal customer tolerances into clear and quantitative functional tolerances. This step involves the use of functional analysis as obtained in the physical structure via axiomatic design (Chapter 9), customer attribute analysis, and competitors' benchmarking. Phase II QFD (Chapter 8) is certainly a valuable tool in translating customers' requirements into functional specifications.

However, most of work in tolerance design involves determination of design parameter tolerances and process variable tolerances given that the functional tolerances have already been determined. In most industries the term *tolerance design* actually means the determination of design parameter tolerances and process variable tolerances.

If a device is complex, the tolerance design is a multiple-stage process. After functional tolerances are determined, system and subsystem tolerances are determined first, and then component tolerances are determined based on system and subsystem tolerances. Finally, process variable tolerances are determined based on component tolerances.

Each stage of the tolerance design can actually be illustrated as in Figure 16.1, where the high-level requirement and tolerance is the requirement and tolerance derived at the preceding stage. For example, functional requirement and tolerance is at a high level compared with the design parameter requirements and tolerances, and system requirement and tolerance is at a higher level compared with component requirements and tolerances. $y = f(x_1, x_2, \ldots, x_n)$ is the transfer function relationship between higher- and lower-level parameters. In a typical stage of tolerance design, given the target requirement of y and its tolerance (i.e., $T_y \pm \Delta_0$), the main task is how to assign the tolerances for each x_i. There are three major issues in tolerance design:

- Managing variability
- Achieving the functional requirements satisfactorily
- Keeping the life-cycle cost of design at a low level

From an economical point of view, it is desirable that the functional requirements be satisfied with minimum variation. From the earlier discussion of customer tolerances, the customer tolerance is defined as the tolerance limits for which 50% of customers will be unhappy if they are exceeded. For each individual customer, tolerance varies from person to person; a very picky customer will not tolerate any deviation of a requirement from its ideal state.

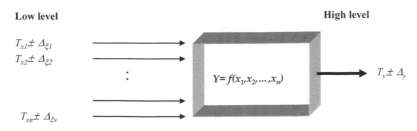

Figure 16.1 Typical stage of tolerance design.

If a design requirement is at boundary of customer tolerance, 50% of customers are already unhappy with the design. Minimizing functional variations will maximize customer satisfaction and will also certainly reduce rework, warranty service cost, and after-sale service cost. On the other hand, it is also highly desirable that design parameter tolerances and process variable tolerances be set at wider intervals. Obviously, loose tolerances of design parameters and process variables will make manufacturing easier and cheaper. Taguchi's parameter design is trying to minimize requirement variation with the presence of noise factors; the noise factors also include piece-to-piece variation. Therefore, a very successful parameter design could "loosen up" some tolerances. However, if a parameter design is insufficient to limit the functional requirement variation, tolerance design is essential.

In tolerance design, cost is an important factor. If a design parameter or a process variable is relatively easy and cheap to control, a tighter tolerance is desirable; otherwise, a looser tolerance is desirable. Therefore, for each stage of tolerance design, the objective is to ensure low functional variation by economically setting appropriate tolerances on design parameters and process variables.

The situation shown in Figure 16.2 is very common in most tolerance design circumstances. However, subject-matter knowledge also plays a role for various circumstances. For example, if the design parameters are all dimensionally related, such as mechanical parts dimensions, there is a full body of knowledge regarding this, called *geometrical dimensioning and tolerancing* (GD&T). In GD&T, the fundamental idea about tolerance design is really the same as that with any other tolerance designs. However, there are lots of special methods and terminologies that are purely dimensionally related.

In this chapter we discuss all major tolerance design methods under the tolerance design paradigm illustrated in Figure 9.1. Subject-matter-related tolerance design aspects such as GD&T are not included here.

There are two classes of tolerance design methods: traditional tolerance design methods and Taguchi's tolerance design method. Traditional methods include worst-case tolerance analysis, statistical tolerance analysis, and cost-based tolerance analysis. Taguchi's tolerance design methods include the relationship between customer tolerance and producer tolerance, and tolerance design experiments. All these methods are discussed in subsequent sections.

16.2.1 Application: Imprecise Measurements

An OEM of a medical device that has an electronic component complained to the supplier that the measurement reported by the supplier on as-delivered items appeared to be imprecise. The supplier undertook to investigate the matter. The supplier's engineers reported that the measurement in question was made up of two components, which we label x_1 and x_2, and the final measurement y was reported according to the following transfer function:

$$y = \frac{Kx_1}{x_2} \tag{16.1}$$

with K a known physical constant. Components x_1 and x_2 were measured separately in the laboratory using two different techniques, and the results were combined by software to produce y. Buying new measurement devices for both components would be prohibitively expensive, and it was not even known by how much the x_1 or x_2 component tolerances should be improved to produce the desired improvement in the precision of y.

Assume that in a measurement of a standard item, the true value of x_1 is $x_{1,0}$ and for x_2 is $x_{2,0}$. Let $f(x_1, x_2) = y$; then the Taylor series expansion

$$f(x_1, x_2) = f(x_{1,0}, x_{2,0}) + (x_1 - x_{1,0})\frac{df}{dx_1} + (x_2 - x_{2,0})\frac{df}{dx_2}$$

$$+ (x_1 - x_{1,0})^2 \frac{d^2 f}{dx_1^2} + (x_2 - x_{2,0})^2 \frac{d^2 f}{dx_2^2} + (x_1 - x_{1,0})(x_2 - x_{2,0})\frac{d^2 f}{dx_1 dx_2}$$

$$+ \text{higher-order terms}$$

$$\tag{16.2}$$

with all the partial derivatives (i.e., df/dx, etc.), evaluated at $(x_{1,0}, x_{2,0})$. Apply formula (16.2) to (16.1) to obtain

$$f(x_1, x_2) = K\frac{x_{1,0}}{x_{2,0}} + (x_1 - x_{1,0})\frac{K}{x_{2,0}} - (x_2 - x_{2,0})\frac{Kx_{1,0}}{x_{2,0}^2} - 2(x_2 - x_{2,0})^2 \frac{K}{x_{2,0}^2}$$

$$- (x_1 - x_{1,0})(x_2 - x_{2,0})\frac{K}{x_{2,0}^2} + \text{higher-order terms} \tag{16.3}$$

It is assumed known from experience that the measurements of x_1 show a distribution with an average value $x_{1,0}$, and a standard deviation $\sigma_{x_1} = 0.003$ x-units. In addition, we assume that the distribution of x_1 is normal. Since 99.74% of a normal distribution's range is covered by 6σ, we take $3\sigma_{x_1} = 0.009$ x_1-unit to be the existing tolerance Δ_{x1} for measurements on x_1. That is, $\Delta_{x1} = \pm 0.009$ x_1-units is the play around $x_{1,0}$ that we expect from the existing measurement system.

It is also assumed known that the x_2 measurements show a normal distribution around $x_{2,0}$, with standard deviation $\sigma_{x_2} = 0.004$ x_2-unit. Thus, $\Delta x_2 = \pm 0.012$. Now $\pm\Delta_{x1}$ and $\pm\Delta_{x2}$ may be thought of as worst-case values for $(x_1 - x_{1,0})$ and $(x_2 - x_{2,0})$. Substituting Δ_{x1} for $x_1 - x_{1,0}$ and Δ_{x2} for $x_2 - x_{2,0}$ in the expanded formula for $f(x_1, x_2)$, we have

$$\Delta_y = K\frac{x_{1,0}}{x_{2,0}} + \Delta_{x1}\frac{K}{x_{2,0}} - \Delta_{x2}\frac{Kx_{1,0}}{x_{2,0}^2} - 2\Delta_{x2}^2 \frac{K}{x_{2,0}^3} - \Delta_{x1}\Delta_{x2}\frac{K}{x_{2,0}^2} + \text{higher-order terms}$$

$$\tag{16.4}$$

an order of magnitude smaller than terms in Δ_{x1} and Δ_{x2}, and for this reason we drop them, so that

$$\Delta_y = K \frac{x_{1,0}}{x_{2,0}} + \Delta_{x1} \frac{K}{x_{2,0}} - \Delta_{x2} \frac{Kx_{1,0}}{x_{2,0}^2} \tag{16.5}$$

Thus, a worst-case Euclidean distance Δ of $f(x_1, x_2)$ from its ideal value $K(x_{1,0}/x_{2,0})$ is approximately

$$\Delta_y = \left[\left(\Delta_{x1} \frac{K}{x_{2,0}} \right)^2 + \left(\Delta_{x2} \frac{Kx_{1,0}}{x_{2,0}^2} \right)^2 \right]^{1/2}$$

$$= \left[\left(0.009 \frac{K}{x_{2,0}} \right)^2 + \left(0.012 \frac{Kx_{1,0}}{x_{2,0}^2} \right)^2 \right]^{1/2} \tag{16.6}$$

This shows the relative contributions of the components to the variation in measurement y.

As $x_{2,0}$ is a known quantity and reduction in Δ_{x1} and Δ_{x2} carries its own price tag, it becomes an economic decision whether one should expend resources to reduce Δ_{x1} or Δ_{x2}, or both.

In this example we used a Taylor series approximation to obtain a simple expression that highlights the benefits of Δ_{x1} and Δ_{x2}. Alternatively, one might simulate values of y, given a specified $(\Delta_{x1}, \Delta_{x2})$ and $(x_{1,0}, x_{2,0})$, and then summarize the results with a model for the variability of y as a function of $(\Delta_{x1}, \Delta_{x2})$.

16.3   WORST-CASE TOLERANCE

The worst-case tolerance is a tolerance design approach that is the worst-case scenario. Specifically, let us assume that the transfer function between a higher-level requirement y with lower-level characteristics $x_1, x_2, \ldots, x_i, \ldots, x_n$ is

$$y = f(x_1, x_2, \ldots, x_i, \ldots x_n) \tag{16.7}$$

and it is further assumed that the target value for y is T and the tolerance limit for y is Δ_y such that y is within specifications if $T - \Delta_y \leq y \leq T + \Delta_y$. Sometimes the tolerance limits are asymmetrical; that is, y is in the specification limit if $T - \Delta_y \leq y \leq T + \Delta_y$, where Δ_y is called the left tolerance limit and Δ_y is the right tolerance limit.

For each x_i, $i = 1$ to n, the target value for x_i is T_i and the tolerance limit for x_i is Δ_i such that x_i is within specifications if $T_i - \Delta_i \leq x_i \leq T_i + \Delta_i$ is satisfied.

Sometimes it is also possible that the tolerance limit for x_i is asymmetrical; that is, x_i is within specifications if $T_i - \Delta_i \leq x_i \leq T_i + \Delta_i$ is satisfied.

The worst-case tolerance design rule can be expressed by the following pairs of formulas:

$$T - \Delta_y = \min_{x_i \in (T_i - \Delta_i, T_i + \Delta_i) \forall i} f(x_1, x_2, \ldots, x_i, \ldots, x_n) \qquad (16.8)$$

$$T + \Delta_y = \max_{x_i \in (T_i - \Delta_i, T_i + \Delta_i) \forall i} f(x_1, x_2, \ldots, x_i, \ldots, x_n) \qquad (16.9)$$

where $\forall i$ means "for all i".

If the transfer function equation is nonlinear [i.e., $y = f(x_1, x_2, \ldots, x_i, \ldots x_n)$] is nonlinear, the tolerance analysis is difficult. From a Taylor expansion formula,

$$\Delta_y \cong \frac{\partial f}{\partial x_1} \Delta x_1 + \frac{\partial f}{\partial x_2} \Delta x_2 + \cdots + \frac{\partial f}{\partial x_i} \Delta x_i + \cdots + \frac{\partial f}{\partial x_n} \Delta x_n \qquad (16.10)$$

According to Chase and Greenwood (1988), the worst-case tolerance limit in the nonlinear case is

$$\Delta_y \cong \left| \frac{\partial f}{\partial x_1} \right| \Delta_1 + \left| \frac{\partial f}{\partial x_2} \right| \Delta_2 + \cdots + \left| \frac{\partial f}{\partial x_i} \right| \Delta_i + \cdots + \left| \frac{\partial f}{\partial x_n} \right| \Delta_n \qquad (16.11)$$

16.3.1 Application: Internal Pressures in Disposable Tubing

Disposable tubing is used in a device used to mix prescribed medicines that contains a drive mechanism that includes a precision actuator, drug container holder, and syringe retention components. This example is concerned with disposable tubing that connects the syringe with a drug container that contains a spike nozzle orifice. The tube internal peak pressure is the output response, the functional requirement (y). Figure 16.2 illustrates the experimental setup of the instrument described above.

Two primary factors contribute to tube internal peak pressure during medical device drug mixing: fluid flow within the drug container spike nozzle,

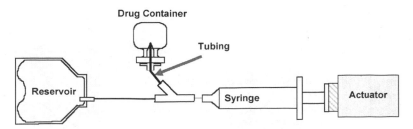

Figure 16.2 Experimental setup for internal pressure of tubing.

and air compression within the tubing circuit. The drug container nozzle lumens act as fluid flow orifices and thereby contribute to a pressure rise in the fluid circuit. The pressure rise from the drug container nozzle lumens occurs only during the portion of the mixing cycle in which fluid flows through the syringe. The contribution to internal tube pressure caused by air compression in the tubing circuit and vial, on the other hand, is always present and increases, during mixing, as the fluid–air boundary advances within the tubing and then the drug container.

The tube internal pressure, then, is simply a combination of the two primary factors of compressed air pressure and the pressure rise across the drug container nozzle:

$$p = p_{gas} + \Delta p_n \qquad (16.12)$$

Quantification of the contribution to tube internal pressure contributed by each of these two primary factors is obtained from well-established principles of physics.

Fluid friction pressure through the nozzle lumens is proportional to the square of the fluid velocity (or, alternatively, the nozzle lumen diameter to the fourth power):

$$\Delta p_n = C v_n^2 \qquad (16.13)$$

where Δp_n is the pressure drop across the nozzle lumens, v_n is the nozzle fluid velocity (calculated based on the actual flow and the actual area), and the proportionality term C is dependent on the nozzle lumen diameter (the lumen being considered as a classic sharp-edged orifice) and the nozzle lumen approach tube diameter.

Air pressure on the air–fluid boundary is determined from a polytropic relationship between the initial air pressure and the initial and final volumes of the air within the tubing circuit:

$$p_{gas} = p_{atm} \left(\frac{V_0}{V_{final}} \right)^k \qquad (16.14)$$

where V_0 is air volume prior to the start of fluid flow (both drug container and tubing air volume), V_{final} is the air volume at the end of fluid flow, k is the specific heat ratio (1.4 for air during an adiabatic process), and the initial tubing air pressure, p_{atm}, is a consequence of venting the tubing circuit to the atmosphere prior to isolation for mixing of drugs.

Nozzle Orifice Parameters Note that each of the two pressure terms in expressions (16.13) and (16.14) depend, in turn, on two system parameters. The pressure rise from fluid acceleration (and friction) in (16.12) depends on the independent parameters of nozzle lumen geometry and fluid velocity through the nozzle. The nozzle lumen geometry is embodied in the expression

$$C = \frac{\rho}{2}\left[\frac{0.25}{K^2}\left(\frac{D}{d}\right)^4 - \frac{1+K^2}{K^2}\right] \tag{16.15}$$

where $K = 0.82$ (as a consequence of orifice length, w, being on the order of three times the approach diameter, that is, $w \approx 3D$) is a well-documented flow correction factor developed from empirical efforts that characterize orifice types, ρ is the fluid density (water was used throughout this study), and the diameters d and D are defined in Figure 16.3.

The form of C in expression (16.15) is developed for use with the nozzle orifice approach tube fluid velocity, where

$$v_n = \frac{Q_n}{(\pi/4)D^2} \tag{16.16}$$

where Q_n is the volumetric fluid flow through the nozzle. For convenient comparison of various nozzle geometries, the nozzle pressure drop can be reformulated in terms of a reference fluid velocity such as the actuator velocity:

$$\Delta p_n = C v_s^2 \tag{16.17}$$

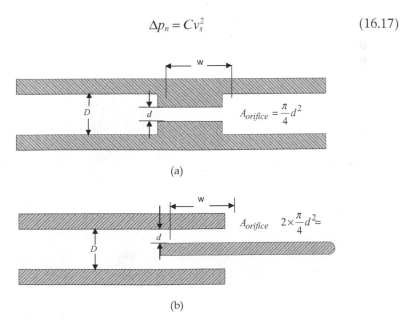

(a)

(b)

Figure 16.3 Nozzle orifice geometry: (a) ideal orifice compared with (b) actual orifice.

where v_s is the actuator velocity (this assumes no air pockets or fluid storage in the fluid circuit) and

$$C = \left(\frac{D_s}{D}\right)^4 C \tag{16.18}$$

Compressed Air Parameters   In the same way, the air pressure, p_{gas}, in (16.14) depends on two parameters, initial and final air volume (assuming that mixing always begins after venting the kit to atmospheric pressure). Initial volume includes the empty volume of the drug container and the volume of unprimed tubing between the fluid–air boundary and the drug container entrance:

$$V_0 = V_{vial} + V_{unprimed\ tubing} \tag{16.19}$$

where currently, V_{vial} = 9.35 mL is the empty volume of the vial and $V_{unprimed\ tubing}$ depends on kit configuration and algorithm architecture (currently, 4.33 mL for mixing). The final air volume, V_f, is the final air volume within the drug container, which is merely the empty drug container volume less its fill volume (the volume of fluid intended to be delivered to the drug container during mixing). Consequently,

$$V_{final} = V_{vial} - V_{fill} \tag{16.20}$$

and V_{fill} is in the range 3 to 5 mL (tentatively).

Pressure Model   In this treatment of tube pressure, the pressure model of expression (16.14), can now be written explicitly in terms of the four parameters that determine the peak pressure:

$$p(d, v_s, V_0, V_f) = p_{atm}\left(\frac{V_0}{V_f}\right)^k + \frac{\rho}{2}\left[\frac{0.25}{K^2}\left(\frac{D}{d}\right)^4 - \frac{1+K^2}{K^2}\right]\left(\frac{D_s}{D}\right)^4 v_s^2 \tag{16.21}$$

where D_s and v_s are the syringe barrel internal diameter (any units consistent with the unit choice for d) and actuator speed, respectively, V_0 is the initial air volume, V_f is the air volume at the maximum drug container fill level, and we have selected the following values for the fixed parameters (fixed for this study):

$D = 2d + 0.028\,\text{in.}$ (assumes nozzle point dimension constant)   (16.22a)

$\rho = 0.001\,\text{g/mm}^3$ (density of water at 70°F)   (16.22b)

$K = 0.82$ (as a consequence of orifice geometry)   (16.22c)

$k = 1.4$ (ratio of specific heats for air)   (16.22d)

$p_{atm} = 14.7\,\text{psi}$ (atmospheric pressure at 70°F)   (16.22e)

Using the numerical values of the fixed parameters in expression (16.21) gives

$$p(d, v_s, V_0, V_f) = 14.7\left(\frac{V_0}{V_f}\right)^{1.4} + \left[\frac{0.026964}{d^4} - \frac{0.18038}{(0.028 + 2d)^4}\right](v_s)^2 \quad (16.23)$$

where the numerical value of d is to be in units of inches and that of v_s in mm/ms. The resulting numerical value of pressure will be in units of psi.

Further analysis was conducted to determine a desirable mixing cycle based on peak tubing pressure. However, peak tubing pressure is not the only design constraint in the mixing cycle. In fact, changing any of the four factors considered in this study (16.23) may well have an effect on the fundamental process of mixing, which seeks to properly mix a powdered form of drug to a liquid form. As an example, if we reduce the actuator speed from 40 mm/s to 30 mm/s while holding the other parameters constant, we will reduce peak pressure by about 18 psi. However, the reduction in actuator speed, and therefore spike nozzle fluid stream speed, may well render the mixing activity less active and, therefore, possibly less effective. Consequently, any interactions between reduced tubing peak pressures and other cycle performance measures must be explored carefully before selecting cycle parameters based on reduced tubing pressures alone.

Design direction for selecting the numerical values of the four factors studied in this report can be determined based on variation analyses of the pressure model. We choose two separate methods to determine the variation of pressure with respect to variation of the four factors in this report. The first method of variation analysis is a sensitivity study in which the partial derivatives of the pressure model are developed with respect to each of the four factors. This analysis provides an immediate determination of the existence of any interactions between the factors. These partial derivatives may also be used for a linearized assessment of peak pressure sensitivity to each of the four factors. However, we defer the sensitivity analysis using this method in favor of the second variation analysis method, the tolerance design of experiments (DOE).

Here is an analysis of the sensitivity. We can use the partial derivatives of the peak pressure function in expression (16.23) to develop expressions that quantify the sensitivity of pressure to each of the four parameters investigated in this report. Note that this is analogous to a study of interactions between the four parameters (factors) when using DOE techniques. Forming the partial derivatives of peak pressure with respect to each of the four parameters of expression (16.23) yields first-order variations of p with respect to each of the parameters:

$$\frac{\partial p}{\partial d} = \left[\frac{1.44304}{(0.028 + 2d)^3} - \frac{0.107856}{d^3}\right]v_s^2 \quad (16.24a)$$

$$\frac{\partial p}{\partial v_s} = \left[\frac{0.053928}{d^4} - \frac{0.36076}{(0.028 + 2d)^3}\right] v_s \qquad (16.24b)$$

$$\frac{\partial p}{\partial V_0} = 20.58 \frac{(V_0)^{0.4}}{(V_f)^{1.4}} \qquad (16.24c)$$

$$\frac{\partial p}{\partial V_f} = -20.58 \frac{(V_0)^{1.4}}{(V_f)^{2.4}} \qquad (16.24d)$$

Inspection of the four sensitivity terms shows that interactions exist between lumen diameter and actuator speed (d and v_s, as both appear in each of the first two sensitivity expressions) and between initial air volume and final air volume (V_0 and V_f).

From the Taylor expansion of (16.23), the worst-case tolerance is given by

$$\Delta p \cong \frac{\partial p}{\partial d} \Delta d + \frac{\partial p}{\partial v_s} \Delta v_s + \frac{\partial p}{\partial V_0} \Delta V_0 + \frac{\partial p}{\partial V_f} \Delta V_f \qquad (16.25)$$

$$\Delta p \cong \left[\frac{1.44304}{(0.028 + 2d)^3} - \frac{0.107856}{d^3}\right] v_s^2 \Delta d + \left[\frac{0.053928}{d^4} - \frac{0.36076}{(0.028 + 2d)^3}\right] v_s \Delta v_s$$

$$+ 20.58 \frac{(V_0)^{0.4}}{(V_f)^{1.4}} \Delta V_0 - 20.58 \frac{(V_0)^{1.4}}{(V_f)^{2.4}} \Delta V_f \qquad (16.26)$$

16.4   STATISTICAL TOLERANCES

The worst-case tolerance design can ensure that high-level tolerance limits are satisfied on all combinations of lower-level characteristics, even in extreme cases. However, this approach will create very tight tolerances for low-level characteristics, and tight tolerance usually means high cost of manufacturing. On the other hand, low-level characteristics such as part dimension and component parameters are usually random variables. The probability that all low-level characteristics are equal to extreme values (all very low or very high) simultaneously is extremely small. Therefore, the worst-case tolerance method tends to overdesign the tolerances and thus is used only if the cost of nonconforming is very high for high-level requirement and the cost to keep tight tolerances on low-level characteristics is low.

The statistical tolerance design method treats both high-level requirements and low-level characteristics as random variables. The objective of statistical tolerance design is to ensure that the high-level requirement will meet its specification with very high probability.

Low-level characteristics are often assumed to be independent random variables. This assumption is quite valid because low-level characteristics such as device dimension and device parameter value often come out of different, unrelated manufacturing processes, and there is usually very little relationship among them. Normal distribution is the most frequently used probability model for low-level characteristics. If a low-level characteristic such as device dimension or component parameter is produced by existing manufacturing process, historical statistical process control data can be used to estimate its mean and standard deviation.

In this chapter we assume that each low-level characteristics (x_i) is a normally distributed random variable [i.e., $x_i \sim N(\mu_i, \sigma_i^2)$ for $i = 1$ to n]. We also assume that the higher-level requirement (y) is also a normally distributed variable, $y \sim N(\mu, \sigma^2)$.

16.4.1 Relationship of Tolerance to Process Capabilities

The process capability, C_p, is given by

$$C_p = \frac{\text{USL} - \text{LSL}}{6\sigma} \qquad (16.27)$$

If the process is centered, or in other words, the target value is equal to the mean of a requirement [say, x_i, $T_i = E(x_i)$, and the specification limit is symmetric, $\Delta_i = \Delta_i'$], it is clear that

$$C_p = \frac{\text{USL} - \text{LSL}}{6\sigma_i} = \frac{\text{USL} - T_i}{3\sigma_i} = \frac{T_i - \text{LSL}}{3\sigma_i} = \frac{\Delta_i}{3\sigma_i} \qquad (16.28)$$

or

$$\Delta_i = 3C_p\sigma_i \qquad (16.29)$$

For each low-level characteristic x_i, $i = 1$ to n.

Similarly, for the high-level requirement (y),

$$\Delta_y = 3C_p\sigma_y \qquad (16.30)$$

If a six sigma quality is required, $C_p = 2$.

16.4.2 Linear Statistical Tolerance

If the transfer function equation between high-level requirements and low-level parameters or variables $x_1, x_2, \ldots, x_i, \ldots, x_n$ is a linear function, that is,

$$y = f(x_1, x_2, \ldots, x_i, \ldots, x_n) = a_1x_1 + a_2x_2 + \cdots + a_ix_i + \cdots + a_nx_n \quad (16.31)$$

then we have the relationship

$$\text{Var}(y) = \sigma_y^2 = a_1^2\sigma_1^2 + a_2^2\sigma_2^2 + \cdots + a_i^2\sigma_i^2 + \cdots + a_n^2\sigma_n^2 \quad (16.32)$$

Equation (16.32) gives the relationship between the variance of a high-level requirement and the variances of low-level parameters. Equations (16.28) and (16.29) provide the relationship between tolerance, variances, and process capabilities of both high- and low-level characteristics. From these equations, we can derive the following step-by-step linear statistical tolerance design procedure.

1. Identify the exact transfer function between a high-level requirement (y) and low-level parameters or variables; that is, identify equation (16.31).

2. For each low-level characteristic, xi, $i = 1$ to n, identify its σ_i, Cp, and Δ_i. This can be done by looking into sampling or historical process control data if x_i is made by an existing process. Otherwise, one should make an initial allocation of its σ_i, Cp, and Δ_i from the best knowledge available.

3. Calculate σ_y^2, the variance of y, using equation (16.32).

4. From equation (16.30) it is clear that

$$C_p = \frac{\Delta_y}{3\sigma_y}$$

which we use to calculate the current C_p value for the high-level requirement. If this C_p is good enough to meet the requirement, stop; if not, go to step 5.

5. Select a desirable C_p level; for example, if a six sigma level is required, $C_p = 2$. Compute the required high-level variance by

$$\sigma_y^2 = \left(\frac{\Delta_y}{3C_p}\right)^2 \quad (16.33)$$

To achieve this high-level variance requirement, we need to scale down the low-level variances. If proportional scaling is used, we can use the following formula to find out the scaling factor p:

$$\sigma_y^2 = p^2 \sum_{i=1}^{n} a_i^2\sigma_i^2 \quad (16.34)$$

so

$$p = \frac{\sigma_y}{\sqrt{\sum_{i=1}^{n} a_i^2 \sigma_i^2}} \tag{16.35}$$

Then the lower-level variance and tolerance can be determined by

$$\sigma_{i_{new}} = p\sigma_i \tag{16.36}$$

$$\Delta_i = 3C_p \sigma_{i_{new}} \tag{16.37}$$

Example 16.1   Consider a medical device assembly of a shaft and a bearing. Let x_1 denote the actual dimension of the shaft and x_2 that of a bearing. Let y denote the clearance between the shaft and the bearing. Then $y = x_2 - x_1$. The tolerance for the clearance, Δ_y, is ±0.05 mm. Determine the tolerances for the shaft and the bearing given they are equal ($\sigma_{x_1} = \sigma_{x_2} = \sigma_x$). Assume that $C_p = 2$.

Solution: From (16.30), the standard deviation of y, σ_y, is given by $\sigma_y = 0.05/3(2) = 0.0083$. We have $p = 1$, and from (16.35) we get

$$\sigma_y = \sqrt{\sum_{i=1}^{n} a_i^2 \sigma_i^2} \Rightarrow 0.0083 = \sqrt{(1)^2 \sigma_{x_1}^2 + (-1)^2 \sigma_{x_2}^2} = \sqrt{2\sigma_x^2}$$

$$= \sqrt{2}\sigma_x \Rightarrow \sigma_x = \frac{0.0083}{\sqrt{2}} = 0.00589 \text{ mm}$$

From (16.29), we have $\Delta_{x_1} = \Delta_{x_2} = \Delta_x = 3(2)(0.00589) = 0.0354 \text{ mm}$.

16.4.3   Nonlinear Statistical Tolerance

If the transfer function equation between high-level requirement y and low-level characteristics $x_1, x_2, \ldots, x_i, \ldots, x_n$ is not a linear function, that is,

$$y = f(x_1, x_2, \ldots, x_i, \ldots, x_n) \tag{16.38}$$

is not a linear function, then we have the following approximate relationship:

$$\mathrm{Var}(y) = \sigma_y^2 \cong \left(\frac{\partial f}{\partial x_1}\right)^2 \sigma_1^2 + \left(\frac{\partial f}{\partial x_2}\right)^2 \sigma_2^2 + \cdots + \left(\frac{\partial f}{\partial x_i}\right)^2 \sigma_i^2 + \cdots + \left(\frac{\partial f}{\partial x_n}\right)^2 \sigma_n^2 \tag{16.39}$$

Equation (16.39) gives the approximate relationship between the variances of high-level requirements and low-level characteristics. Equations (16.29) and (16.30) can still provide the relationship between tolerance, variances, and process capabilities of both high- and low-level characteristics.

It is very often that the transfer function $y = f(x_1, x_2, \ldots, x_i, \ldots, x_n)$ is not a closed-form equation. In the design stage, computer simulation models are often available for many products and processes: for example, the FEA model for a mechanically related design and electrical circuit simulator for electronic designs. Many of these computer simulation models can provide sensitivities, which is essentially $\Delta y/\Delta x_i$. These sensitivities can be used to play the roles of partial derivatives, $\partial f/\partial x_i$.

Here we can develop the following step-by-step procedure for nonlinear statistical tolerance design.

1. Identify the exact transfer function between high-level requirement y and low-level characteristics; that is, identify equation (16.38). If the equation is not given in closed form, we can use a computer simulation model or an empirical model derived from a DOE study.

2. For each low-level characteristic (parameter) x_i, $i = 1$ to n, identify its σ_i, C_p, and Δ_i. This can be done by looking into historical process control data if xi is made by an existing process. Otherwise, make an initial allocation of its σ_i, C_p, and Δ_i from the best knowledge available.

3. Calculate σ_y^2, the variance of y, using equation (16.39). Sensitivities can be used to substitute partial derivatives.

4. From equation (16.30) it is clear that

$$C_p = \frac{\Delta_y}{3\sigma_y}$$

Use this equation to calculate the current C_p value for the high-level requirement. If this C_p is good enough to meet the requirement, stop; if not, go to 5.

5. Select a desirable C_p level. For example, if a six sigma level is required, $C_p = 2$. Compute the high-level variance required by (16.33).

To achieve this high-level variance requirement, we need to scale down low-level variances. If proportional scaling is used, we can use the following formula to find out the scaling factor p:

$$\sigma_y^2 = p^2 \sum_{i=1}^{n} \left(\frac{\partial f}{\partial x_i} \right)^2 \sigma_i^2 \qquad (16.40)$$

so

$$p = \frac{\sigma_y}{\sqrt{\sum_{i=1}^{n} (\partial f/\partial x_i) \sigma_i^2}} \qquad (16.41)$$

Then the lower–level variance and tolerance can be determined by

$$\sigma_{i_{\text{new}}} = p\sigma_i \tag{16.42}$$

$$\Delta_i = 3C_p\sigma_{i_{\text{new}}} \tag{16.43}$$

Example 16.2 A medical device circuit has two resistances in parallel, as given in Figure 16.4. The value of each resistance is a random variable. We know that $\mu_{R_1} = 100\,\Omega$, $\mu_{R_2} = 200\,\Omega$, $\sigma_{R_1} = 10\,\Omega$, and $\sigma_{R_2} = 15\,\Omega$. Determine the equivalent resistance mean, μ_R, and its standard deviation, σ_R, and the tolerance of R as given in (16.40).

Solution: From circuit theory, the transfer function is given by

$$R = \frac{R_1 R_2}{R_1 + R_2} \tag{16.44}$$

From the Taylor series,

$$E(R) \approx f(R_1, R_2) = \frac{\mu_{R_1}\mu_{R_2}}{\mu_{R_1} + \mu_{R_2}} = \frac{100 \times 200}{100 + 200} = 66.7\,\Omega$$

Differentiating, we have

$$\frac{\partial f}{\partial R_1} = \frac{R_2^2}{(R_1 + R_2)^2} \tag{16.45}$$

$$\frac{\partial f}{\partial R_2} = \frac{R_1^2}{(R_1 + R_2)^2} \tag{16.46}$$

$$\left.\frac{\partial f}{\partial R_1}\right|_{\mu_{R_1}, \mu_{R_2}} = \frac{200^2}{(100 + 200)^2} = 0.444 \tag{16.47}$$

$$\left.\frac{\partial f}{\partial R_2}\right|_{\mu_{R_1}, \mu_{R_2}} = \frac{100^2}{(100 + 200)^2} = 0.111 \tag{16.48}$$

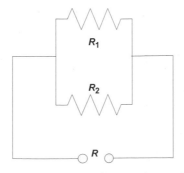

Figure 16.4 Two resistances in parallel.

The variance is given by (16.40) as

$$\sigma_R^2 = p^2[(0.444)^2(10)^2 + (0.111)^2(15)^2]$$
$$= 22.4858 p^2 \Omega^2$$

(16.49)

When $p = 1$, we have

$$\sigma_R = 4.74 \Omega$$

(16.50)

16.5 TAGUCHI'S LOSS FUNCTION AND SAFETY TOLERANCE DESIGN

Robust design is a disciplined engineering process that seeks to find the best expression of a system design. *Best* is carefully defined to mean that the design is the lowest-cost solution to the specification, which itself is based on the customer needs identified. Taguchi has included design quality as one more dimension of cost. High-quality systems minimize these costs by performing, consistently, at targets specified by the customer.

Taguchi's philosophy of robust design is aimed at reducing loss due to variation of performance from the target value based on a portfolio of concepts and measures such as quality loss function (QLF), signal-to-noise (SN) ratio, optimization, and experimental design. *Quality loss* is the loss experienced by customers and society and is a function of how far performance deviates from target. The QLF relates quality to cost and is considered a better evaluation system than the traditional binary treatment of quality (i.e., within or outside specifications). The quality loss function, $L(y,T_y)$, of a functional requirement y has two components: mean (μ_y) deviation from targeted performance value (T_y), and variability (σ_y^2). It can be approximated by a quadratic polynomial of the functional requirement y, as shown in Figure 16.4.

Taguchi developed a unique approach to tolerance design and tolerance analysis. His tolerance design approach includes a cost-based tolerance design and allocation. The most important consideration in cost is the quality loss due to requirement deviation from the ideal requirement level.

16.5.1 Nominal-the-Best Tolerance Design

The quality loss can be expressed by the Taguchi quality loss function that we discussed in detail in Chapter 15. Figure 16.5 is the quadratic curve for the quality loss function for the "nominal the best" case. The quality loss function can be expressed as

$$L(y, T_y) = \frac{A_0}{\Delta_0^2}(y - T)^2$$

(16.51)

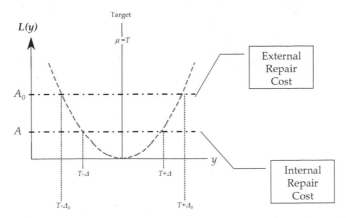

Figure 16.5 Quality loss function, customer tolerance, and producer tolerance.

where Δ_0 is the customer tolerance limit and A_0 is the cost incurred to the customer when the requirement level y is at the boundary of the customer tolerance limit. In Taguchi's view, if the design can be repaired or fixed before shipping to customers at a lower cost, say, A and $A < A_0$, then the producer tolerance, which comprises the internal tolerance limits for shipping inspection, called the producer tolerance limit, or Δ should be set at a narrower level than the customer tolerance limits. Taguchi proposes that the specific producer tolerance limit Δ should be set based on the quality loss function. Specifically, he thinks that at producer tolerance, the quality loss should break even with the internal repair cost. That is, when $y = T + \Delta$ or $y = T - \Delta$, by Equation (16.51), the quality loss

$$L(y, T_y) = \frac{A_0}{\Delta_0^2} \Delta^2 \tag{16.52}$$

But if the quality loss $L(y, T_y)$ is equal to the repair cost A, then

$$A = \frac{A_0}{\Delta_0^2} \Delta^2 \tag{16.53}$$

Therefore, the producer tolerance limit Δ can be computed by

$$\Delta = \sqrt{\frac{A}{A_0}} \Delta_0 = \frac{\Delta_0}{\sqrt{A_0/A}} = \frac{\Delta_0}{\phi} \tag{16.54}$$

where the safety factor

$$\phi = \sqrt{\frac{A_0}{A}}$$
$$= \sqrt{\frac{\text{loss of exceeding functional limit}}{\text{loss at factory for exceeding factory standard}}} \qquad (16.55)$$

From Figure 16.5 we can see that if a medical device company does not have after-sale customer service, the cost for customers due to poor quality will follow a quadratic curve. If the company cannot control the variation in design requirement, the cost for customers will be high and may be fatal, depending on the application. Clearly, this is very bad for customers as well as for the company. Actually, the company may lose even more than the quality loss cost, because customer dissatisfaction, bad reputation, and bad publicity will hurt the company even more than it hurts the customers. For example, if a famous restaurant chain had one incidence of food poisoning, the loss to the customer will be medical cost, a few days or a few weeks of pay, and so on, but the cost for the restaurant chain will be bad publicity, litigation, loss of consumer confidence, big losses in sales, and so on, which very easily reaches a magnitude higher than the customer loss.

Having customer tolerance limits Δ_0 and after-sale service, the company can reduce the maximum customer loss to below the external repair cost A_0. If the company can set a tighter producer tolerance limit Δ, and practice preventive repair at cost A, the maximum loss to the customers will be reduced to repair cost A.

Example 16.3 Assume that a touch screen on a medical instrument, say the Auto 3D device covered in the case study in Chapter 20, has a customer tolerance limit Δ_0 for color density y equal to 7 units. If y is either greater than $T + 7$ or less than $T - 7$, 50% of customers would be unhappy and will demand a screen replacement, at a cost (A_0) of \$98. However, if the screen is repaired by adjustment within the factory, the repair cost would be \$10, and then the producer tolerance Δ should be

$$\Delta = \sqrt{\frac{A}{A_0}}\Delta_0 = \sqrt{\frac{10}{98}}\Delta_0 = \frac{\Delta_0}{\sqrt{98/10}} = \frac{\Delta_0}{3.13} = \frac{7}{3.13} = 2.24$$

That is, the producer tolerance Δ should be 2.24, and the safety factor ϕ in this example is 3.13.

16.5.2 Smaller-the-Better Tolerance Design

For the smaller-the-better requirement, the quality loss function is

$$L(y, T_y) = \frac{A_0}{\Delta_0^2} y^2 \qquad (16.56)$$

If the internal repair cost is A at producer tolerance Δ, by setting repair cost equal to quality loss,

$$A = \frac{A_0}{\Delta_0^2} \Delta^2 \tag{16.57}$$

Therefore,

$$\Delta = \frac{\Delta_0}{\sqrt{A_0/A}} = \frac{\Delta_0}{\phi} \tag{16.58}$$

Example 16.4 Clearly the bacteria count y within a low-cost medical device is a smaller-the-better requirement. Assume that if the bacteria count is more than 6 logs, a user of the device could become contaminated. Suppose that the average cost of medical treatment and lost pay is \$5000. If the count is determined to exceed the limit within the device packaging facility, the device will be discarded, at a cost of \$3.00. We can suggest the internal inspection limit for bacteria count Δ to be

$$\Delta = \frac{\Delta_0}{\sqrt{A_0/A}} = \frac{6}{\sqrt{5000/3}} = \frac{6}{40.825} = 0.147$$

That is, the packaging facility will inspect the device package, and if the package contains a bacteria count above 0.147 logs, the device will be discarded. The safety factor is 40.825.

16.5.3 Larger-the-Better Tolerance Design

For the larger-the-better requirement, the quality loss function is

$$L(y, T_y) = A_0 \Delta_0^2 \frac{1}{y^2} \tag{16.59}$$

If the internal repair cost is A at producer tolerance Δ, by letting the repair cost equal the quality loss,

$$A = A_0 \Delta_0^2 \frac{1}{\Delta^2}$$

Therefore,

$$\Delta = \sqrt{\frac{A_0}{A}} \Delta_0 = \phi \Delta_0 \tag{16.60}$$

16.6   HIGH- VS. LOW-LEVEL REQUIREMENTS' TOLERANCE RELATIONSHIPS

Given the transfer function of a high-level requirement y and low-level characteristics, $x_1, x_2, \ldots, x_i, \ldots, x_n$:

$$y = f(x_1, x_2, \ldots, x_i, \ldots, x_n)$$

Taguchi tolerance design also has its own approach to determining low-level tolerances. If the transfer function above can be linearized, or sensitivities can be found, then for each low-level characteristic x_i, for $i = 1$ to n, we have

$$y - T_y \approx \frac{\partial f}{\partial x_i}(x_i - T_i) \cong a_i(x_i - T_i) \tag{16.61}$$

Then the Taguchi loss function is approximately

$$L(y, T_y) = \frac{A_0}{\Delta_0^2}(y - T_y)^2 \approx \frac{A_0}{\Delta_0^2}[a_i(x_i - T_i)]^2 \tag{16.62}$$

Assume that when a low-level characteristic x_i exceeds its tolerance limit, Δ_i, the cost for replacing it is A_i. Equating A_i with quality loss in equation (16.62), we get

$$A_i = \frac{A_0}{\Delta_0^2}(a_i \Delta_i)^2 \tag{16.63}$$

$$\Delta_i = \sqrt{\frac{A_1}{A_0}} \frac{\Delta_0}{|a_i|} \tag{16.64}$$

Example 16.5   The specification of the output voltage of a medical device power supply circuit is $9 \pm 1.5\,V$. If the power supply circuit is out of specification, the replacement cost is $2.00. The resistance of a resistor affects its output voltage; every 1% change in resistance will make output voltage vary by $0.2\,V$. The replacement cost for a resistor is 15 cents. What should be the tolerance limit for the resistor (in percentage)?

Solution: Using equation (16.64), we get

$$\Delta_i = \sqrt{\frac{A}{A_0}} \frac{\Delta_0}{|a_i|} = \sqrt{\frac{0.15}{2.0}} \frac{1.5}{0.2} = 2.05$$

So the tolerance limit for the resistor should be set at about ±2%.

16.6.1 Tolerance Allocation for Multiple Parameters

Assume that the transfer function $y = f(x_1, x_2, \ldots, x_i, \ldots, x_n)$ is given. If we want to design tolerance limits for all low-level characteristics, $x_1, x_2, \ldots, x_i, \ldots, x_n$, in Taguchi's approach, we can simply apply equation (16.64) to all parameters:

$$\Delta_1 = \sqrt{\frac{A_1}{A_0}} \frac{\Delta_0}{|a_1|}, \quad \Delta_2 = \sqrt{\frac{A_2}{A_0}} \frac{\Delta_0}{|a_2|}, \quad \ldots, \quad \Delta_n = \sqrt{\frac{A_n}{A_0}} \frac{\Delta_0}{|a_n|} \qquad (16.65)$$

Therefore, the square of the range of the output y caused by the variation of $x_1, x_2, \ldots, x_i, \ldots, x_n$, is

$$
\begin{aligned}
\Delta^2 &= (a_1\Delta_1)^2 + (a_2\Delta_2)^2 + \cdots + (a_n\Delta_n)^2 \\
&= \left(\sqrt{\frac{A_1}{A_0}}\Delta_0\right)^2 + \left(\sqrt{\frac{A_2}{A_0}}\Delta_0\right)^2 + \cdots + \left(\sqrt{\frac{A_n}{A_0}}\Delta_0\right)^2 \\
&= \frac{A_1 + A_2 + \cdots + A_k}{A_0}\Delta_0 \qquad (16.66)
\end{aligned}
$$

or

$$\Delta = \sqrt{\frac{\sum_{i=1}^{n} A_n}{A_0}}\Delta_0 \qquad (16.67)$$

If $x_1, x_2, \ldots, x_i, \ldots, x_n$, are n components that form a device, then in equations (16.67) and (16.69), A_0 stands for the cost to make the system back to specification, and $A_1 + A_2 + \ldots + A_n$ stands for the total cost of purchasing these n components. This leads to the following three cases:

- *Case 1:* $A_1 + A_2 + \cdots + A_n \ll A_0$

    This means that the total cost of components is much smaller than the cost of rectifying the system. This could certainly happen if the entire system has to be scraped when it is out of specification. From equation (16.68) it is clear that Δ, the actual producer tolerance for the assembly, will be much smaller than the customer tolerance Δ_0. For example, if

$$A_1 + A_2 + \cdots + A_n = \frac{1}{4} A_0 \qquad (16.68)$$

    That is, the total component cost is one-fourth of the system replacement cost; then, by equation (16.68),

$$\Delta = \sqrt{\frac{1}{4}}\Delta_0 = \frac{1}{2}\Delta_0 \qquad\qquad (16.69)$$

That is, the producer tolerance should be half of the customer tolerance.

- *Case 2:* $A_1 + A_2 + \ldots + A_n \gg A_0$

    It means that the total cost of components is much larger than the cost of rectifying the system, and this could certainly happen if the system can easily be adjusted back to specification. From equation (16.68) it is clear that Δ, the actual producer tolerance for the assembly, will be much larger than the customer tolerance Δ_0.

- *Case 3:* $A_1 + A_2 + \ldots + A_n \approx A_0$.

    This means that the total cost of components is about the same as the cost of rectifying the system. This case does not happen very often. From equation (16.68) it is clear that Δ, the actual producer tolerance for the assembly, will be about the same as the customer tolerance Δ_0.

We can see clearly that there is a fundamental philosophical difference between traditional and Taguchi tolerance allocation. Traditional tolerance allocation will assign tolerances, $\Delta_1, \Delta_2, \ldots, \Delta_n$ for low-level characteristics $x_1,$ $x_2, \ldots, x_i, \ldots, x_n$ such that the actual tolerance for y, say Δ, is about the same as that of customer tolerance Δ_0. On the other hand, Taguchi tolerance allocation will assign tolerances, $\Delta_1, \Delta_2, \ldots, \Delta_n$ for low-level characteristics $x_1, x_2, \ldots,$ $x_i, \ldots, x_n$, such that the actual tolerance for y, say Δ, could be either much smaller than the customer tolerance Δ_0 if the cost of correcting error at high levels is much bigger than that at low levels; or Δ could be much larger than the customer tolerance Δ_0 if the cost of correcting error at high levels is very small.

16.7 TAGUCHI'S TOLERANCE DESIGN EXPERIMENT

The Taguchi tolerance design approach is generally used when a transfer function is not available but can be approximated after a parameter design (Chapter15) is conducted. In a system a high-level requirement y is related to a group of low-level characteristics, $x_1, x_2, \ldots, x_i, \ldots, x_n$, with an unknown transfer function $y = f(x_1, x_2, \ldots, x_i, \ldots, x_n)$. The tolerance design methods discussed in Section 16.6 cannot be applied directly. In this case, Taguchi (1986) proposed using a tolerance design experiment to determine the impact of the variability of low-level characteristics, or factors $x_1, x_2, \ldots, x_i, \ldots, x_n$, on the high-level requirement y. The experimental data analysis is able to prioritize the low-level factors' tolerance adjustments based on their impact and cost.

A tolerance design experiment is conducted after the parameter design experiment. After parameter design experiment, the nominal level of control factors, that is, the target values of $x_1, x_2, \ldots, x_i, \ldots, x_n$, have already been determined. In a tolerance design experiment, Taguchi (1986) recommended that the experimental factor levels be set by the following rules:

- *Two-level factors:*
  First level = target value $(T_i) - \sigma_i$
  Second level = target value $(T_i) + \sigma_i$
- *Three-level factors:*

$$\text{First level} = T_i - \sqrt{\frac{3}{2}}\sigma_i$$

$$\text{Second level} = T_i$$

$$\text{Third level} = T_i + \sqrt{\frac{3}{2}}\sigma_i$$

Using these settings, for two-level factors the two levels are located at the 15th and 85th percentile points in the variation range. For three-level factors, the three levels are located at the 10th, 50th, and 90th percentile points in the variation range. Clearly, these levels are set at reasonable ends of the variation range.

Tolerance design is a regular orthogonal array design experiment in which a regular functional requirement (y) is observed at each run of the experiment. Looking at the equation

$$\text{var}(y) = \sigma_y^2 \approx \sum_{i=1}^{n}\left(\frac{\delta y}{\delta x_i}\right)^2 \sigma_i^2 \tag{16.70}$$

if we set $\delta x_i \approx \sigma_i$, then

$$\sigma_y^2 \approx \sum_{i=1}^{n}(\delta y)_i^2 \tag{16.71}$$

Equation (16.71) actually indicates that the total mean square estimate in a DOE is a good statistical estimator of var*(y)*. The percentage contribution of each factor for a total sum of squares can be used to prioritize the tolerance reduction effort. If a factor makes a large percentage contribution to the total sum of squares and it is also cheap to reduce the tolerance, that factor is a good candidate for variation reduction. We illustrate the Taguchi tolerance design experiment in the following example.

16.7.1 Application: Tolerance Design

This example is an extension of the example in Section 16.3.1. A two-level DOE using an L_{16} orthogonal array (resolution V) was performed on the response function, which is the peak pressure of expression (16.23), repeated here:

$$p(d, v_s, V_0, V_f) = 14.7 \left(\frac{V_0}{V_f} \right)^{1.4} + \left[\frac{0.026964}{d^4} - \frac{0.18038}{(0.028 + 2d)^4} \right] (v_s)^2 \quad (16.72)$$

The numerical values of the four factors (the four parameters discussed above) were selected to be the numerically extreme bounds for the factors according to current design, as best determined by the authors, and are listed in Table 16.1.

Using the level calculations for a two-level factor, we have $T_1 = (0.031 + 0.039)/2 = 0.035$ in. and $\sigma_1 = (0.039 - 0.031)/2 = 0.004$ in. The reader is encouraged to calculate the target and variance for all other factors.

The mean performance of the response function is $\mu_p = 52.25$ psi (gauge) and the standard deviation of the response is $\sigma_p = 22.31$ psi (gauge). The main factor effects for each of the four factors are shown in Figure 16.6. Note that the final air volume (recall that the vial fill volume is 9.35 mL – final air volume) has the largest effect on pressure followed by actuator speed, initial

TABLE 16.1 DOE Factors and Their Levels

Factorial Level	Lumen Diameter, d (in.)	Actuator Speed, v_s (mm/s)	Initial Air Volume, V_0 (mL)	Final Air Volume, V_f (mL)
1	0.031	20.0	10.3	4.35
2	0.039	40.0	13.7	6.35

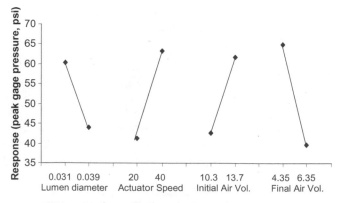

Figure 16.6 Main factor effects for peak pressure.

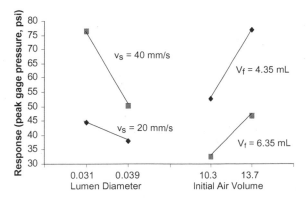

Figure 16.7 Interaction effects.

air volume, and finally, lumen diameter. Of course, this ordering is also a function of the numerical values selected for the levels.

Figure 16.7 shows the effects for the two interactions predicted by this simple model of peak pressure. Note that a mild interaction occurs for speed and lumen diameter and also for initial and final air volume, as predicted by the sensitivity terms in expressions (16.24a) to (16.24d). Since the interactions are mild (the factor effect lines in Figure 16.6 do not cross), the choice of values for the factors that cause the interactions is clear. We merely pick the combination of factors that yield the minimum values shown in Figure 16.6. From the figure the factor values that minimize the response (peak pressure) are

$d = 0.039\,\text{in.}$

$v_s = 20\,\text{mm/s}$

$V_0 = 0.3\,\text{mL}$ (primed fluid circuit, or alternatively, short tubing circuit)

$V_f = 6.35\,\text{mL}$ (3 mL vial fill volume)

The relative contribution of each factor to the total response variability is as follows:

lumen diameter (d)	14.1%
actuator velocity (v_s)	25.9%
initial air volume (V_0)	19.7%
final air volume (V_f)	33.91%
diameter and velocity interaction	5.1%
initial and final air volume interaction	1.3%

Using ANOVA, we leave the verification of these calculations as an exercise for the reader. Note that the relative contributions of the main factor

effects listed above agree with the results of the main factor effects shown in
Figure 16.5.

16.8 SUMMARY

In this chapter we develop several analytical approaches for medical tolerance
design and tolerancing of our medical device DFSS approach. Tolerance
design is the science of predicting variations in device performance caused by
variations in component values or the environment. In this chapter we show
how tolerance design and tolerancing approaches can be used to predict and
improve the quality of a device before even one prototype has been built.
Using these methods allows new devices to be developed rapidly and introduced with fewer unexpected problems. The examples in this chapter are
simple to enhance comprehension. The analytical and statistical tolerance
design methods may be used successfully for any device engineering problem
where a transfer function can or cannot be derived.

17

MEDICAL DEVICE DFSS VERIFICATION AND VALIDATION

17.1 INTRODUCTION

The final aspect of DFSS methodology that differentiates it from the prevalent "launch and learn" method is design verification, design validation, software validation, and process validation. The FDA design control perspective of design verification and validation is discussed in Section 2.6.5. In this chapter we cover in detail the verify/validate phase of the DFSS (ICOV) project road map (Figure 7.1). Design verification, process validation, and design validation helps identify unintended consequences and effects of design and process, develop plans, and reduce risk for full-scale commercialization to all stakeholders, including all customer segments. There is a degree of overlap with Chapter 18 and readers are encouraged to read these chapters in sequence.

At this final stage before full-scale production stage (see Section 1.3.6), we want to verify that device performance is capable of achieving the requirements specified for them and we also want to validate that those devices met the expectations of customers and stakeholders at six sigma performance levels. We need to accomplish this assessment in a low-risk, cost-effective manner. This chapter covers the medical device–relevant aspects of DFSS design verification and design validation, including process validation, software validation, prototyping, testing, and assessment.

Medical device manufacture's [original equipment manufactures (OEMs)] are still finding it somewhat difficult to meet the requirements of

Medical Device Design for Six Sigma: A Road Map for Safety and Effectiveness,
By Basem S. El-Haik and Khalid S. Mekki
Copyright © 2008 John Wiley & Sons, Inc.

both verification and validation. Some medical device OEMs and suppliers still confuse the two and struggle to distinguish them. Medical device verification and validation requirements have been mandated for over 10 years through quality system regulation. In the United States the Food and Drug Administration (FDA) does not prescribe how manufacturers should conduct verification and validation activities because there are so many ways to go about it, developed through mechanisms such as in-house knowledge. The FDA's intent is not to constrain manufacturers but to allow them to adopt definitions that satisfy verification and validation terms which they can implement with their particular design processes. In this chapter we provide a design for six sigma (DFSS) recipe for device verification and validation. Customization is warranted by an industry segment and by device application.

In 2005, design verification was cited in 41% of 49 warning letters with design control violations, while design validation was noted in 27% of the letters compared to 37% (design validation) and 9% of (design control violations) of 54 warning letters in 2004. The picture may be even worse than is conveyed by these statistics. The complexities of risk management and software make it more difficult for FDA investigators to uncover deficiencies and thus produce fewer warning letter citations. The warning letter statistics seem to show that design verification is tougher than other violations for OEMs to avoid. Design verification violations appear in more warning letters because it's an easier observation for FDA investigators to make when conducting a facility inspection. However, our observations are that many OEMs have the same, if not more, problems with design validation. In addition, because many OEMs are often under budget pressure and schedule deadlines, there's always a motivation to compress that schedule, sacrificing verification and validation more than any other activities in the development process.

Medical device Design verification [QSR Section, 21 CFR 820.30(f)] is intended to ensure that design outputs meet design inputs. According to the FDA, verification can be performed at all stages of the design process. The requirement instructs firms to review, inspect, test, check, audit, or otherwise establish whether or not components, subsystems, systems, the final device, processes, services, and documents conform to requirements or design inputs. Typical verification tests may include biocompatibility testing for material, bioburden testing or microbial limit testing, risk analysis, package integrity testing, testing for conformance to standards, and reliability testing. In some cases design verification can be done by analysis where physical tests are impractical or inappropriate. Finite element analysis, worst-case condition analysis, mechanical and electrical tolerance analysis, clinical evaluation analysis, and software codes analysis are considered acceptable design verification.

Medical device design validation [QSR Section, 21 CFR 820.30 (g)] ensures that a device meets defined user needs and intended uses. Validation includes testing of production units under simulated and/or actual-use conditions, and clinical trials may be conducted. Validation, is which basically the culmination of risk management, of the software, and of proving user needs and intended uses, is usually more difficult than verification. As the DFSS team goes upstream and links to the abstract world of customer and regulation domains, the validation domain, things are not black and white as in the engineering domain, the verification domain. Software validation and process validation are considered part of design validation. To emphasize the importance of software and process validation in the context of this book, we decided to include them in separate sections of this chapter. Typical validation tests may include clinical trials, clinical studies, clinical investigations, risk analysis, and labeling and packaging external evaluation. In some cases design validation can be done by analysis where physical tests are impractical or inappropriate. Clinical evaluation analysis, benchmark and historical product comparison analysis, product risk analysis, and scientific literature review are some examples.

We find it very beneficial in the context of this section to reproduce Figure 1.2 here as Figure 17.1, to emphasize the differentiation between

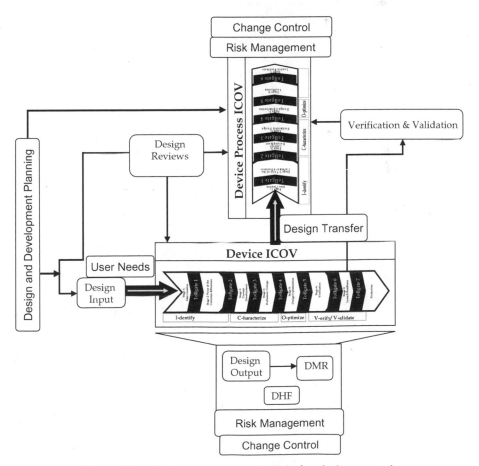

Figure 17.1 Design process: medical device design controls.

QSR Section 820.30(f), "Design verification":

Each manufacturer shall establish and maintain procedures for verifying the device design. Design verification shall confirm that the design output meets the design input requirements. The results of the design verification, including identification of the design, method(s), the date, and the individual(s) performing the verification, shall be documented in the design history file.

QSR Section 820.30(g), "Design validation":

Each manufacturer shall establish and maintain procedures for validating the device design. Design validation shall be performed under defined operating conditions on initial production units, lots, or batches, or their equivalents. Design validation shall ensure that devices conform to defined user needs and intended uses and shall include testing of production units under actual or simulated use conditions. Design validation shall include software validation and risk analysis, where appropriate. The results of the design validation including identification of the design, method(s), the date, and the individual(s) performing the validation, shall be documented in the design history file.

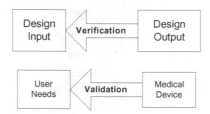

Figure 17.2   Quality system regulation definition.

design verification and design validation coupled with the FDA definition of both (Figure 17.2). It will be useful to refer to both figures in the following sections.

In following sections we describe a high-level process for design verification, process validation, software validation, and design validation. It is not intended to cover every aspect, but rather, to provide a DFSS verification and validation algorithm to design teams to help them understand and plan verification and validation activities when combined with common industry practices.

17.2   DESIGN VERIFICATION PROCESS

Design verification process can take on many different forms, depending on the magnitude of the design change and the complexity of the environment in which the design will operate. Typically, it is desirable to understand the performance of the new device (newly designed or redesigned) as early as possible in the development process with the highest confidence achievable. In our DFSS methodology we accomplish this objective from several perspectives. In the characterize phase, we use axiomatic design, the theory of inventive problem solving (TRIZ/TIPS), and other creativity tools to reduce conceptual vulnerabilities while cascading design inputs and other requirements. In the optimize phase, we employ aggressive optimization tools to reduce operational vulnerabilities, via functional requirement variability optimization and mean shift to target, to enable device-inherent capability to desensitize the effect of noise factors in manufacturing and use environments. We can rely on the design of experiments methods detailed in Chapters 14 and 15. Often, the DOEs are specialized around a subset of input significant factors and not a full functional test. Transfer functions are often obtained. When we think of medical device–specific verification, it often means building prototypes and testing them in a *beta environment*, one in which real end users utilize the new device in their actual application and provide feedback. The process is similar to having people proofread a draft of this book to provide valuable feedback. In a beta environment end users are willing to test the new design because they are offered something of value in return, such as free product or early access to new technologies. For beta testing to provide useful feedback to the design team, frequent debriefings on the experience and detailed notes on the operating environment are necessary.

As we move into a medical device verification environment, many of the same concepts are directly applicable from a traditional product verification environment, but often it is just as easy to run the new medical device or process parallel to the legacy device design.

In the medical device verification flowchart introduced in Figure 17.3 we see that the first thing to be done is to reassess the makeup of the design team. Often at this stage the team needs to be expanded to members who have practical operations experience or who can mentor customers as they use the new device. The next step is to ensure that all team members are up to date with the design intent, background, and objectives. The key activity during the review of background information is to begin planning and coordinating the production of prototypes (which will increase in levels of complexity) and to establish the corresponding measurement and testing facilities that will be required. The DFSS team in this step should begin reviewing information with a focused examination of the program test plan. This test plan should suggest a specific progression of tests for components and integrated subsystems through the device level. This will initiate development of the comprehensive test plan matrix that is required during this step.

During the course of this activity, it is recommended that the team give specific attention to identifying the acceleration and correlation properties for

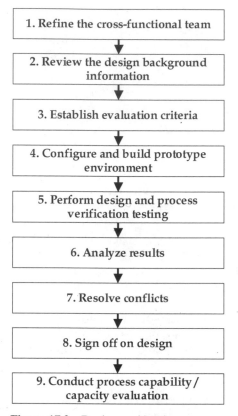

Figure 17.3   Design verification process.

the individual tests. This is typical for development of the key life test[1] (KLT), and a review of our knowledge about these tests is a must.

Engineering specifications for component, subsystem, and device levels need to be understood by the working team. Included in these reviews are the manufacturing process control plans, as these are systems that will experience verification testing. The team needs to look to databases of internal information systems so that previous lessons learned are not overlooked.

The DFSS core team, which consists of both product and manufacturing area personal, will continue to be a common feature of verification activity. Verification is a simultaneous activity in which both the design and manufacturing processes go through verification and problem-solving stages of development concurrently. Team leadership and relative levels of participation from the design and manufacturing arenas will change as the focus varies between these two aspects of verification.

---

[1]KLT uses test parameters that accelerate failure modes under consideration at an established rate, allowing for the test to be completed in a significantly reduced time frame.

Special expertise is always an important consideration, and for the amount of testing that will be conducted here we strongly suggest support from people knowledgeable in these areas: prototype development, test method development, development of testing plans, regulatory and clinical affairs, and measurement instrumentation. Since there will be an emphasis on data analysis and problem solving, persons skilled in descriptive statistical methods and six sigma will be a valuable addition for certain activities.

There will also be a changing dimension according to prototype level. Activity at the component level will progress logically toward the device level as various subsystems become integrated. The very act of integration at the prototype stage requires the same level of horizontal and vertical organization and cooperation that was required to move from component optimization into system optimization in the DFSS optimize phase.

The team may be refined and strengthened for verification activities by including the following individual customers: plant manufacturing and process engineers, service engineers, suppliers, material control personnel, system and subsystem engineers, purchasing and procurement personnel, machine tool suppliers, test engineers and specialists, and others.

In step 3 (Figure 17.3), the team defines the evaluation criteria and the associated budgets and schedules. This should be a compilation of a multitude of tools, such as QFD, axiomatic design, and test method development[2] (TMD). This step simply specifies what will be measured and the minimum levels of measurement performance attributes required to declare successes.

Step 4 consists of establishing the prototype environment such that it is as close to the production environment as possible, considering cost and risk factors. This requires the following:

a. *Determine affected components and subsystems.* Identify parts and assemblies for test. Note which are carryover and which are the result of new designs or optimization. This list is known as the *test parts list.*

b. *Identify related component, subsystem, and device tests.* Utilize design specification and FMEA information (Chapter 11), especially robust design FMEA (Mekki, 2006), which is valuable at this point to identify tests normally performed to verify functional performance. Begin developing total test matrix.

c. *Identify test variances (new or nonstandard tests).* Document nonstandard tests. Identify all new KLTs[3] applicable to optimized or non-carryover device technology. Record key feature dimensions and characteristic features for analysis of degradation during and after verification tests.

---

[2]Test method development is a documented process that is a design process, a systematic collection, and an analysis of sufficient information that will give a high degree of assurance that a test method will consistently meet the requirements expected for the intended application.

[3]KLTs use test parameters that accelerate failure modes under consideration at an established rate, allowing the test to be completed in a significantly reduced time frame.

d. *Identify testing acceptance criteria.* Use engineering specifications and teardown analysis[4] guides for acceptance criteria. In the case of teardown and dimensional analyses (including wear-related degradation), non-performance-related criteria can be referenced from device (assembly) prints and control plans.

e. *Develop a comprehensive testing schedule with budget elements.* Examine the availability of facilities for component and combined systems testing. Create a timing schedule for prototype construction, measurement and documentation, test application, and analysis of results. Identify details such as the number of samples required at component and successive levels of assembly within the device.

f. *Establish a similar-to-production plan.* Develop a specific coordinated plan for building representative device prototype examples (preferably at limits of dimensional and performance specifications). Where possible, plan for the use of actual production-level tooling and processes even if coordinated multiple-site processing and assembly are required.

g. *Assemble a total test plan.* Identify the minimum number of tests for each level of the system (component, subsystem, etc.). Cross-reference and coordinate time and resources and related costs and constraint issues. We need to verify the device design in the following aspects:

- *Functional performance verification.* This is to verify if the device can deliver all its design output and functional requirements. For example, for a device monitor set, functional performance verification will verify if the monitor set can emit signals and alarm sound effects, and so on.
- *Operation environmental requirements verification.* This is to verify if the device can deliver its function under diverse environmental conditions such as high and low temperatures, shocks and vibrations, humidity, wind, salt, and dust.
- *Reliability requirements verification.* This is to verify whether the device can perform its functions in an extended period of use. Many devices are designed for use over an extended period of time. This verification should include useful life and functional degradation verification.
- *Usage requirements verification.* This is to verify if the device can deliver its functions under various usage conditions, sometimes foreseeably abusive usage conditions.
- *Safety requirements verification.* This is to verify if the device can meet the safety requirements.
- *Interface and compatibility verification.* If a device has to work with other equipment, we need to verify whether they can work well together.

---

[4]As the name implies, teardown analysis is a complete teardown of device components and assemblies for analysis.

- *Maintainability requirement verification.* This is to verify if the necessary maintenance work can be performed conveniently, how well the maintenance can "refresh" the product, the benchmark mean time between maintenance, the mean corrective maintenance time, the mean preventive maintenance time, and so on.

h. *Secure test plan approval.* Secure approval by all responsible design and manufacturing supervisors and their respective managers to proceed with the plan after you've received a commitment by management to resolve identified constraints.

i. *Order parts and coordinate the test process.*

j. *Build device prototypes.* Procure prototype and production parts and system assemblies, as necessary, to support design verification testing on the dates scheduled. Preinspect assemblies according to specification-related documentation. See Sections 17.2.1 and 17.2.2 for more details on prototype issues and the discussion of the production part approval process in Chapter 18.

In step 5, device testing is run and observed based on the evaluation criteria and environmental factors determined. The objective is to conduct a progressive sequence of verification tests to quantify the ability of the device to satisfy performance requirements under conditions that approximate the conditions of actual use and accumulated stress. The team needs to make initial adjustments to the test and measurement equipment and to verify and record initial conditions according to the test plan matrix, device verification specification, and design verification project plan. They need to begin collecting data for tests that are designed to analyze performance or device requirement degradation, collect all data according to test matrix plan, and record any abnormalities that may occur during test and may facilitate subsequent concern resolution.

Next, the team needs to evaluate and verify device performance that involves a hierarchical testing program as part of the test strategy to enable functional verification at progressive levels of device configuration. The first tier is associated with component-level testing. The second tier is associated with subsystem assemblies. The third tier of testing is for systems that combine the functional subsystems. The final tier consists of device-level tests similar to Figure 17.4, the Six Sigma Professionals, Inc. (www.SixSigmaPI.com) application of the W-model.[5]

---

[5]The W-model of verification testing, introduced by Paul Herzlich in 1993 for software, attempts to address shortcomings in the V-model. The specific purpose of the test activity is to determine whether the objectives of the DFSS ICOV process have been met and the deliverable meets its requirements. In its most generic form, the W-model presents a hierarchical development with every hierarchical level mirrored by a test activity.

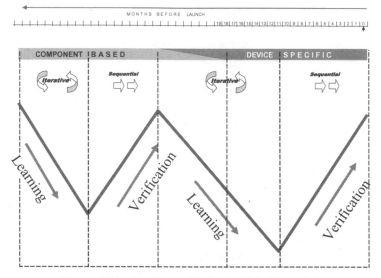

Figure 17.4   Six Sigma Professionals's W-model.

This process should be planned over the product development cycle and should be iterative. Once any verification testing results are available, the results are analyzed. It is important to note that the team should not wait until the end of all testing, as the team will want to be sensitive to any initial defects as soon as possible and make go/no-go decisions at each completed cycle. If design modifications are made, a decision must be made whether to loop back to the characterize phase.

Functional insensitivity to the testing environment (reliability) will be the most quantifiable at the device's component and subsystem tier levels. This is due in part to the number of tests that can be performed effectively and to the greater ability to measure functional performance at lower levels of device complexity. The issue just noted is not a hard-and-fast rule but is certainly observable in the greater number of tests that are run (hence, the improved quantification) at the component and subsystem levels. Testing costs at the component level are typically one-tenth those at the device level.

The team then finalizes packaging, sterilization, shipping, service instruction manual, use labeling, operator manual, and delivery systems with actual shipping and delivery functions for each component, subsystem level, and the total device. To verify service procedures and time studies for the subsystem design work performed earlier, the team provides effective service for all systems and key components. Supplier service review of the device and supporting service documentation will verify the functionality of the service.

The purpose of verification activities is to quantify all meaningful aspects of functional performance and key dimensional characteristic values after severe testing has been completed. This information can then be used to isolate any concerns. The isolation of these problems should follow six sigma formats for describing the problem in quantifiable ways through the use of statistical methods wherever applicable.

In step 6 the team conducts analyses such as inspection and teardown of hardware to enable comparison to specifications, related performance, and/or dimensional requirements. Where previously established degradation analysis has been planned, utilize the teardown phase to complete this data collection. Another type of analyses is degradation analysis using graphical and analytical techniques conducted by modeling functional (or dimensional characteristics) degradation as a result of accumulated stress. Data are collected at scheduled inspection points and on completion of the test. Various software scenarios can be used to create stress. Ideally, the measurement strategy will not require teardown of the test product and possible compromise of the test validity. The team should consider whether it is feasible, during the test planning phase, to perform a practical precorrelation of internal degradation levels to external measurables. Reliability prediction can be modeled from either the degradation data or from pass/fail data if the sample size is sufficient for this purpose.

The risk assessment for each test, which is based on comparisons of reliability predictions (or obvious issues) to reliability targets (if applicable), is entered into inspection results and risk assessment documentation. All problems should be representative of a possible customer concern and hence require corrective action in either design or manufacturing activities, or both. The team then updates the documentation (in the design history file) accordingly to reflect these issues in order to facilitate the necessary action and analytical models. The efficiency and relevancy of analytical tools such as FEA and CAD will benefit from updates derived from hardware testing.

Conflicts and problems that arise from the various verification tests will require resolution (step 7). Resolution of such problems is best approached in a systematic way using six sigma as a proven statistical problem-solving method. Most problems at this stage of development should be the result of unexpected prototype execution issues and/or unwanted or unplanned testing conditions. The reasoning is as follows: After systematic device development and functional optimization at the component and system levels (characterize and optimize phases of DFSS methodology), all problems should have been discovered or anticipated and subsequently removed from the design. It is expected, however, that the best, or optimized, design may produce interface issues that have gone undiscovered and now manifest themselves as process verification failures. The team will need to distinguish less-than-adequate optimization from poor prototype execution. A systematic approach will clarify this issue so that appropriate action can be taken.

Once the team is satisfied that the new device design is correct, the documentation should be formally signed off, which concludes step 8. The last step (step 9) is to conduct process capability analysis and any capacity planning. This will be the advent of the process validation activities.

17.2.1   Building a Verification Prototype

To produce a useful prototype of the new device that is sufficient to allow for evaluation; consideration must be given to the completeness and stability of the elements that make up the device. These elements can be classified as design parameters that are manifested into components and subsystems as well as the production process variables with all steps and subprocesses. We can look at components, subsystems, and systems to determine the lack of knowledge of performance and the interaction of preexisting (carryover) subsystems into a new device. To assist in determining if the prototype is complete enough and relevant for testing, it is helpful to assess the elements as being:

- Current design
- Analogous design
- New design, low risk
- New design, high risk

Risk can be assessed from FMEA and technology road maps or other sources (e.g., design history file) and/or DFSS tool use. If any of the elements are of the new design, high-risk category, they should not be compromised and must be included in the prototype.

The prototype in any product environment may not be produced on production equipment or with production process and people. The same can happen in a medical device environment. For example, software may be months away and you want to know if the new device will perform. Often, the configured device or a part of it is built as nonproduction hardware and tested under test script scenarios.

Prototypes usually involve some trade-off between the final completed design and some elements that are not available until later in the development cycle (see Figure 17.4). Prototype designs are tested off-line under controlled conditions. Some examples are:

- Initial mock-up hardware that is created in a lab environment.
- New device software
- A modified version of the current design tested in parallel with the actual system prior to pilot testing

Prototypes should be evaluated using objective and robust analytical techniques to demonstrate objectively design performance for the device pilot. The testing method is critical in accomplishing objective decision making and obtaining this information in the most cost-effective manner. See the discussion of the production part approval process in Chapter 18.

Several principles of prototyping are useful in guiding the use of prototypes in the product development process (Yang and El-Haik, 2003):

1. Analytical prototypes are generally more flexible than physical prototypes because it is usually much easier to adjust the design parameters in a mathematical or computer model and compute new output values. It usually takes much longer to build a physical prototype, and once build it is usually quite difficult to change the design parameters.

2. Physical prototypes are required to detect unexpected phenomena: An analytical prototype can only display the properties within the assumptions, mathematical models, and mechanism on which the analytical prototypes are based. It can never reveal phenomena that are not part of its assumptions and mechanism. For example, a Monte Carlo simulation prototype for a clinic is based on a stochastic process model and given probability distributions; it can never represent true doctor–patient interactions. No matter how well a computer simulation model works, testing on true physical prototypes often detects some unexpected bugs.

3. A prototype may reduce the risk of costly iterations: Analytical prototypes can be analyzed conveniently, design change can be simulated, and improvements can be made. Physical prototypes can be tested and unexpected phenomena, good or bad, can be revealed. Eliminating design disadvantage in a timely manner will definitely shorten the product development cycle time.

However, building prototypes also takes time and costs money, so planning of prototyping activities should be based on the balance of risk and development cost. Usually, for a item that is inexpensive, has a low failure cost, and/or with a known technology, less effort should be spent in prototyping. For an item that is expensive, with a high failure cost, and/or with a new or unknown technology, more effort should be spent on prototyping activities.

17.2.2 Prototype Testing

When testing prototypes, it is vital to follow a rigorous process to assess the performance and learn from any unusual observances. Many times, unexpected results may occur, and without the correct approach these will have to be written off as unusual observations, when in fact they may be significant events that can either differentiate the new design or plague it. The key elements of a rigorous test plan are as follows, in order of performance:

- Assign individual names to each role.
- Confirm that the test environment has been established and is ready for use.
- Finalize or confirm testing estimates.
- Estimate the hours to be spent by each person.
- Plan the calendar duration of all testing.

- Test the milestones (target dates).
- Finalize the test cases.
- Finalize test scenarios.
- Describe the input and expected results.
- Implement defect-tracking mechanisms.
- Confirm issue resolution procedures, which should include decisions to defer, fix, or withdraw.
- Finalize acceptance test criteria or comparison tests.
- Perform cycle tests.
- Carry out a performance test.
- Carry out an integration test.
- Carry out a regression test.
- Carry out a biocompatibility test.

17.2.3 Confidence Interval of Small-Sample Verification

When testing in a preproduction environment, the scope of the samples or resources available is often very small, due to cost or time factors. Proof of concept is usually determined after a single successful transaction, but robust performance can be determined only after significant learning cycles have been experienced. It is recommended that the legacy system be baselined for statistical parameters and the new device design be verified to a degree of statistical significance. Power and sample-size calculations can be made based on the underlying variation assumptions and the change in performance expected. If a medical device will experience only a few cycles in the period of a year, it is very unlikely that you will be able to validate the device statistically. Many new processes or medical devices experience many cycles of operation per week, and it is reasonable to validate these with 95% confidence intervals.

The statistical factors that affect the sample size are the confidence interval desired, the system noise (standard deviation), and the delta change between the signals (averages). The sample size (n) is given by

$$n = \left(\frac{Z_{\alpha/2}\sigma}{\delta} \right)^2 \tag{17.1}$$

where δ = error = $|\bar{y} - \mu|$

Take, for example, an apheresis[6] device that processes 24 red blood cell collections per day with a 22-minute average processing time and a standard deviation of 4.7 minutes. How many samples would we need to have 95%

---

[6]In apheresis, the blood of a donor or patient is passed through an apparatus that separates out a particular constituent and returns the remainder to circulation.

confidence that there was a statistically significant difference between two different designs? If we take the cases of a difference in average processing time of 2, 6, and 15 minutes, we find the following required sample sizes:

2-minute change	22 samples
6-minute change	3 samples
15-minute change	1 sample

The factors that affect sample size are the confidence interval desired, the system noise (standard deviation), and the delta change between signals (averages).

If in your verification process you are unable to achieve such a level of test confidence, it is recommended that the team roll out the verification plan gradually and incrementally. They need to start out with typical users who are less sensitive to any issues and pulse them for performance. As they feel more comfortable with the performance, the scope should be increased while continuing to ramp up the new medical device testing (Figure 17.4).

In Section 17.3 we list a high-level process for device production process validation. It is not intended to cover every aspect but rather, to provide a DFSS validation algorithm to design teams to help them understand and plan such activities when combined with common industry practices. It is highly recommended that the same concept and activities be utilized for device servicing, packaging, and labeling processes.

17.3 PRODUCTION PROCESS VALIDATION

The objective of production process validation activities is to confirm manufacturing and assembly processes capable of achieving device design intent. The same activities can be applied for service, packaging, and labeling processes. This step provides a rapid, smooth confirmation of the device manufacturing and assembly capability, with a need for only minimal refinements. Design verification and process specifications are completed and released before the start of this confirmation step.

Production process validation is part of the integrated requirements of a quality management system (21 CFR 820 and ISO 13485:2003). It is conducted in the context of a system that includes design and development control, quality assurance, process control, and corrective and preventive action. For some technologies the interrelationship of design control and process development may be very close. For others the relationship may be remote. The product should be designed robustly enough to withstand variations in the manufacturing process, and the manufacturing process should be capable and stable, to assure continued safe products that perform adequately.

Process validation is used in the medical device industry to indicate that a process has been subject to such scrutiny that the result of the process (a product, a service, or other outcome) can be practically guaranteed. The FDA defines process validation as follows: "Process validation is establishing documented evidence which provides a high degree of assurance that a specific process will consistently produce a product meeting its pre-determined specifications and quality characteristics."

The validation of a process is the mechanism or system used to plan, obtain data, record data, and interpret data. These activities may be considered to fall into three phases: (1) an initial qualification of the equipment used and provision of necessary services, also know as *installation qualification* (IQ); (2) a demonstration that the process will produce acceptable results and establishment of limits (worst case) of the process parameters, also known as *operational qualification* (OQ); and (3) and establishment of long-term process stability, also known as *performance qualification* (PQ). Refer to GHTF/SG3/N99–10:2004 for more information on process validation.

Process validation is to verify if the manufacturing process can produce devices that meet design intent with sufficient process capability. Manufacturing process validation includes at least the following activities:

1. *Product specification validation:* used to verify if the manufacturing process can produce devices that satisfy the design input
2. *Process capability validation:* used to verify if the manufacturing process can produce devices with satisfactory process capability

From a production standpoint, we need to confirm that the final mass production can deliver good products with low cost, high throughput, and six-sigma quality. Production validation may include at least the following activities:

1. *Process capability validation:* used to verify that satisfactory process capability can be achieved in mass production
2. *Production throughput validation.* used to verify that the mass production process can produce devices with sufficient quantity and productivity and a satisfactorily low level of downtime and interruptions
3. *Production cost validation:* used to verify if mass production can produce the product at sufficiently low cost

Prior to in-house installation, processes (i.e., manufacturing/assembly processes, measurement processes) have already been optimized in the presence of potential sources of manufacturing and customer "noise" and have demonstrated potential capability at the supplier location. These activities have involved significant simulated production (manufacturing and assembly) runs and form the basis for a low-risk installation at the intended manufacturing location. Daily measuring and monitoring activities are conducted as specified by the process control plan, which is often developed largely during process validation.

Unanticipated installation or manufacturing trial concerns are identified, and corrective actions are implemented prior to launch production. Production capability is assessed and the process is exercised in a manner that would be expected for normal production operation (i.e., shift changes/tool changes, operator variability, etc.).

Training programs should include a focus on the transfer of knowledge from design and process development experts to the on-site production personnel, including standby labor. This transfer of knowledge enables the DFSS team to add and improve on the control plan as they add their individual skills to the production planning.

Figure 17.5 provides a validation high-level map. In step 1, the skills and expertise necessary to confirm manufacturing capability and to initiate an effective production launch can be found in a refined cross-functional DFSS team. Much of the earlier planning work done for quality control and maintainability of the process will be executed during the launch phase of production. The new DFSS team members who will participate in the launch now have to prepare themselves by reviewing the process documentation and control plans. This documentation, combined with supporting discussion by

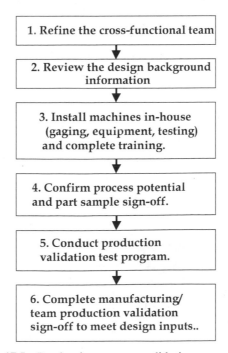

Figure 17.5 Production process validation process map.

the other team members, will provide new members with the knowledge the team has accumulated and will align them with the team's operating philosophy. Members suggested for the launch team should include machine (equipment) suppliers, purchased parts/material suppliers, maintenance/skilled tradespeople, production and marketing personnel, customers, design engineers on site (resident engineers), and quality department and manufacturing engineers. Once the validation team has been formed, the next step is to plan the approach and define the requirements. Many manufacturers develop what is referred to as a *master validation plan*, which identifies those processes to be validated, the schedule for validations, interrelationships between processes requiring validation, and timing for revalidations.

In step 2 (Figure 17.5), the team should access the relevant program information that defines the design and manufacturing intent. Ideally, information sources should be presented by team members who were involved in development of the information to ensure understanding of intent. Complete understanding will only be the result of participation in using various operational plans that will occur during device launch. Evaluation of process data collected during machine trials and from preliminary testing will assist the team in understanding. Suggested information sources can include manufacturing launch plans, control plans, axiomatic design zigzagging to process domain, historical machining/gauging issues (process FMEAs), manufacturing layout plans, machine specifications, prints, software, advance product quality planning (APQP; see Chapter 18) documentation, valuation/acceptance standards, correlation to customer use, process validation test plan, vendor sign-off data, and engineering specifications.

For step 3 the team needs to establish a satellite information center at the plant to coordinate manufacturing concerns. A satellite center should be established because manufacturing personnel must have easy access to device information concerning design and manufacturing intent, the current status of concerns and issues; timing and training plans, and so on. Device status review meetings and presentations with operators and others, all the way up to senior management, should be focused within this location to ensure that the common vision and relevant up-to-date information are transferred at all levels.

The location and availability of process history and control documentation should be organized based on the prioritization of operator needs and documented in the design history file as part of the device master records[7] (DMRs). Process instructions, operator instruction aids, the process control plan, and reaction plans should be readily accessible in the operator workstation area.

---

[7]Section 820.3(j) of the QS regulation define a device master record as a compilation of records containing the procedures and specifications for a finished device. The detailed requirements for device master records are contained in Section 820.181, as well as throughout the regulation (see Chapter 18).

The team should establish how to identify and locate specialists in case operators require assistance with special process adjustments or with the reaction plan. Design and manufacturing experts in the team should be available and should recognize their two major roles:

1. To enable efficient and effective decision making and identification of actions to resolve issues
2. To maximize transfer of their knowledge to operations personnel

Issues are to be identified and evaluated for their potential effect on the critical and significant performance characteristics. Unresolved issues should be evaluated for their inclusion as a source of variation (noise) in later capability studies.

Also in this step, the team conducts machine setup and gauging capability studies. Based on gauging repeatability and reproducibility (GR&R), control plan procedures developed by the team, operators, machine setup personnel, and maintenance personnel should conduct short-term versions of these procedures for all process gauge systems, including off-line. The performance of these gauges needs to be quantified subsequent to machine and gauge installation, and prior to processing potential studies which will depend on these measurement systems.

Quality support personnel should be available to assist with (but not perform) these studies. This will reinforce the learning that needs to take place on the part of the operators and related maintenance personnel who have to utilize system-related gauge systems.

As a reminder, the gauge capability studies will need to address/quantify the following potential sources of variation:

- What effect do multiple operators have on measurement capability? (Reproducibility)
- What is the effect of multiple measurements of the same characteristic on the same master part? (Repeatability)
- How well is the gauge calibrated to read the expected value of the characteristic on the master part? (Accuracy)
- What is the quantified variation of the gauge when used repeatedly over several trials? (Stability over time)

Ideally, overall gauge capability should be in the neighborhood of not more than 10% of the characteristic tolerance (up to 30% is not uncommon). The target for gauge system improvement should always be zero error. This issue becomes more critical as the gauging systems become a vital element of continuous process improvement moving forward. The ultimate level of acceptability will be a point of team review and agreement.

Vendor-supplied materials and parts should be used in preliminary (trial) process runs. During these runs, data should be collected for all important performance- and assembly-related purchased materials to determine the range in variation. This information can be used by the team to construct the trial runs so that when known incoming variability is imposed on the process, the in-process performance indicators can be studied to determine process insensitivity to input variation.

These activities can be performed for various subprocesses in preparation for the initial sample production runs and process capability studies. These runs will enable operators to become familiar with data collection and process control analysis and the related reaction activities. During this step, special support from quality personnel in the use of statistical methods (descriptive techniques) is suggested. An assessment of vendor capability, and any subsequent process potential capability, will be the output of these activities. Performance to target should be the primary emphasis of the launch team and a big part of the vendor capability assessment.

The following guidelines from the control plan characterize a process potential study (P_p and P_{pk}):

- The study includes as many measurements as possible, but at least 20 subgroups of three to five samples are necessary.
- If fewer than 50 samples are available, an individuals or run chart must be used to provide a sense of process movement over time.
- In all cases, simulate production cycles from setup through steady state. A tool or die change, process adjustment, or operator change can mark the end of a cycle. Collect data through at least two cycles and include worn tools in the run.
- Analyze data statistically. Estimate the process P_{pk} (and assess process centering). A P_{pk} (see Section 18.5) of less than 1.67 is a reason for concern and should be investigated by the launch team for corrective actions.

In step 3 (Figure 17.5) the team also implements process sheets, a work plan, and a control plan. Process control documentation should be finalized after the vendor capability assessment. During these trials, the team should consider any necessary adjustments to the control plan. If it is not clear to the operator how to respond to indications of an out-of-control process, now would be a good time to review and practice the necessary process adjustments and study the corresponding effects. Autonomous maintenance should be initiated by the operators at this stage to review that aspect of work plan documentation, measurement, and record keeping.

The production team training should be completed. The team should provide an environment that maximizes the transfer of knowledge from the team's temporary experts to on-site operations personnel. Process training should include making people aware of process development history, process and illustration sheets, control plans and gauging, and previous concerns and the actions taken to resolve them. Temporary or standby labor must be trained and certified for each operation.

As the production team is formed, the project team should evaluate and ensure optimization of skills/functions mix (specialists) versus production team requirements. Temporary or relief operators and backup (afternoon and midnight shift labor) should be evaluated, trained, and selected for specific operation assignments. Persons with key skills should be selected and the use of their skills optimized across all production shifts.

In step 4 (Figure 17.5) the team should include known noise factors (Chapter 15) in the validation trials. Typical sources of variation to the manufacturing process should be included in the manufacturing capability study trials. Anticipate how the process capability may be affected by these issues (i.e., shift changes, breaks, temperature variation, line speed, tool and vendor differences, etc.) and induce them into the capability study. If common sources of variation are not introduced during the production sample runs, the parts produced will not be representative of typical production. Satisfactory performance under these conditions should not be an issue if the device design and key processes have been optimized in the presence of anticipated sources of variation.

In addition to process gauging and tooling frequencies, additional areas requiring observation during the trials should be considered and systems or methods agreed upon for data collection. Studies should consider not only the individual process operation but also the interprocess steps. For the trials the team should consider whether the total manufacturing environment is in line with the process sheets as intended for mass production runs at line speed.

Gauge reproducibility and repeatability (GR&R) studies should be conducted in preparation for the validation trials. Confidence in the capability of measurement systems should be high due to previous potential studies and team-initiated corrective actions. Operators and maintenance personnel should also be familiar with gauging systems and their use.

The validation significant production run should consist of a continuous production run which would be representative of between "one hour" and "one shift" of production. Should this not be possible, conduct a production run of sufficient length to produce a sample of 300 devices. Parts, materials, assemblies, and process data from the run will be used for the following:

- To produce engineering specification test data
- To conduct and confirm process potential (P_{pk}) for all critical and significant characteristics (according to process control plan)
- To evaluate and obtain dimensional and material data per print
- To verify assembly feasibility

Prior to validation sign-off, the team should agree that all validation requirements are met. Refer to the current validation process documentation manual to ensure documentation compliance of test results and demonstration of control plan requirements and process capability.

In step 5 (Figure 17.5), significant dimensional or functional attributes which are linked to customer satisfaction were identified and toleranced accordingly during the characterize phase of the DFSS process. To support the posttest analyses of the process validation tests and the customer testing results, teardowns in certain applications are used to evaluate dimensional and functional deterioration over time.

Degradation data generate important information continuously to improve analytical models regarding stress–strain relationships and material behavior. In addition, improved correlation between testing environments and actual use may be possible where the degradation data have been collected as a result of fleet testing.

The planning for degradation analysis must include initial values for all characteristics of interest (as many dimensions and related functional/performance characteristics as possible). To emphasize this point, consider that the characteristic of interest in degradation analysis is the differential value, not the absolute value of the requirement. It is desirable for knowledge and estimation purposes to assess trends of degradation for each characteristic of interest. That is, a single (absolute) data point is not of much use for estimation purposes; two data points provide only a linear estimate of degradation (not a close approximation for typical material- and use-related degradation); and three (or more) data points are required to approximate nonlinear degradation.

It is useful that the design verification life test is essentially repeated using validation components and assemblies. The key initiative here is to fully evaluate the device and mass production capability to meet customers' wants and the design intent by verifying that design outputs meet design inputs.

1. *Dimensional evaluation.* The team must perform the necessary measurements to determine conformance with all drawing specifications, including assembly levels. Identify critical characteristics and include process potential or capability results for all critical and significant characteristics. Indicate the date of the engineering drawing and engineering level and the dates when these measurements were made. Any results that are out of specifications are cause for the team to reject and not submit the initial sample. Indicate these results in the documentation.

2. *Materials tests.* These tests are to be performed for all parts and device materials for specified chemical, physical, and metallurgical requirements. Samples that are tested must be retained (and marked "laboratory samples") unless other regulations prevail. Indicate the name of the laboratory where the samples were tested and the number and date of the specifications to which the material was tested.

3. *Engineering specification tests.* These tests are to be performed when performance and functional requirements are referenced on the part drawing.

The team must perform the necessary testing in accordance with all requirements of the control plan and the production validation requirements of the engineering specification. All specification test requirements are to be listed along with the quantity tested and the test results. As noted previously, indicate the date of the part drawing, the date and number of the specifications, and the name of the laboratory where the samples were tested. Parts should be retained (and marked "test samples") for a predetermined period from the date of first production shipment unless other regulations prevail.

The team to conduct the degradation data collection and teardown analysis according to the previous plan and identify performance (reliability) risks and take corrective action based on knowledge and best judgment. The team is advised not to disregard unusual degradation and failures or to predetermine "outlier" performance. Customer team members now evaluate device performance in the "newest" condition. This potentially displays, for example, the highest performance efforts or the poorest performance levels.

The delivery process can affect device performance, particularly where multiple on/off truck loadings occur, or where trains and ships are involved, and within differing climates. These effects were considered and incorporated in the optimize phase and evaluated for possible effects and improvement actions in the design and process FEMA. A final evaluation of the validation production-level device should be performed in the delivery environment.

The final action associated with design and manufacturing confirmation involves team sign-off that the production validation-level products and processes meet design intent (step 6, Figure 17.5). Any open issues are communicated to management with the appropriate risk-level assessment (minor or major) and planned activities for resolution. All documents and reports are included the design history file.

Validation planning should begin early in the design process starting with the DFSS characterize phase. It is most important to integrate validation activities early in the design rather than as an afterthought. Significant design issues must be reviewed, understood, and accepted by the extended DFSS team before progressing too far into detail design. Validation continues as a monitoring activity through the vehicles of control plans and statistical process control.

17.3.1 Device Verification Analysis

The basic objective of the device verification is to confirm that all the design requirements, such as functional performance requirements, operation environmental requirements, and reliability requirements, are confirmed. The methods for confirmation can be classified into two categories: design analysis and testing. Device design analysis is to use analytical means, such as a mathematical model, computer model, or conceptual model (such as FMEA) to verify some aspects of the device requirements. For many device situations, testing is the hardware test, in which physical prototypes or actual device will be put into well-designed tests. For software development, testing is a well-planned rigorous testing on the testing or final version of the software.

Device design analysis usually starts in the characterize phase. Testing is conducted in the later phases. Compared with testing, design analysis is usually easier, cheaper, and quicker to perform, but it may not be able to give a sufficient confirmation for the device requirements. Testing may give a sufficient confirmation with respect to some requirements, but it is usually more difficult to perform, more expensive, and more time consuming.

Design analysis and testing are related. If design analysis is very effective on a device requirement, the final confirmation testing on that requirement might be reduced in test sample size, changed to a cheaper testing, or simply canceled. On the other hand, if the design analysis reveals some potential weaknesses in the design, we may also conduct more testing on that concern to make sure that potential weakness gets resolved in redesign.

Design analysis is the first pass for verification; usually, design analysis can only partially confirm the device output requirements. Testing is the next step in verification. Sometimes, the verification process (Figure 17.5) can go backward as well. A design analysis or test may indicate that the current design is not able to meet a device requirement, so we have to either redesign or adjust the design requirement. Past results, another source of knowledge, are also very important in verification process.

There is no need to reinvent the wheel. Past test results on a similar product, relevant knowledge in the public domain, government publications, and university research results can all be part of the knowledge base. More relevant information on the knowledge base for a design requirement will lead to less design analysis and less testing on that requirement.

17.4   SOFTWARE VALIDATION

In this section we list a high-level process for software validation. It is not intended to cover every aspect but rather, to provide a DFSS verification and validation algorithm to design teams to help them understand and plan the verification and validation activities when combined with common industry practices. The FDA's analysis of 3140 medical device recalls conducted between 1992 and 1998 reveals that 242 of them (7.7%) are attributable to software failures. Of those 242 software-related recalls, 192 (or 79%) were caused by software defects that were introduced when changes were made to the software after its initial production and distribution. Software validation and related good software engineering practices are a principal means of avoiding such defects and resulting recalls using the DFSS ICOV· process. Software validation is not done in a vacuum. Software development and its relation to DFSS verification are depicted in Figure 7.5.

Software validation is a requirement of the quality system regulation [21 CFR 820.3(z) and (a) and 820.30(f) and (g)]. Validation requirements apply to software used as any of the following three different scenarios: (1) components in medical devices, (2) software that is itself a medical device, and (3) software used in production of the device or in implementation of the device manufacturer's quality system. Software validation is accomplished through a series of activities and tasks that are planned and executed at various stages of the design and development life cycle. In scenarios (1) and (3), the medical device life-cycle activities, vetted with DFSS concepts, can be used to establish verification, testing, and other tasks that support software validation.

In scenario (2), software developers should establish a software life-cycle model (e.g., waterfall, spiral, rapid prototyping, incremental development) that is appropriate for their product and organization. Below are activities in which verification testing and other tasks that support software validation occur that can be used in a typical software life-cycle model during each activity.

- Quality planning
- System requirements definition
- Detailed software requirements specification
- Software design specification
- Construction or coding
- Testing
- Installation
- Operation and support
- Maintenance
- Retirement

17.5 DESIGN VALIDATION

Now that we have covered design verification and production process and software validation, it is becoming clear that validation is addressing a different issue, where validation can be summarized as a set of activities which ensure that the right product was built from a customer point of view. This is accomplished through a series of activities and tasks that are planned and executed at various stages of the design and development life cycle. Design validation includes testing of production units under simulated and/or actual-use conditions, and clinical trials may be conducted. Validation—basically, the culmination of risk management, the culmination of the software, the culmination of proving the user needs and intended uses—is usually more difficult than verification. As the DFSS team goes upstream and links to the abstract world of customer and regulations domains, the validation domain, things are not as black and white as in the engineering domain, the verification domain. Typical validation tests may include clinical trials, clinical studies, clinical investigations, risk analysis, and labeling and packaging external evaluation. In some cases, design validation can be done by analysis where physical tests are impractical or inappropriate: clinical evaluation analysis, benchmark and historical product comparison analysis, product risk analysis, and scientific literature review. The results of the design validation must be documented in the design history file.

17.6 SUMMARY

Design verification and process validation are critical steps in the DFSS road map (Chapter 7) and need to be thought out well in advance of final production of a new device. Verification often requires prototypes that need to be close to the final design but are often subject to trade-offs in scope and completeness, due to cost or availability. Assessing the components and subsystems of any new device against the type of design risk assists in determining when a prototype is required and what configuration must be available. Once prototypes are available, a comprehensive test plan should be followed to capture any special event and to populate the design scorecard. Any go/no go decision should be based on statistically significant criteria, and all lessons learned, if appropriate, should be incorporated into the final design.

The validation activities provide a rapid, smooth confirmation of the device and manufacturing capability, with the need for minimal refinements. Design and process specifications are completed and released before the start of these activities. Before handing off to the production environment, the process stability and capability should be assured.

18

DFSS DESIGN TRANSFER

18.1 INTRODUCTION

Design transfer simply encompasses clear establishment of a relationship between design engineering and production and service during the product life cycle. In the DFSS process this is an ongoing activity that will gain more momentum as the device design matures in the DFSS ICOV process (Chapter 7). According to FDA regulations and to avoid duplication of effort on the part of the DFSS team, we strongly advocate use of the device master record (DMR) as the documented DFSS knowledge institutionalization. Depending on the project scope, the DFSS part may partially or fully overlap with the DMR. That is, DMR is sufficient and necessary documentation of any device, or a subset of such documentation.

Our approach in this chapter is to complement current medical device industry practices (e.g., use of the device master record) through two value-added tracks: First, we extend the DFSS ICOV process to another new and complementary process such as advanced product quality planning (APQP; see Section 18.6) and production part approval process (PPAP; see Section 18.6) and second, we lace current practices with DFSS standard operating procedures (SOPs) where appropriate.

Design transfer is a process in which the device design is translated correctly into production and service specifications and the finished device is transferred successfully from design to production and service. The FDA,

Medical Device Design for Six Sigma: A Road Map for Safety and Effectiveness,
By Basem S. El-Haik and Khalid S. Mekki
Copyright © 2008 John Wiley & Sons, Inc.

along with other regulatory bodies and standards, set forth the requirement for a successful design transfer. We will use the FDA definition as stated in 21 CFR 820.30(h) in the context of this chapter: "Each manufacturer shall establish and maintain procedures to ensure that the device design is correctly translated into production specifications."

The FDA's intent is not to constrain the manufacturers and allow them to adopt definitions that satisfy design transfer which they can implement with their particular product development processes. In this chapter we provide a design for six sigma recipe for successful device design transfer as the design team transfers the technology and the design detail to the production and service sectors (internal or external). Successful transfer of this information implies that the engineering knowledge has been developed completely. In doing so, the team needs to pay special attention to identified risks, incidental or minor, particularly if they remain unresolved. In a DFSS tollgate review (Chapter 7), management needs to review and confirm that all major and critical risks have been effectively removed and that tangible plans are in place for unresolved minor risks. Failure to achieve this has a negative impact on device quality and unnecessary delays in program launch.

In the following sections we list a high-level process for elements of successful design transfer to manufacturing and service. It is not intended to cover every aspect but rather, to provide a DFSS design transfer algorithm to design teams to help them understand and plan such activities when combined with common industry practices.

18.2   DESIGN TRANSFER PLANNING

Design transfer planning should begin early in the design process, starting with a characterise DFSS phase. It is most important to integrate design transfer activities early in design rather than as an afterthought. Significant design issues must be reviewed, understood, and accepted by the extended DFSS team progressing too far into detail design. The key activity for successful design transfer is to involve production and service early in the planning for prototype production and also in establishing the corresponding testing measurement required.

The device master record[1] (DMR) contains a comprehensive list of design output elements critical to successful design transfer. The authors selected a subset of the list below to explore. All, however, require extra attention and need to be evaluated by the DFSS team, including production and service representatives:

---

[1]See Section 18.7. Section 820.3(j) of the QS regulation defines a device master record as a compilation of records containing the procedures and specifications for a finished device. The detailed requirements for device master records are contained in Section 820.181 as well as throughout the regulation.

- Hazard analysis
- Design and process FMEA
- Design verification and validation
- Process validation plan and report
- Design reviews (especially design transfer review)
- Bill of materials
- Supplier approval process
- Design specifications and drawings
- Process control plans
- Statistical process control
- Process capability
- In-process and final inspection plans
- Production plan
- Service design (see El-Haik and Roy, 2005) plan
- Advanced product quality planning, including the production part approval process[2]

Doing each DMR element justice would require several volumes. Here we chose to cover a few that are most relevant, new, or misused. The process control plans, statistical process control, and advanced product quality planning including PPAP will be expanded in the following sections as (the remainder of the design elements are covered elsewhere).

18.3 PROCESS CONTROL PLAN

As we build on the DOE transfer functions in the DFSS optimize phase, (see Chapters 13 to 15) and finalize the process capability, then update the design scorecard, we are now cognizant of the key design parameters and their key process variables, which are critical for monitoring and controlling in the production environment. One of the best tools to start the process of implementing process control is the control plan depicted in Figure 18.1. We take the key process input variables and key process output variables and list them in the column labeled "Specification Characteristic." In the columns labeled "Subprocess" and "Subprocess Step" we input the corresponding labels. The next required element is the "Specification/Requirement." In this cell the upper and lower specification limits (USL and LSL) are typically entered. In some processes only one limit may be required, or for attribute-type requirements, the target value. The next cell is "Measurement Method."

---

[2]Used in the automotive supply chain to establish confidence in component suppliers and their production processes.

Process Control Plan

Process Name: _____   Prepared by: _____   Page: ____ of ____
Customer _____ Int/Ext ____   Approved by: _____   Document No: _____
Location: _____   Approved by: _____   Revision Date: _____
Area: _____   Approved by: _____   Supercedes: _____

Sub Process	Sub Process Step	CTQ		Specification Characteristic	Specification/Requirement		Measurement Method	Sample Size	Frequency	Who Measures	Where Recorded	Decision Rule/Corrective Action	SOP Reference
		KPOC	KPIV		USL	LSL							

Figure 18.1 Process control plan.

In the cell labeled "Sample Size" are entered how many measurements will be required at the specified frequency. This comes back to the underlying statistical significance that is required to capture the variation. In an injection molding process we define the sample collection frequency required. This can be, for example, every hour, shift, day, or week, depending on the stability of the molding process and the nature of the characteristic measured. The column labeled "Who Measures" is for the person(s) assigned to collect the measurement. "Where Recorded" is the location where the collected measurement is documented for referral or audit purposes. The "Decision Rule/Corrective Action" column is to list the rules regarding what action to take if a measurement is outside the specification requirement. This can be either a set of actions or a reference to a policy or procedure. The column labeled "SOP Reference" is for the document name or number that is the standard operating procedure for the subprocess or subprocess step.

Of special note is that if the design team has followed all of the optimization and validation steps and the design is operating at a very low defect rate (approaching six sigma capability), there should be relatively few key process input variables (KPIVs) and the key process output characteristics (KPOCs) should be the prioritized from the DFSS optimize phase.

18.4 STATISTICAL PROCESS CONTROL

When the data measurements are collected as prescribed in the control plan, the method for charting the data should be determined. Since statistical process control (SPC) is a well-developed subject and there are many textbooks on the subject, we do not covering the methodology in any detail in this book. We do, however, feel that in the business world of medical devices there is little evidence of the use of SPC, so a brief coverage of the subject will be provided. We cover the selection of the charting method and some of the basic rules of interpretation.

18.4.1 Choosing the Control Chart

Figure 18.2 shows the decision tree for choosing what type of SPC method to use. To follow this chart to the correct method, you enter at the start and determine if the data you are collecting are attribute or variable measures. *Attributes* are counts or categorical designations (pass/fail, go/no-go), and *variables* are measures that typically can have many values in a continuous mode. For example, if we measure go/no go data, this is attribute, whereas if we measure time to complete in minutes, this is variable. If we follow the variables side of the chart, the next decision point is: Are we measuring individual values or rational subgroups? The answer to this comes directly from the sample size cell in the control plan. If we are measuring individuals, the most common chart method is the individual moving-range (IMR) chart, which is useful when the value being measured is changing slowly. If the process is changing rapidly, a moving-average (MA) chart is used. If the measure is rational subgroups (sample size greater than 1), we enter another

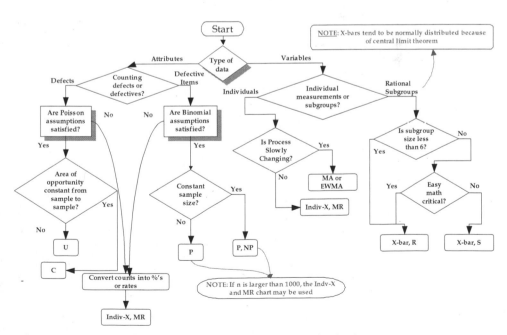

Figure 18.2 SPC charting method selection.

decision point for whether the subgroup size is less than 6. Again, the subgroup size is answered by the sample size cell on the control plan. For subgroups below 6 the chart of choice is the $\bar{X}$ (called *X-bar*) moving range ($\bar{X}$ MR); if the subgroup size is greater than 6, the chart recommended is the $\bar{X}$ standard deviation chart ($\bar{X}$ S). Moving back to the top decision point and following the attribute side to the left, the first decision point is whether we are measuring defects or defectives. We are counting defects when we count the number of defects in a device. We are counting defectives when we count a device defective regardless of the number of defects that the device contains. Let's assume that we are measuring defects. The first check is if the Poisson assumptions are satisfied. You have Poisson data when the data meet the following conditions:

- The data are counts of discrete events (defects) that occur within a finite area of opportunity.
- The defects occur independent of each other.
- There is an equal opportunity for the occurrence of defects.
- The defects occur rarely (compared to what could be possible).

Assuming that the assumptions are satisfied, the next decision point is whether the area of opportunity is constant from sample to sample, or variable. A changing opportunity occurs if we measure the number of items per device; this would definitely be nonconstant. With the constant opportunity, the *C*-chart is the correct method; if nonconstant, the *U*-chart is the proper method.

Returning to the first decision point for attribute data, we move to the defectives path on the right-hand side. The first check is if the binomial assumptions are satisfied. You have binomial data when they meet the following conditions:

- Each item is the result of identical conditions.
- Each item results in one of two possible outcomes (pass/fail, go/no-go).
- The probability of success (or failure) is constant for each item.
- The outcomes of the items are independent.

Assuming that these assumptions are met, we need to determine whether or not the sample size is constant. With a constant sample size the *P*-chart is the correct method; for a nonconstant sample size the NP-chart or *P*-chart is the correct method. You may note from Figure 18.2 that the most robust chart is the I-MR chart, which can be used for individual variable measures and for the defects or defectives if the number of data points is large or the results are converted to percentages.

18.4.2   Interpreting the Control Chart

When the proper charting method is selected the data are plotted and the charts are interpreted for stability. A process that is in control exhibits only random variation. In other words, the process is stable or consistent. There is no evidence of special-cause variation.

Control charts assess statistical control by determining whether the process output falls within statistically calculated control limits and exhibits only random variation. A process is classified as in control if the data demonstrate stability on the control chart. The typical indicators that a process is unstable or out of control is when there are definitive trends upward or downward (usually seven consecutive points), evidence of cyclical behavior, either by shift, supplier, or even season. Figure 18.3 depicts the distribution that occurs on most control charts.

The diagram is symmetrical about the centerline, which is the mean. The zone defined by the two C's is called zone C and is ±1 standard deviation about the mean. The area encompassed by the two B's (and the previous C's), called zone B, encompasses ±2 standard deviations. The final zone, called zone A, encompasses ±3 standard deviations.

The specific tests used are (the Nelson test):

- Any point outside the control limits (outside zone A)
- Nine points in a row on the same side of the centerline
- Six points in a row, all increasing or all decreasing
- Fourteen points in a row, alternating up and down
- Two out of three points in the same zone A or beyond
- Four out of five points in the same zone B or beyond
- Fifteen points in a row in either zone C
- Eight points in a row: more outside zone con the same side of the centerline

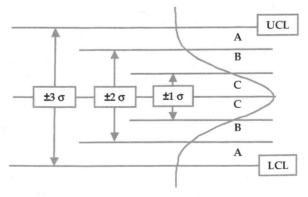

Figure 18.3   Control chart zones and distribution.

18.4.3 Taking Action

When interpreting control charts, if they are in control, everything is fine and processing should continue. If one of the stability rules is violated, a decision must be made. These rules indicate that a special-cause situation has occurred. Every attempt must be made to discover the underlying cause of the special-cause situation. This does not mean that the process is not producing acceptable devices.

18.5 PROCESS CAPABILITY

A process can be in control and still have poor capability. SPC on a process with poor capability will only assure us that the process will not degrade further; it will not prevent defects. It is also necessary to determine if the process is meeting customer requirements. The control chart has little relationship to the voice of the customer (VOC); it is strictly the voice of the process (VOP). The last step in validation is to ensure process capability. Before we get to this point we must ensure that we have adequate measurement capability and that the process is in a state of stability as indicated by the control chart.

Process capability can be assessed in either the short long term. In the short term this is a condition without variation between the rational subgroups; this is the best the process can perform under ideal situations. The customer can get glimpses of the short-term capability but more likely will experience the full variation. Therefore, the long-term capability is a better gauge of what the customer will experience.

Capability can be measured using several indices. There are the traditional methods defined by C_p and C_{pk} and there are the sigma values that correspond to the part per million defects. Each of the methods utilizes the specification limits assigned by the customer and can be defined as USL − LSL. We are interested in how many times the process variations can fit within these limits. Obviously, the more times the process spread can fit in the specification limits, the less chance there is that a defect will be experienced.

The following are several process capability indices that are widely used:

- C_p = process capability index, a simple and straightforward indicator of process capability:

$$C_p = \frac{\text{USL} - \text{LSL}}{6\sigma} \tag{18.1}$$

where σ can be calculated using the following formula for an overall long- or short-term sample of size n:

$$\sigma = \sqrt{\frac{\sum_{i=1}^{n}(x_i - \bar{x})^2}{n-1}} \qquad (18.2)$$

- C_{pk} = process capability index, basically an adjustment in C_p for the effect of noncentered distribution:

$$C_{pk} = \min\left(\frac{\text{USL} - \bar{x}}{3\sigma}, \frac{\bar{x} - \text{LSL}}{3\sigma}\right) \qquad (18.3)$$

- P_p = process performance index, which differs from C_p in that process performance applies only to a specific batch of material. Samples from the batch may need to be quite large to be representative of the variation in the batch. Process performance is used only when process control cannot be evaluated.
- P_{pk} = process performance index, adjustment of P_p for the effect of non-centered distribution.

18.6   ADVANCED PRODUCT QUALITY PLANNING

Advanced product quality planning (APQP) is a structured method for defining and executing the actions necessary to ensure that a product satisfies both the internal and external customers. APQP specify three phases: development, industrialization, and product launch. There are 23 elements (Table 18.1) in the APQP process: design robustness, design testing and specification

TABLE 18.1   APQP Elements

No.	APQP Element	No.	APQP Element
1	Sourcing decision	13	Measurement systems evaluation
2	Customer input requirements	14	Manufacturing process instructions
3	Craftsmanship	15	Packaging specifications
4	Design FMEA	16	Production trial run control plan
5	Design verification plan and report	17	Production trial run
6	Prototype build control plan	18	Preliminary process capability study
7	Prototype build(s)	19	Production validation plan and report
8	Drawings and specifications	20	Production control plan
9	Manufacturing feasibility commitment	21	Production part approval process
10	Manufacturing process flowchart	22	Design and manufacturing review(s)
11	Facilities, tools, and gauges	23	Subcontractor APQP status
12	Process FMEA		

compliance, production process design, quality inspection standards, process capability, production capacity, product packaging, product testing, and others. Some of the benefits of APQP are:

- Focuses on the customer through prevention and improvement
- Promotes early identification of required changes
- Reduces planning complexity
- Improved customer–supplier communication

18.6.1 APQP Procedure

The DFSS teams should follow the following steps to deliver the 23 elements required for APQP:

1. The first step in the APQP process is to assign responsibility to a cross-functional team. Effective APQP requires the involvement from all areas within a corporation. The team includes representatives from engineering, manufacturing, supply chain, purchasing, marketing, regulatory, medical, quality, sales, field service, subcontractors, and customers as appropriate.

2. Next, the team meets to:

- Select a project team leader responsible for overseeing the planning process and define the roles and responsibilities of each area represented.
- Identify the customers, internal and external.
- Define customer requirements.
- Select the disciplines, personnel, and/or suppliers that must be added to the team and those not required.
- Understand customer expectations (i.e., requirements definition).
- Assess the feasibility of the proposed design requirements, performance requirements, and manufacturing process.
- Identify costs, timing, and constraints that must be considered, and determine the assistance required from the customer.
- Determine the assistance required from suppliers.
- Identify the documentation process or method.

3. After this meeting, the DFSS black belt as a team leader documents the roles and responsibilities of each team member.

4. The team's first order of business following the organizational activities described above is the development of a quality plan using the APQP status tracking matrix (Figure 18.4). The purpose of APQP status tracking matrix is to establish:

- Common APQP expectations for internal and external suppliers
- Common APQP process metrics

Supplier: \
Location: \
Supplier Code: \
Contact Name/Tel: \
Review Date: \
Project \
Part Name: \
Part Number: \
User Plant:

I-dentify   C-haracterize   O-ptimize   V-erify/ V-alidate

APQP ELEMENT	S1	S2	S3	S4	S5	S6	S7	Responsibility
1 Sourcing Decision								DFSS Team
2 Customer Input Requirements								DFSS Team
3 Craftmanship								DFSS Team
4 Design FMEA								DFSS Team/Supplier
5 Design Verification Plan & Report (DVP&R)								DFSS Team/Supplier
6 Prototype Build Control Plan								DFSS Team/Supplier
7 Prototype Build(s)								DFSS Team/Supplier
8 Drawings & Specifications								DFSS Team/Supplier
9 Manufacturing Feasibility Commitment								DFSS Team/Supplier
10 Manufacturing Process Flowchart								Supplier
11 Facilities, Tools & Gages								Supplier
12 Process FMEA								Supplier
13 Measurement Systems Evaluation								Supplier
14 Manufacturing Process Instructions								Supplier
15 Packaging Specifications								Supplier
16 Production Trial Run Control Plan								Supplier
17 Production Trial Run								Supplier
18 Preliminary Process Capability Study								Supplier
19 Production Validation Plan & Report(PVP&R)								Supplier
20 Production Control Plan								Supplier
21 Production Part Approval Process (PPAP)								Supplier
22 Design and Manufacturing Review(s)								DFSS Team/Supplier
23 Subcontractor APQP Status								DFSS Team/Supplier
OVERALL APQP STATUS RATING (GYR)								

Figure 18.4 APQP status tracking matrix.

- A common program status reporting format to be used in the DFSS meetings and tollgate reviews
- Roles and responsibilities for APQP elements
- A better understanding of how the APQP elements relate to the DFSS ICOV process, design control SOP, and timing

The APQP time line will be used to track the deliverables status of the 23 APQP elements. The matrix integrates several interim reviews and tollgates. These interim milestones track progress toward completion of the APQP elements.

5. A color-coded scale of green (G), yellow (Y), and red (R) is used as a rating format for tracking status of the 23 elements of APQP deliverables listed in Table 18.1. GYR status communicates the progress toward successful

completion of an APQP element by the project time line. Definitions and risk factors for green, yellow, and red are listed in Table 18.2. The purpose of the risk assessment is to determine what elements in the APQP process a supplier, organization, or program team must work on to meet the project time line.

TABLE 18.2   APQP Project Time Line Risk Assessment

Risk	Color	Definition
High	Red	Target dates and/or deliverables are at risk. A recovery work plan is not available and/or implemented, or the work plan does not achieve program targets.
Moderate	Yellow	Target dates and/or deliverables are at risk, but a resourced recovery work plan has been developed to achieve program targets and has been approved by the appropriate management team.
None	Green	Target dates and deliverables are on track and meeting objectives.

Supplier: _____   Project: _____
Location: _____   Part Name: _____
Supplier Code: _____   Part Number: _____
Contact Name/Tel: _____   User Plant: _____

Element / Activity		Issue(s) for Red/Yellow Elements	Corrective Action / Resolution Plan	Timing		Responsibility	
#	Activity	(summarize the concern & resulting risk)	(e.g. revise timing, allocate resources)	Open	Close	Baxter	Supplier

Figure 18.5   APQP problem resolution sheet.

6. An APQP problem resolution sheet (Figure 18.5) is used to document issues regarding those elements that are assessed as yellow or red at any of the interim program reviews. The problem resolution sheet should be used to report, analyze, resolve, and record any issues on the APQP deliverables. A corrective action/resolution plan must be identified and recorded for each issue with associated timing and responsible person(s).

7. The team discusses each APQP element and determines:

- The applicability to the program
- The timing for start and completion
- The lead responsibility for completing the element and associated team members' risk assessment associated with completion of the item indicated
- An assignment of a G, Y, or R rating based on risk assessment
- Initiation of a problems resolution sheet for Y or R ratings

Note: A separate APQP status tracking matrix is initiated for each subsystem [i.e., subsystem design teams, subsystem manufacturing processes (internal and external suppliers)] of the DFSS project or program.

8. After approval, the team works to complete each APQP element. As a minimum requirement in assuring completion and assessing the status of each APQP deliverable, the team prepares quality of event checklists. The checklists cover the basic requirements for successful completion of the elements, but may not be all-inclusive. Expectations for each element are described in the checklists. The checklists are used to plan for the element and understand the element's association with the project milestone timing assess status (G,Y,R).

9. In conjunction with the milestones on the status tracking matrix, the supplier or customer conducts status review meetings with the team as needed. The customer provides the supplier with a list of all scheduled program status review dates. The supplier submits supporting documentation upon customer request. GYR ratings for each element are reviewed at these meetings and adjusted as appropriate. The issues resolution sheet is updated.

10. The system team will then complete the status report for their product as above, with their subsystem supplier status summarized on the subcontractor APQP status line. The system team submits the data to their customer, the project team.

11. The project team submits an updated status tracking matrix at all major program reviews.

APQP is an integrated quality planning tool that is well integrated in both product and manufacturing process design toward meeting or exceeding customer, FDA, and corporate requirements in such areas as quality and reliability, safety, cost, and time line. Figure 18.6 shows a generic APQP process map.

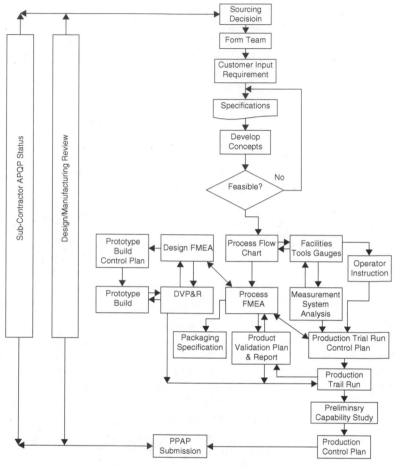

Figure 18.6   APQP process map.

18.6.2   Product Part Approval Process

PPAP is used to determine if all the customer engineering design record and specification requirements are met by the supplier and if the process can, based on statistical studies, produce product meeting these requirements during an actual production run. Success will result in overall quality improvements and cost savings to customers, suppliers, and business.

It is important to understand the minimum acceptance level of a DFSS project device during the ICOV phases. The production part approval process (PPAP) is a procedure for qualifying purchased material for production. The objectives of PPAP are:

- To verify design requirements
- To verify design quality and process capability

- To validate the measurement system
- To demonstrate process control and capability at the supplier

Due to PPAP activities, the DFSS membership should be extended to the supplier quality engineer and the buyers. The ideal PPAP is a vertical process where the supplier, in concert with the DFSS team, progress through each sequential step necessary to meet all the requirements to obtain approval to ship production parts. Past experience reveals that PPAP is more often an iterative process. Much of this repetition is a result of problems attributed to inadequate planning. Successful use of the APQP process, the prototype planning and execution, are prerequisite for approaching the ideal PPAP conclusion. An ideal PPAP has three stages.

PPAP Stage 1: Confirmation Prototype   In this stage, all device prototypes should be fully confirmed with production tooling using the intended manufacturing process and run at normal production speeds with the following provisos:

- Samples must conform to all dimensional requirements as detailed on the drawing.
- The testing of samples to determine conformance to all engineering specifications (optimize phase) and material specification requirements as referenced on the drawing must have begun.
- Statistical process capability (SPC) studies, including measurement systems analysis on measuring equipment on all identified significant and critical characteristics, must have been conducted.
- Sample stock for evaluation must be labeled in accordance with details as defined in packaging SOPs.

Quantities required to support this build phase will be provided by the DFSS team to a company buyer with quantities of sample parts required for engineering and functional evaluation noted on the purchase order.

PPAP Stage 2: Initial Submission   The primary objective is to permit special submissions to support the prelaunch and launch stages (Chapter 1). Any use of special submissions may require approval of a formal engineering deviation prior to shipment of stock. The purpose of special submission is to test the assembly process at the plant using parts representative of the final design and of the part quality that will be supplied for ongoing production, with certain requirements:

- Samples are to be completely off production tooling, using the final manufacturing process, and run at normal production speeds at the quoted rate.

- Samples must conform to all dimensional and engineering specification test and material requirements as detailed on the device drawing.
- All significant and critical characteristics from each major process stream must have been studied and completed to identify and verify dimensional conformance using statistical techniques (SPC).
- Shipping and handling processes must be approved.
- Sample stock for evaluation must be labeled in accordance with respective packaging SOPs.
- Quantities required to support this build phase will be provided by the DFSS team to a company buyer with quantities of sample parts required for engineering and functional evaluation noted on the purchase order.

PPAP Stage 3: Customer Validation Units   Devices from this stage will be used to design validation. Quantities required to support this build phase will be provided by DFSS team. All stock to be used is to be identified:

- Sample stock for evaluation must be labeled in accordance with respective packaging SOPs.
- A label is to be affixed to the stock packaging for all shipments for the duration defined.

A generic PPAP process map is shown in Figure 18.7.

18.7   DEVICE MASTER RECORD

The design master record is the documentation aspect of the device product development and DFSS ICOV process and output. *Device master record* (DMR) is the term used in the quality system (QS) regulation for all of the routine documentation required to manufacture devices that will meet company requirements consistently. Section 820.3(j) of the QS regulation (21 CFR 820) defines a device master record as "a compilation of records containing the procedures and specifications for a finished device." The detailed requirements for device master records are contained in Section 820.181 as well as throughout the regulation.

The definition of design output in 820.3(g) gives the basis and/or origin of the device master record for all class II and III devices as "Design output means the results of a design effort at each design phase and at the end of the total design effort." The finished design output is the basis for the device master record. The total finished design output consists of the device, its packaging and labeling, and the device master record.

For some devices, many of the design output documents are the same as the device master record documents. Other device output information is used to create a DMR drawing such as for a test or an inspection procedure.

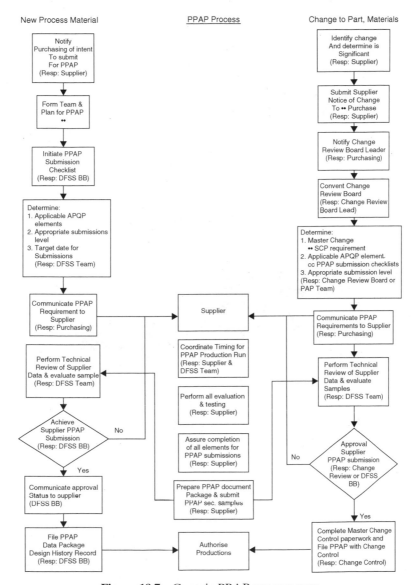

Figure 18.7 Generic PPAP process map.

Figure 18.8 shows the close relationship between design output and the device master record within a device and its manufacturing DFSS ICOV processes.

The definition for design output [820.3(g)] and requirements for design output [820.30(d)] do not apply to most class I devices. Therefore, the requirements for the DMR for most class I devices are in 820.181 device master record. Of course, a manufacturer of class I devices may use the design output sections of the GMP as guidance.

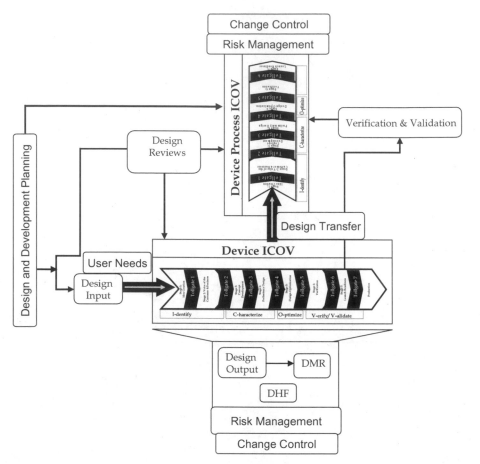

Figure 18.8   DMR in the DFSS process.

However, almost all sections of the QS regulation have requirements related to the device, master record. The device master record contains specifications for the device, accessories, labeling, and packaging, and contains a full description of how to procure the components and manufacture the device, including specifications for facilities, environment, and production equipment. In addition to the device specifications, a device master record contains documents that cover typical manufacturing activities, such as procurement and PPAP, assembly, labeling, test and inspection, packaging, and where applicable, sterilization.

Note that the activities and records or documents listed are required to produce any product medical, industrial, or consumer. There is nothing special about device master records except the name! Also, note that in common usage, the term *device master record* refers to the total record or to any of its individual records. Therefore, the term is singular for the total record, singular for a single document, and plural for a group of single documents. The term also may refer to an original record or to a copy of a record.

Device master records should be technically correct, contain and/or reflect the approved device and process designs, be under change control, contain the release or other control date, contain an approval signature, and be directed toward the intended user. These requirements are in the QS regulation because the device master record is the "beginning and end" of product errors, so the DMR will have a serious impact on the state of control of the manufacturing operation and also, perhaps, on the safety and performance of the device. The device master record, should be accurate and complete because the essence of the QS regulation is a quality system based on designing a device to meet user needs, documenting the design and production procedures in the device master record, and then producing a finished device that meets the DMR requirements. Thus, the device master record must accurately reflect the device intended to be produced by a manufacturer.

18.7.1 Document for Intended Employees

The content, style, language, graphics, and so on, of device master records should be directed toward the needs of employees, and if the record is a specification or text for labeling, it should be directed toward users. Similarly, installation instructions should be directed to installers. Labeling is often prepared by the same employees who draft device master records, and these employees should also be aware that labeling must meet the needs of the user as directed by 21 CFR 809.10, 801.6, and 820.30.

In any manufacturing activity (e.g., assembly, labeling, processing, testing), achieving and maintaining a state of control is enhanced by appropriate personnel who know:

- What task is to be done
- How to do the task
- Who is to do the task
- What task is being done
- What task was done and/or the results of the activity

For employees to perform a job correctly, they must know exactly what is to be done and exactly how to do the work. Section 820.181 requires that what is done be documented in the device master record. The device master record also contains test and inspection procedures and data forms that are used to help determine and record what was done.

Documents that instruct people how to fabricate, assemble, mix, label, test, inspect, and operate equipment should:

- Be directed toward the needs of the employees who will be using them and not directed toward the draftsperson or designer

- Match the tools and equipment to be used
- Be correct, complete, and current
- Depend on part numbers and basic drawings to transfer information rather than almost-photographic drawings

If a component is changed, the representations on pictorial or photographic drawings are no longer correct and may be very confusing to employees, particularly new employees.

The "how to manufacture" instructions should be correct for the intended operation and adequate for use by employees. In a mediumiszed to large company, the instructions tend to be extensive technical (engineering) drawings and written procedures. In any company, particularly small manufacturers, the work instructions may take several forms:

- Engineering drawings may be used if employees are trained to read and use them. Some of the "how to" information comes from employee training rather than from drawings.
- Assembly drawings may contain parts lists and quality acceptance criteria. A separate quality acceptance test and/or inspection procedure is not always necessary.
- Exploded-view drawings are used when employees cannot read plan view engineering drawings. Exploded-view drawings tend to be more "how to" than plan view drawings but they are expensive to draft. In some cases it may cost less to teach employees how to read and use ordinary plan view drawings.
- Step-by-step written procedures may be used to detail how to perform specific tasks with check-off blanks to show that each specific task was performed. This type of procedure is commonly used for critical operations and where there is little or no visual indication of what has been done, such as for cleaning operations or for mixing chemicals.

Documentation may be supported by production aids such as labeled photographs, videotapes, slide shows, sample assemblies, or sample finished devices. All of these perform device master record functions and should be identified, and be current, correct, and approved for the operation intended.

The most commonly used aids are models or samples. Two conditions should be satisfied in order to use these aids. First, a written specification for the sample should be contained in the device master record. This specification may, of course be the same as the specification for the assembly or finished device to be manufactured. This specification is subject to a formal change control procedure. Even though a model is available, the specification is needed for present and future product development and for production control purposes. The second condition includes the following elements:

- The sample should adequately reflect the device master record specification.
- The sample should be identified as an approved acceptable representative sample; that is, it should meet the company' required workmanship standards. The sample need not be a working model if the nonworking condition is not misleading to employees being guided by the sample.
- When appropriate, containers are to be tagged with a drawing number, revision level, and control number (lot, serial, and batch).

A card or tag may be used to identify and help control the use of samples of assemblies or finished devices. Such tags are usually covered by a clear plastic pouch and attached to the model or sample.

Samples and other aids, such as photographs, are subject to normal wear and tear in a production environment. Therefore, such aids should be adequately protected by a suitable means, such as being located in a protected area or being covered by a protective pouch or container. Production aids should be audited periodically to make sure that they continue to be suitable for the use intended. Section 820.100 contains requirements for corrective action, which may involve the use of samples, changes in the samples, or changes in control of the samples.

18.7.2 Adequate Information

Although a manufacturer tries to document for the employees, there is a need to audit periodically to see how well the goal is being met. There are various means of determining if information in the device master record, production tools, and other production elements are adequate for a given operation and associated employees. These include analyzing:

- The assistance required by new employees
- The assistance required when a new device is introduced into production
- Any confusion and hesitation
- The information exchanged among employees
- The "homemade" documentation drafted by line employees
- Rework
- The products produced (productivity)
- Complaints from departments that subsequently process the device
- Customer complaints

If any of these factors persist and are out of line with industry norms or with previous production experience, the manufacturer should take corrective action. Management should review the quality system as directed in Section

820.20 and be aware of device quality problems or quality system problems such as those listed above. The corrective action may include, for example, changes in supervision or documentation, adding new documentation, modifying the design, using different tools, and modifying the environment.

18.7.3 Preparation and Signatures

A separate device master record is required for each type or family of devices. A separate device master record may be needed for accessories to devices when these are distributed separately for health care purposes. Such accessories are considered to be finished devices. In practice, if the device and accessories are made by the same manufacturer, the device master record for the accessory may be incorporated into the device master record for the primary device.

Within a family of devices, variations in the family may be handled by dash-number extensions on drawing and procedure numbers. Usually, a top assembly or other major drawing contains a table or list of the devices in the family and lists the variable parameters for each member of the family.

Section 820.40 of the QS regulation requires that an individual(s) be designated to review, date, and approve all documents required by the QS regulation, including the device master record, and authorize changes. Those with the necessary technical training and experience should be designated to prepare and control device master records. In addition to requiring approval signatures on device master records, the QS regulation requires individual identification for a few other activities. These activities, together with the section numbers that designate them, are as follows:

820.30(b)	Approval of design plans
820.30(c)	Approval of design input
820.30(d)	Approval of design output
820.30(e)	Results of design review
820.30(f)	Results of design verification
820.30(g)	Results of design validation
820.40	Approval of device master record of changes
820.70(g)	Equipment maintenance and inspection activities performed
820.72(b)	Calibration performed
820.75(a)	Approval of process validation
820.75(1)(2)	Performance of validated process
820.80(d)	Release of finished devices
820.80(e)	Acceptance of activities conducted
820.90(b)	Authorization to use nonconforming product
820.120(b)	Labeling inspection
820.180(c)	Audit certification
820.198(b)	Decisions not to investigate complaints

The list is self-explanatory except for audit certification. When a manufacturer certifies in writing to the FDA that quality system audits have been performed, the certification letter is signed by those managers who have responsibility for the matters audited. Also note that the records in 820.70, 820.72, 820.80, 820.90(b), 820.120(b), and 820.160 are not part of the device master record but, rather, are part of the device history record. Records in 820.198(b) are part of the complaint files.

If a record that requires a signature is maintained on a computer, it is best if the designated person(s) maintains an up-to-date signed printout of the record. Where it is impracticable to maintain current printouts, computer-compatible identifiers may be used in lieu of signatures as long as there are adequate controls to prevent improper use, proper employee identification, inaccurate data input, or other inappropriate activity.

18.8 SUMMARY

The process of the medical device design transfer involves a close working relationship among product development team (i.e., design, manufacturing, service, etc.). Comprehensive planning early in the product development life cycle is required to develop high confidence in transferring the design to production and service personnel with no or few problems. Tracking and managing the various design transfer elements utilizing risk assessment helps in reducing project risk.

DFSS teams and suppliers should strengthen their relationship during design transfer activities. In particular, APQP and PPAP processes will not be successful without a strong relationship.

19

DESIGN CHANGE CONTROL, DESIGN REVIEW, AND DESIGN HISTORY FILE

19.1 INTRODUCTION

The *change control process* (CCP) is a process for managing change in order to ensure that any changes in a device's design, labeling, packaging, device master record (DMR; or see Section 18.7), or design inputs prior to or after design transfer are identified; documented; validated or, where appropriate, verified; reviewed; and approved prior to implementation; and finally, closed and documented in the design history file (DHF). The change control process must ensure that every change has appropriate quality oversight and confirms to regulatory requirements such as (but not limited to) 21 CFR 820.30(i) and ANSI/ISO/ASQC Q9001-2000 7.3.7.

Design reviews are one of the key design control elements in the quality system regulation 21 CFR 820.30(e). They are intended to assure that the design meets the requirements definition, and they also act as a mechanism for identification of a potential development weaknesses associated with safety, reliability, efficacy, manufacturability, service, implementation, and customer misuse of a device. A design review is a documented, comprehensive, systematic examination of the design or subject under review to adequately meet the requirements and to identify potential problems. These reviews are not to be confused with the DFSS project tollgate reviews discussed in Chapter 7. Design reviews are to be performed at major decision points or milestones in the product development process. They include a

Medical Device Design for Six Sigma: A Road Map for Safety and Effectiveness,
By Basem S. El-Haik and Khalid S. Mekki
Copyright © 2008 John Wiley & Sons, Inc.

review of the device and its subsystems and components, including software, labeling, packaging, manufacturing, installation, and service requirements as applicable. Design review results are documented in the product design history file.

A *design history file* (DHF) is a compilation of records that describe the design history of a finished device. The quality system regulation 21 CFR 820.30(j) requires that each manufacturer establish and maintain a DHF for each type of device. "Each type of device" means a device or family of devices that are manufactured according to one DMR. That is, if the variations in the family of devices are simple enough that they can be handled by only one DMR, then a single DHF is adequate. The quality system regulation also requires that the DHF contains or references all records necessary to demonstrate that the design is developed according to the approved design and development plan.

The following sections list a high-level process for design change process, design review, and design history file. It is not intended to cover every aspect, but rather, to provide the DFSS team with the necessary steps for change control of their design: in particular, in the last stages of the device development cycle presented in Chapter 1. The objective is to help them understand and plan those activities when combined with common industry practices.

19.2 DESIGN CHANGE CONTROL PROCESS

During any product design and development life cycle, changes occur. The change control process is mandated by the quality system regulation (QSR) as part of design control (21 CFR 820.30). Inadequate change control exposes a company to product liability actions and results in a serious violation of the QSR and leads in product recalls. Changes in a device's design, labeling, packaging, device master record, or design inputs can happen prior to transferring the design to production and service, or it can happen after the design transfer has occurred. In several incidents and in the predesign transfer stage, design change control process is always compromised and left without rigorous attention, and the focus is usually shifted to postdesign transfer. In the following sections we cover aspects of the change control process in both pre- and postdesign transfer to production and service. We would like to emphasize that although the change control process in essence is the same for both cases, differences in input, application rigor, and attention are usually noticed in the industry based on our experience.

19.2.1 Pre- and Postdesign Transfer CCP

Note that the change control process for design is mandated under 21 CFR 820.30(i), which is only effective when the first set of product requirement is approved. It is highly recommended that some sort of change control on engineering and documentation activities be implemented prior to design control [design activities at the characterize and optimize phases (Chapter 7) are predesign control activities], to act as a lessons-learned information base for future DFSS projects and team members. Changes in a product prior to approval of the first set of user/customer needs are not mandated by the design control regulations and standards, as at that point the concept design is changing rapidly. It is our experience that a less rigorous or informal change control process is of great value for maintaining consistency among working teams and to capture lessons learned for future projects.

To aid in the daily use of a change control process, many medical device companies use forms in conjunction with a change control procedure. Examples of these forms include a request for engineering action, an engineering change order, and an engineering change notice. The use of such forms simplifies the design change process and encourages consistency among projects. The forms are usually controlled through unique sequential numbers that facilitate tracking. All completed forms need to be reviewed and document controlled as required by the regulation.

The steps shown in Figure 19.1 represent the change control process prior to and following design transfer. Inputs to change control process are also shown. The postdesign transfer change control process differs from predesign transfer in input requirements. The additional inputs include product holds, a material management system, and postmarket analysis that occur only after design transfer to production and service.

Step 1: Identify proposed change. Identify the changed device, assembly, component, labeling, packaging, software, process, procedure, manufacturing material, and any related items or documents. Identify the design for which the change is requested within the DFSS project, such as (but not limited to) program name, project name, or whatever the configuration for the device or document to which the changes will be made. Define an effective date for the change, usually the proposed completion date.

Step 2: Initiate design change record. The design change record is generally a form or a procedure that contains the change information. The following is some information that can be used in the form: design identification, description of change, reason for change, justification for change, change risk assessment, action plan, and approval list.

Step 3: Review and preapprove design change record. Review and preapprove the change and make sure the record contains the tracking number, program and project name, and date the record was preapproved for tracking purposes.

Step 4: Execute and complete design change record. Execute action plan activities and update and complete documentation of the design change record.

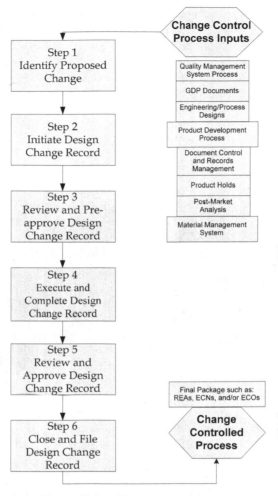

Figure 19.1   Change control process.

Step 5: Review and approve design change record. Review and approve the
   change after completion of the plan and make sure that the record is
   adequate.
Step 6: Close and file design change record. Submit the design change
   records to document control to be referenced in the design history file.

19.3   DESIGN REVIEW

Design reviews are conducted to identify deficiencies in the product development life cycle as early as possible (see Figure 1.2). These reviews are intended

to assure that the design meets the requirements definition and to identify any potential development weaknesses associated with safety, reliability, efficacy, manufacturability, service, implementation, and potential customer misuse of the product. The primary purpose of design reviews is to have different subject matter experts review a design or the subject under review to eliminate or minimize the risk of any significant deficiency. A design review can be initiated as early as during the identify phase of the DFSS ICOV process. There should be at least one design review prior to any major decision point or milestone in the device life cycle (Chapter 1). Equivalently, under 21 CFR 820.30, design controls, we need to have a design review after completing the design input deliverables (such as product requirements and system requirements) in order to close or sign off on these design input deliverables and prior to proceeding in the product development process. The same thing applies to design output deliverables (the optimize phase) prior to proceeding to design verification and validation. The number of design reviews depends on the company culture; some companies try to limit the number of design reviews to a minimum. It is our recommendation that there be at least one design review prior to any major decision point or milestone and as many informal reviews or DFSS team meetings as possible. The following steps define a generic design review structure (see Figure 19.2).

> *Step 1: Design review plan.* The DFSS team first scopes and defines the objectives of the design review. Place the document or subject information to be reviewed in a specific location to which all team members invited to the review has access. Next, identify reviewers or subject matter experts to be invited to the review. A potential list of functional areas from which to include reviewers: technology development, design engineering, quality assurance, quality engineering, manufacturing, marketing and sales, regulatory, reliability, service, and supplier quality. Independent reviewers are mandated at every design review. The team moves to develop a review communication plan of the review time and location, indicating the review leader, moderator, recorder, reader, and reviewer, and to define their roles and responsibilities. It should also be noted if a reviewer must attend the review or if it is optional to attend.
>
> *Step 2: Design review execution.* The design review leader sends documents or review subject information to be reviewed to the review team members two to three days prior to the time scheduled for design review. The reviewers review the documents or the subject information and send feedback to the review leader prior to review time. The review leader summarizes and prioritizes all issues in preparation for the review. The design review team meets and discusses the prioritized issues in sequence. The moderator should postpone the meeting if no reviewers are present or if the "must attend" reviewers are not available. After the meeting, the leader collects and documents in a design review report all issues and resolutions and the time spent at the review.

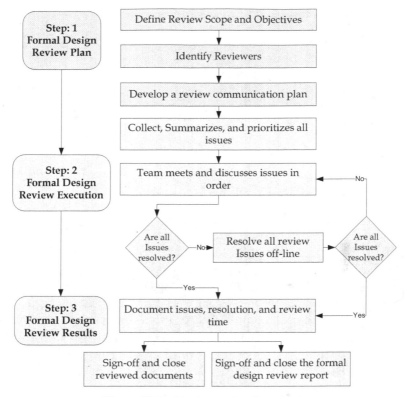

Figure 19.2 Design review flowchart.

Step 3: Design review results. The design review leader tracks and drives all
design review unresolved issues off-line after each review conclusion and
then signsoff and closes the documents reviewed, the design review report,
and the product design history file. In some cases, major or significant
issues may arise from a design review and can require a second or follow-
up review for the DFSS team to resolve. *All actions identified in the design
review need to be resolved; otherwise, the review leader needs to go back
and restart the process from the beginning.* If any of the issue resolution
is beyond the design review team's responsibility, the difficulties need to
be forwarded to the appropriate level of management for resolution.
Responsible management will be included as tollgate reviewers (Chapter
7) as well as being identified in the earlier stakeholder analysis.

19.4 DESIGN HISTORY FILE

The design history file (DHF) is a compilation of records that describe the
design history of a finished device. The quality system regulation [21 CFR

TABLE 19.1   Design History File Candidate Documents

DHF Documents	Design Control Elements
Design and development plans	Design and development planning
Products and systems requirement documents	Design input
Sketches and drawings	Design output
Design and development procedures	Design output
Engineering notebooks	Design output
Design review notes and report	Design review
Verification and validation reports	Design verification
	Design validation
Device master record	Design transfer
Design transfer deliverables	Design transfer
Risk management file	Risk management
Design change control records	Design change control

820.30(j)] requires that each manufacturer establish and maintain a DHF for each type of device. "Each type of device" implies a device or family of devices that are manufactured according to one design master record (DMR). That is, if the variations in the family of devices are simple enough that they can be handled by only one DMR, a single DHF is adequate. The quality system regulation also requires that the DHF contain or reference all records necessary to demonstrate that the design has been developed according to the approved design and development plan. The documents/deliverables listed in Table 19.1 are candidates to be positioned or referenced in the design history file together with their link to quality system regulation 21 CFR 820.30. The DHF needs to be maintained within the time frame defined by the quality records retention policy.

The DHF, which contains the "institutional" memory of previous design activities, is of great value in helping DFSS teams troubleshoot design problems when they occur or in preventing problems from repeating as well as preventing bad design ideas, already tried, from reoccurring.

19.5   SUMMARY

In this chapter we provide a quick overview of design change control informal and formal processes. We emphasize the necessity of controlling design changes informally prior to entering the design control stage. We divide the formal change control process into two stages: pre- and postdesign transfer to production and service. We link the change control process to the DFSS road map (Chapter 7) and the requirements of 21 CFR 820.30(i) and ANSI/ISO/ASQC Q9001-2000 7.3.7.

In addition, we initiate a high-level overview of design review steps and emphasized their importance to assure that a design meets the requirements definition and in acting as a mechanism for identification of a potential development weaknesses associated with safety, reliability, efficacy, manufacturability, service, implementation, and customer misuse of the product. In the last part of the chapter we review the design history file, containing the institutional memory of previous design activities, which is of great value in helping DFSS teams troubleshoot design problems when they occur or in preventing problems from repeating as well as preventing bad design ideas, already tried, from reoccurring.

20

MEDICAL DEVICE DFSS CASE STUDY

20.1 INTRODUCTION

In this chapter we present the development of an automatic dissolving and dosing device (Auto 3D), described briefly as a system of hardware, disposables, and software used by a nurse, pharmacist, and/or a caregiver at home to automatically dispense a prescribed dose of medication to be administered in one or multiple doses. The system goal is to dissolve and dose the required pharmaceutical consistently, safely, and effectively. Figure 20.1 is a schematic of the Auto 3D.

20.2 DFSS IDENTIFY PHASE

Early on, the design team segmented the external customer base into the following groups:

1. Hospital product evaluation committee
2. Physicians and clinical specialists
3. Pharmacists, nurses, and others

The pharmacists and nurses are the closest to the patient. In this segment, the customer needs for the Auto 3D device were defined based on marketing

Medical Device Design for Six Sigma: A Road Map for Safety and Effectiveness,
By Basem S. El-Haik and Khalid S. Mekki
Copyright © 2008 John Wiley & Sons, Inc.

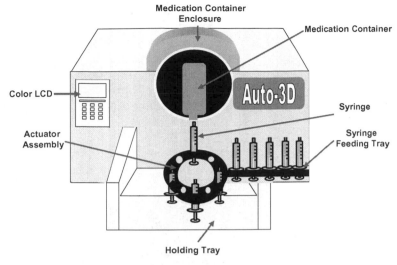

Figure 20.1 Auto 3D schematic.

research (through interviews laced with common sense), and the following list of needs was obtained:

- Safety and effectiveness
- Medication security
- Device ease of use
- Device reliability and availability
- Device value cost
- Device visual appearance

The high-level wants were prioritized using the analytical hierarchy process[1] (AHP) shown in Figure 20.2. In the first step in AHP, the team breaks down the customer wants, the "whats" in Chapter 8, into their constituent elements, progressing from the general to the specific. In its simplest form, this structure comprises a goal, criteria, and alternative levels. Each set of alternatives would then be further divided into an appropriate level of detail, recognizing that the more "whats" criteria are included, the less important each individual criterion may become.

Next, assign a relative weight to each. Each "what" has a local (immediate) and a global priority. Its global priority shows its relative importance within

[1] Developed by Thomas Saaty, AHP provides a proven, effective means to deal with complex decision making and can assist with identifying and weighting selection criteria, analyzing the data collected for the criteria and expediting the decision-making process (see chapter 8).

the overall model. Finally, after the criteria are weighted and the information is collected, the DFSS team puts the information into the model. Scoring is on a relative, not an absolute basis, comparing one choice to another. Relative scores for each choice are computed within each leaf of the hierarchy. Scores are then synthesized through the model, yielding a composite score for each choice at every tier, as well as an overall score. This process is depicted in Figure 20.2. The importance column will be used in Auto 3D QFD for all customer segments.

The list of "whats" is not actionable directly and needs further detailing using affinity diagramming (see Chapter 8). Figure 20.3 shows the affinity diagram that was used to determine these high-level needs. The DFSS development team then used the affinity diagram in a brainstorming session and defined the set of "whats" shown in Figure 20.3. In applying the affinity process, the team collected a list of Auto 3D "whats," clarified the list, recorded them on small Post-It notes, and laid the notes out randomly on a table. Without speaking, the team sorted the notes into "similar" groups based on their gut reactions. If a team member didn't like the placement of a particular note, he or she moved it until consensus was reached. Later, header notes consisting of a concise three- to five-word description were created as the unifying concept for each group and placed at the top of each group. The team discussed

Analytical Hierarchy Process			Safety and effectiveness	Medication security	Ease of use	Reliability and availability	Value cost	Visual appearance	Total	Importance
			A3D Needs							
			1	2	3	4	5	6		
A3D Needs	1	Safety and effectiveness	1.0	5.0	10.0	10.0	10.0	10.0	46.0	5.0
	2	Medication security	0.2	1.0	10.0	5.0	10.0	10.0	36.2	4.0
	3	Device ease of use	0.1	0.1	1.0	5.0	10.0	10.0	26.2	1.0
	4	Device reliability and availability	0.1	0.2	0.2	1.0	1.0	5.0	7.5	1.0
	5	Device value cost	0.1	0.1	0.1	1	1.0	5.0	6.3	1.0
	6	Device visual appearance	0.1	0.1	0.1	0.2	0.2	1.0	1.7	0.0
		Total	1.6	6.5	21.4	22.2	32.2	41.0		
		Importance	5.0	4.0	3.0	1.0	1.0	0.0		

Figure 20.2 Auto 3D prioritized need using AHP.

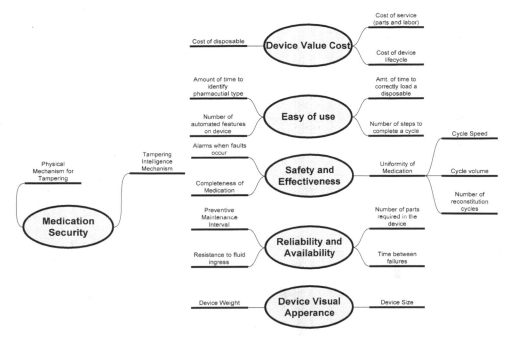

Figure 20.3 Auto 3D affinity diagram.

the groupings and understood how the groups related to each other. The output of the affinity diagramming is depicted in Figure 20.3.

We take the these affinity elements and begin to build our house of quality (HOQ 1) as we did in Chapter 8 (HOQ 2 is omitted in this chapter). Figure 20.4 shows the completed HOQ 1 that was built. From QFD house of quality phase 1, the critical-to-satisfaction (CTS) requirements were determined to be:

- Uniformity of medication
- Completeness of medication
- Tampering Intelligence mechanism
- Number of automated features on the device
- Amount of time to load a disposable correctly
- Number of steps to complete a cycle
- Time between failures
- Resistance to fluid ingress
- Number of parts required in the device
- Preventive maintenance interval
- Cost of device life cycle
- Cost of disposable part

Legend:

Symbol	Meaning	Value
●	Strong	9
○	Moderate	3
▽	Weak	1

(a) Rooms 1 to 7

	Importance	1 Uniformity of Medication	2 Completeness of Medication	3 Tampering Intelligence Mechanism	4 Number of automated features on device	5 Amt. of time to correctly load a disposable	6 Number of steps to complete a cycle	7 Time between failures	8 Resistance to fluid ingress	9 Number of parts required in the device	10 Preventive maintenance interval	11 Cost of device lifecycle	12 Cost of disposable	13 Cost of service (parts and labor)	14 Device Size	15 Device Weight	Competitor 1	Competitor 2	Competitor 3
1 Safety and effectivness	5	9	9	3	3	3			3								5	5	5
2 Medication security	4			9	3				3								3	5	2
3 Device ease of use	3			3	9	9	9										2	2	2
4 Device reliability and Availbility	1			3	1	3	3	9	9	9	9						2	3	1
5 Device value cost	1											9	9	9	3	3	2	2	1
6 Device visual apperance	1	3	3												9	9	1	1	1
Technical Importance		48	48	63	55	45	30	9	36	9	9	9	9	9	12	12			

Competitive Benchmark "Technical Importance Value on Hows": Competitor 1, Competitor 2, Competitor 3

Targets and Limits

	1	2	3	4	5	6	7	8	9	10	11	12	13	14	15
Metric	Siemens (mS)	% transferd	% caught	Count	Seconds	Count	Months	% Leaked	Count	Months	$	$	$	in^3	lbs
USL	440	N/A	99%	10	26	6	36	99%	11	18	2000	3.2	110	50	22
Target		95%	N/A	7	15	3	24	N/A	7	12	1600	2.5	90	40	18
LSL	350	90%	95%	N/A	N/A	N/A	N/A	95%	N/A	N/A	N/A	N/A	N/A	N/A	N/A

(b) Room 8 (conflict)

Correlation:
Enter a value from '-5' to '5'
'-5' implies large negative correlation.
'5' implies large positive correlation.
'0' implies no correlation.

LIB= larger is better
NIB= nominal is best
SIB= samll is better

	Direction	1	2	3	4	5	6	7	8	9	10	11	12	13	14
1 Uniformity of medication	HIB														
2 Completeness of medication	HIB	0													
3 Tampering intelligence mechanism	NIB	0	0												
4 Number of automated features on device	NIB	0	0	0											
5 Amt. of time to correctly load a disposable	SIB	0	0	0	0										
6 Number of steps to complete a cycle	SIB	0	0	0	0	0									
7 Time between failures	LIB	0	0	0	0	0	0								
8 Resistance to fluid ingress	LIB	0	0	0	0	0	0	0							
9 Number of parts required in the device	SIB	0	0	0	0	0	0	-5	0						
10 Preventive maintenance interval	LIB	0	0	0	0	0	0	5	5	-5					
11 Cost of device lifecycle	SIB	-3	-3	-5	-3	0	0	-5	-3	-5	-5				
12 Cost of disposable	SIB	0	0	0	0	0	0	0	0	0	0	-5			
13 Cost of service (parts and labor)	SIB	0	0	0	0	0	0	-5	0	-3	-5	-5	0		
14 Device size	NIB	0	0	0	0	0	0	0	0	0	0	-5	0	0	
15 Device wei ght	NIB	0	0	0	0	0	0	0	0	0	0	-5	0	0	-5

Direction row (Hows): HIB, HIB, NIB, NIB, SIB, SIB, LIB, LIB, SIB, LIB, SIB, SIB, SIB, NIB, NIB

Figure 20.4 Auto 3D house of quality: (a) rooms 1 to 7; (b) room 8 (conflict).

- Cost of service (parts and labor)
- Device size
- Device weight

Those CTSs are further cascaded to QFD phase 2 based on the process presented in Chapter 8. A partially completed QFD phase 2 is shown in Figure 20.5. This will be used later in the DFSS optimize phase.

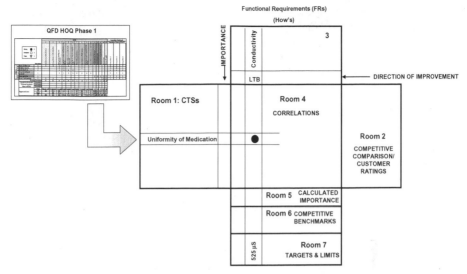

Figure 20.5 Partially completed QFD phase 2.

20.3 DFSS CHARACTERIZE PHASE

The Auto 3D device concept contains a drive mechanism that includes a precision linear actuator, holder, and syringe retention components under an actuator assembly. For control of this drive mechanism as well as all other functions, the device incorporates microprocessor-based electronics. These electronics contain embedded software that executes monitoring, control, configuration, maintenance, diagnostic, security, and safety functions. The device is powered mainly by standard ac but can be powered by a rechargeable lithium ion battery. The electronics, electrical wiring, and battery are part of the under electrical and power subsystem. The impeder and interface software are part of the software subsystem.

The user interface is a small color LCD touch-screen display. This display provides the user with output from the Auto 3D device as well as the ability to provide input. Optional features in the device include:

- A locking cover with a switch for detecting door status, to discourage unauthorized access
- A security code, required to operate the device
- A frangible breaker assembly and dispensing subsystem to fully automate the reconstitution process
- Speakers for audible alarm proposes

The structural decomposition above was developed using axiomatic design principles (Chapter 9). The team used the axiomatic design zigzagging process for cascading through requirements. The zigzagging process input is the house of quality (Figure 20.5), using the "hows" (room 3, Figure 8.3) which will be used as a hierarchical level in the zigzagging analysis. In this phase, we present only the decomposition of two functional requirements as follows:

FR0 = mix medicine to ready-to-use state
DR0 = Auto 3D system

We map to the design parameters (DP domain) as a next step:

$$\{FR0\} = [X]\{DP0\}$$

where X denotes a mapping relationship between an FR and a DP. Level 1:

FR1 = Auto 3D system provides a uniform mixing of medication
FR2 = Auto 3D system provides a complete dosing of medication
FR3 = Auto 3D system provides controllability

With DP0 in mind, we map to the design parameters (DP domain) as a next step, a zig step. At this step, DPs that satisfy the FRs were established, and some are depicted in the P-diagram (Mekki, 2006) of Figure 20.6. The control factors are also defined as design parameters in the P-diagram. The following DPs have been selected to satisfy level 1 FRs:

DP1 = actuator assembly (Figure 20.6)
DP2 = electrical and power subsystem
DP3 = software commands

The next logical step is to determine the corresponding design matrix [DM] that provides the relationships between the FR and DP elements in the same level. It is critical to ensure that the [DM] satisfies the independence axiom. The design matrix is given as:

$$\begin{Bmatrix} FR1 \\ FR2 \\ FR3 \end{Bmatrix} = \begin{bmatrix} X & X & X \\ 0 & X & X \\ 0 & 0 & X \end{bmatrix} \begin{Bmatrix} DP1 \\ DP2 \\ DP3 \end{Bmatrix} \tag{20.1}$$

A quick look at (20.1) indicates a decoupled design and also shows that the independence axiom is satisfied. In the [DM] above, an "X" represents a strong relationship between the corresponding FR–DP pair, and "0" represents no relationship.

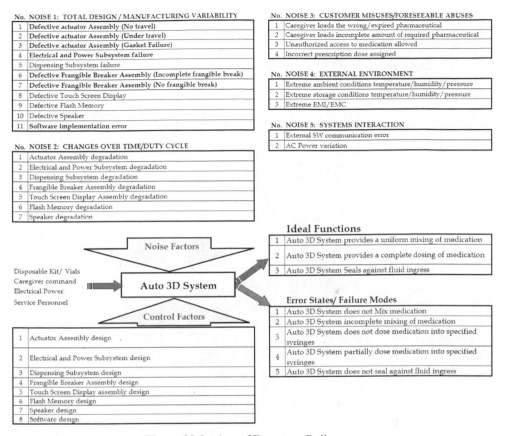

No.	NOISE 1: TOTAL DESIGN / MANUFACTURING VARIABILITY
1	Defective actuator Assembly (No travel)
2	Defective actuator Assembly (Under travel)
3	Defective actuator Assembly (Gasket Failure)
4	Electrical and Power Subsystem failure
5	Dispensing Subsystem failure
6	Defective Frangible Breaker Assembly (Incomplete frangible break)
7	Defective Frangible Breaker Assembly (No frangible break)
8	Defective Touch Screen Display
9	Defective Flash Memory
10	Defective Speaker
11	Software implementation error

No.	NOISE 2: CHANGES OVER TIME/DUTY CYCLE
1	Actuator Assembly degradation
2	Electrical and Power Subsystem degradation
3	Dispensing Subsystem degradation
4	Frangible Breaker Assembly degradation
5	Touch Screen Display Assembly degradation
6	Flash Memory degradation
7	Speaker degradation

No.	NOISE 3: CUSTOMER MISUSES/FORESEEABLE ABUSES
1	Caregiver loads the wrong/expired pharmaceutical
2	Caregiver loads incomplete amount of required pharmaceutical
3	Unauthorized access to medication allowed
4	Incorrect prescription dose assigned

No.	NOISE 4: EXTERNAL ENVIRONMENT
1	Extreme ambient conditions temperature/humidity/pressure
2	Extreme storage conditions temperature/humidity/pressure
3	Extreme EMI/EMC

No.	NOISE 5: SYSTEMS INTERACTION
1	External SW communication error
2	AC Power variation

Noise Factors

Disposable Kit/ Vials
Caregiver command
Electrical Power
Service Personnel

Auto 3D System

Control Factors

1	Actuator Assembly design
2	Electrical and Power Subsystem design
3	Dispensing Subsystem design
4	Frangible Breaker Assembly design
5	Touch Screen Display assembly design
6	Flash Memory design
7	Speaker design
8	Software design

Ideal Functions

1	Auto 3D System provides a uniform mixing of medication
2	Auto 3D System provides a complete dosing of medication
3	Auto 3D System Seals against fluid ingress

Error States/ Failure Modes

1	Auto 3D System does not Mix medication
2	Auto 3D System incomplete mixing of medication
3	Auto 3D System does not dose medication into specified syringes
4	Auto 3D System partially dose medication into specified syringes
5	Auto 3D System does not seal against fluid ingress

Figure 20.6   Auto 3D system P-diagram.

The zigzagging process continues and the first-level DPs (DP1, DP2, and DP3) need to zigzag by going from the physical to the functional domain again, a zig step, to produce their corresponding DPs. DP1 (the actuator assembly) is decomposed as follows:

FR11 = travel back and forth to transport diluent to pharmaceutical at specified speed

FR12 = pause between travel

DP11 is a cycling mechanism (number of actuation cycles × duration of pause between actuation cycles) and DP12 is the actuator push-pull velocity.

The next step is to determine the second-level design matrix [DM], which provides the relationships between the FR and DP elements above. The design matrix is given as

$$\begin{Bmatrix} FR11 \\ FR21 \end{Bmatrix} = \begin{bmatrix} X & 0 \\ X & X \end{bmatrix} \begin{Bmatrix} DP11 \\ DP12 \end{Bmatrix} \tag{20.2}$$

In this DFSS phase, the design risk assessment started with risk estimation, which establishes the linkage between requirements and hazards and ensures that safety requirements are complete. A preliminary hazard analysis (PHA) or a system robust design FMEA can be used to assess product risk. PHA and robust design FMEA are mentioned in Chapter 11. The DFSS team decided to perform a robust design FMEA and began a brainstorming session to develop a system-level P-diagram (Mekki, 2006), as shown in Figure 20.6. The brainstorming information gathered from generating the P-diagram was surrogated, analyzed, and flowed appropriately down to the robust system FMEA as shown in Figure 20.7.

20.4 DFSS OPTIMIZE PHASE

In this section we do not intend to list all possible Auto 3D optimization studies. Rather, a glimpse of such studies is presented here. We chose the uniformity requirement as an example.

The uniformity of the medication, FR1, is a critical functional requirement as outlined in the Auto 3D first house of quality. The DFSS team would like to investigate the impact on medication uniformity by changes in a set of parameters identified in the characterize phase. The DFSS team develops a set of potential factors that can affect the uniformity of medication, output FR1. Eight primary factors contribute to uniformity of medication during the dissolving process:

1. Diluent temperature
2. Air volume
3. Cycle volume
4. Number of cycles
5. Actuator push velocity
6. Actuator pull velocity
7. Duration of pause between cycles
8. Duration of pause during cycles

One approach to investigating the impact of the factors listed above is to design an optimization experiment that allows the DFSS team to study a widely feasible range for each factor. Three levels were selected for each factor so that the product development team can check for nonlinear behavior of a given factor, as shown in Table 20.1.

The uniformity of the medication, FR1, which is the response of this experiment, is best measured by conductivity, G, a surrogate metric with the designa-

Project Number: 12345
Project Name: Auto 3D System
Part Number: 1234567890
Part Name: Auto 3D System
Core Team: TBD

Design Responsibility: TBD
Key Date: TBD

FMEA Number: XXXX-FMEA-1234
Page of:
Prepared by: Khalid Mekki
FMEA Date (Orig.): TBD
(Rev.) 0.0

Item/Function	Potential Failure Mode	Potential Effect(s) Of Failure	SEV	Potential Cause(s) Mechanism (s) Of Failure	Current Design Controls Prevention and/or Detection	OCC	DET	CLASS	RPN	Recommended Actions	Responsibility & Target Completion Date	Action Taken	SEV	OCC	DET	Class
1.1 Auto 3D System provides a uniform mixing of medication	Auto 3D System does not Mix medication	Disposable Kit loss Procedure Time Delays (Operation) Clinical person manually mixes the medication Customer Dissatisfaction Requires Field Service	8	Defective actuator Assembly (No travel)	Actuator Assembly is defined as a Key Product in the key product Characteristics sheet, Prototype control plan check, Implement Advanced Product Quality Planning process on actuator assembly manufacturer	5	2	R3	80	Initiate DVP&R, Initiate process FMEA and Control plan, Continue APQP process, Continue Design/Mfg Reviews	Design & Process Engineers TBD Date					
				Electrical and Power Subsystem failure	Electrical and Power Subsystem is defined as a Key Product in the key product Characteristics sheet, Prototype control plan check.	3	2	R2	48	Initiate DVP&R, Initiate process FMEA and Control plan, Continue APQP process, Continue Design/Mfg Reviews	Design & Process Engineers TBD Date					
				Defective Frangible Breaker Assembly (No frangible break)	Frangible Breaker Assembly is defined as a Key Product in the key product Characteristics sheet, Prototype control plan check, Implement Advanced Product Quality Planning process on Frangible Breaker assembly manufacturer	5	2	r3	43	Initiate DVP&R, Initiate process FMEA and Control plan, Continue APQP process, Continue Design/Mfg Reviews	Design & Process Engineers TBD Date					
				Software implementation error	See Software FMEA Design/Mfg Reviews	5	3	R3	120	Continue Design/Mfg Reviews	Design & Process Engineers TBD Date					

Project Number: 12345
Project Name: Auto 3D System
Part Number: 1234567890
Part Name: Auto 3D System
Core Team: TBD

Design Responsibility: TBD
Key Date: TBD

FMEA Number: XXXX-FMEA-1234
Page of:
Prepared by: Khalid Mekki
FMEA Date (Orig.): TBD
(Rev.) 0.0

Item/Function	Potential Failure Mode	Potential Effect(s) Of Failure	SEV	Potential Cause(s) Mechanism (s) Of Failure	Current Design Controls Prevention and/or Detection	OCC	DET	CLASS	RPN	Recommended Actions	Responsibility & Target Completion Date	Action Taken	SEV	OCC	DET	Class
1.2 Auto 3D System provides a uniform mixing of medication	Auto 3D System incomplete mixing of medication	Potential hazard on patient (under dose) Procedure Time Delays (Operation) Customer Dissatisfaction Requires Field Service	10	Defective actuator Assembly (under travel)	Actuator Assembly is defined as a Key Product in the key product Characteristics sheet. Prototype control plan check. Implement Advanced Product Quality Planning process on actuator assembly manufacturer	3	2	R4	60	Initiate DVP&R, Initiate process FMEA and Control plan, Continue APQP process, Continue Design/Mfg Reviews	Design & Process Engineers TBD Date					
				Electrical and Power Subsystem failure	Electrical and Power Subsystem is defined as a Key Product in the key product Characteristics sheet, Prototype control plan check.	3	2	R4	60	Initiate DVP&R, Initiate process FMEA and Control plan, Continue APQP process, Continue Design/Mfg Reviews	Design & Process Engineers TBD Date					
				Defective Frangible Breaker Assembly (incomplete frangible break)	Frangible Breaker Assembly is defined as a Key Product in the key product Characteristics sheet. Prototype control plan check. Implement Advanced Product Quality Planning process on Frangible Breaker assembly manufacturer	3	2	R4	60	Initiate DVP&R, Initiate process FMEA and Control plan, Continue APQP process, Continue Design/Mfg Reviews	Design & Process Engineers TBD Date					
				Actuator Assembly degradation/fatigue	Actuators Assembly evaluation/ benchmark. Manufacturer Spec. actuator life for 5000KM. Application requires 60KM. Design/Mfg Reviews	2	2	R3	40	Initiate Assembly DVP&R, Continue Design/Mfg Reviews	Design & Process Engineers TBD Date					
				Software implementation error	See Software FMEA Design/Mfg Reviews	3	3	R4	90	Initiate Assembly DVP&R, Continue Design/Mfg Reviews	Design & Process Engineers TBD Date					
				EMI/ESD/RFI	Design/Mfg Reviews	3	5	R4	150	Initiate Assembly DVP&R, Continue Design/Mfg Reviews	Design & Process Engineers TBD Date					

Figure 20.7 Auto 3D robust system FMEA.

Project Number: 12345
Project Name: Auto 3D System
Part Number: 1234567890
Part Name: Auto 3D System
Core Team: TBD

Design Responsibility: TBD
Key Date: TBD

FMEA Number: XXXX-FMEA-1234
Page of:
Prepared by: Khalid Mekki
FMEA Date (Orig.): TBD
(Rev.) 0.0

Item/ Function	Potential Failure Mode	Potential Effect(s) Of Failure	SEV	Potential Cause(s) Mechanism (s) Of Failure	Current Design Controls Prevention and/or Detection	OCC	DET	CLASS	RPN	Recommended Actions	Responsibility & Target Completion Date	Action Taken	SEV	OCC	DET	Class
2 Auto 3D System provides a complete dosing of medication	Auto 3D System does not dose medication into specified syringes	Potential hazard on patient (delay of medication) Procedure Time Delays (Operation) Customer Dissatisfaction Requires Field Service	10	Defective actuator Assembly (No travel)	Actuator Assembly is defined as a Key Product in the key product Characteristics sheet, Prototype control plan check, Implement Advanced Product Quality Planning process on actuator assembly manufacturer	3	2	SC	60	Initiate DVP&R, Initiate process FMEA and Control plan, Continue APQP process, Continue Design/Mfg Reviews	Design & Process Engineers TBD Date					
				Electrical and Power Subsystem failure	Electrical and Power Subsystem is defined as a Key Product in the key product Characteristics sheet, Prototype control plan check,	3	2	SC	60	Initiate DVP&R, Initiate process FMEA and Control plan, Continue APQP process, Continue Design/Mfg Reviews	Design & Process Engineers TBD Date					
				Defective Frangible Breaker Assembly (No frangible break)	Frangible Breaker Assembly is defined as a Key Product in the key product Characteristics sheet, Prototype control plan check, Implement Advanced Product Quality Planning process on Frangible Breaker assembly manufacturer	3	2	SC	48	Initiate DVP&R, Initiate process FMEA and Control plan, Continue APQP process, Continue Design/Mfg Reviews	Design & Process Engineers TBD Date					
				Software implementation error	See Software FMEA Design/Mfg Reviews	3	3	SC	90	Continue Design/Mfg Reviews	Design & Process Engineers TBD Date					
	Auto 3D System partially dose medication into specified syringes	Potential hazard on patient (under dose) Procedure Time Delays (Operation) Customer Dissatisfaction Requires Field Service	10	Defective actuator Assembly (under travel)	Actuator Assembly is defined as a Key Product in the key product Characteristics sheet, Prototype control plan check, Implement Advanced Product Quality Planning process on actuator assembly manufacturer	3	2	R4	60	Initiate DVP&R, Initiate process FMEA and Control plan, Continue APQP process, Continue Design/Mfg Reviews	Design & Process Engineers TBD Date					
				Actuator controller malfunction	Actuator controller is defined as a Key Product in the key product Characteristics sheet, Prototype control plan check, Implement Advanced Product Quality Planning process on actuator controller manufacturer	3	2	R4	60	Initiate DVP&R, Initiate process FMEA and Control plan, Continue APQP process, Continue Design/Mfg Reviews	Design & Process Engineers TBD Date					
				Defective Frangible Breaker Assembly (incomplete frangible break)	Frangible Breaker Assembly is defined as a Key Product in the key product Characteristics sheet, Prototype control plan check, Implement Advanced Product Quality Planning process on Frangible Breaker assembly manufacturer	3	2	R4	60	Initiate DVP&R, Initiate process FMEA and Control plan, Continue APQP process, Continue Design/Mfg Reviews	Design & Process Engineers TBD Date					
				Actuator Assembly degradation/fatigue	Actuators Assembly evaluation/ benchmark. Manufacturer Spec. actuator life for 5000KM, Application requires 60KM, Design/Mfg Reviews	2	2	R3	40	Initiate Assembly DVP&R, Continue Design/Mfg Reviews	Design & Process Engineers TBD Date					
				Software implementation error	See Software FMEA Design/Mfg Reviews	3	3	R4	90	Initiate Assembly DVP&R, Continue Design/Mfg Reviews	Design & Process Engineers TBD Date					
				EMI/ESD/RFI	Design/Mfg Reviews	3	5	R4	150	Initiate Assembly DVP&R, Continue Design/Mfg Reviews	Design & Process Engineers TBD Date					

Figure 20.7 *Continued*

TABLE 20.1 Experiment Factors and Their Levels

No.	Input/Independent	Low	Medium	High	Measurement Unit
			Factor Level		
1	Dilument temperature	4/40	21/70	30/86	°C/°F
2	Air volume	9	5	2	mL air
3	Cycle volume	3	4	5	mL
4	Number of cycles	4	8	12	
5	Actuator push velocity	20	30	40	mm/s
6	Actuator pull velocity	20	30	40	mm/s
7	Duration of pause between cycles	1	2	3	s
8	Duration of pause during cycles	1	2	3	s

TABLE 20.2 Experiment Response and Its Designation

No.	Response/Dependent	Measurement Unit	Low	Medium	High
1	Conductivity	μS	395	525	600

tion given in Table 20.2. Conductivity can be formulated as a static or dynamic response. The DFSS team decided to use the static conductivity measure as a response of this experiment, as the dynamic conductivity is very sensitive to temperature variation and can skew the experiment results. The basic unit of conductivity is the siemens (S), formerly called the mho.

Conductivity is the ability of a material to conduct electric current. The principle by which instruments measure conductivity is simple. Two plates are placed in the sample, a potential is applied across the plates (normally, a sine-wave voltage), and the current is measured. Conductivity (G), the inverse of resistivity (R), is determined from the voltage and current values according to Ohm's law. Since the charge on ions in any solution facilities the conductance of electrical current, the conductivity of a solution is proportional to its ion concentration. In some situations, however, conductivity may not correlate directly to concentration and uniformity. Figure 20.8 illustrates the relationship between conductivity and ion concentration for two medicine solutions. Notice that the graph is linear for medicine solution (a) but not for highly concentrated medicine solution (b). Ionic interactions can alter the linear relationship between conductivity and concentration in some highly uniformly concentrated solutions. This linear relation is maintained for medicines of uniformity in the interval 395 to 600 μS.

To investigate all possible combinations of the eight factors in three levels, each team would need 6561 unique runs, which is a completely unrealistic sample size. The L_{27} orthogonal array is chosen to investigate the factors. The team decided to replicate the array once, which leads to totally unique experimental combinations of 54 runs. See Table 20.3 for the experiment matrix.

TABLE 20.3 Experiment Matrix Array

	1		2		3		4	
	Diluent Temperature		Air Volume		Cycle Volume		Number of Cycles	
Exp. No.	A	Check	B	Check	C	Check	D	Check
1	1		1		1		1.	
2	1		1		1		2	
3	1		1		1		3	
4	1		2		2		1	
5	1		2		2		2	
6	1		2		2		3	
7	1		3		3		1	
8	1		3		3		2	
9	1		3		3		3	
10	2		1		2		1	
11	2		1		2		2	
12	2		1		2		3	
13	2		2		3		1	
14	2		2		3		2	
15	2		2		3		3	
16	2		3		1		1	
17	2		3		1		2	
18	2		3		1		3	
19	3		1		3		1	
20	3		1		3		2	
21	3		1		3		3	
22	3		2		1		1	
23	3		2		1		2	
24	3		2		1		3	
25	3		3		2		1	
26	3		3		2		2	
27	3		3		2		3	

			Low	Medium	High	Units
1	A	Diluent temperature	4/40	21/70	30/86	°C/°F
2	B	Air volume	9	5	2	mL air
3	C	Cycle volume	3	4	5	mL
4	D	Number of cycles	4	8	12	
5	E	Actuator push velocity	20	30	40	mm/s
6	F	Actuator pull velocity	20	30	40	mm/s
7	G	Duration of pause between cycles	1	2	3	s
8	H	Duration of pause during cycles	1	2	3	s

| 5 | | 6 | | 7 | | 8 | | |
| Actuator Push Velocity | | Actuator Pull Velocity | | Duration of Pause Between Cycles | | Duration of Pause During Cycles | | Response |
E	Check	F	Check	G	Check		Check	Conductivity
1		1		1		1		
2		2		2		2		
3		3		3		3		
2		2		3		3		
3		3		1		1		
1		1		2		2		
3		3		2		2		
1		1		3		3		
2		2		1		1		
2		3		2		3		
3		1		3		1		
1		2		1		2		
3		1		1		2		
1		2		2		3		
2		3		3		1		
1		2		3		1		
2		3		1		2		
3		1		2		3 .		
3		2		3		2		
1		3		1		3		
2		1		2		1		
1		3		2		1		
2		1		3		2		
3		2		1		3		
2		1		1		3		
3		2		2		1		
1		3		3		2		

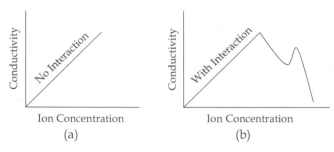

Figure 20.8 Conductivity as a function of ion concentration.

Note the check columns after each factor array; the check column is intended for quality verification purpose.

20.4.1 DOE Optimization Analysis[2]

In this section we list linear models, ANOVA, response tables, response graphs, and residual plots for both the signal-to-noise ratio (SN) and the conductivity mean. The SN analyses are given first in Table 20.4 and Figure 20.9.

20.4.2 DOE Optimization Conclusions

SN ratio analysis indicates that there are a group of factors that are statistically significant from a variability perspective [i.e., have a large "delta" gain (Table 20.4)]. The rule of thumb is that any SN gain of less than 1 dB is considered in significant. The rank of each factor and the delta gains are listed in Table 20.4 and depicted graphically in Figure 20.9. The "number of cycles" is the most significant factor, with a gain of 7.78 dB (i.e., flipping between this factor's levels will give us over a 50% reduction in variability). From the SN ratio perspective, the recommended factorial levels are as follows:

1. Diluent temperature at 30°C (level 3)
2. Air volume at 2 mL of air (level 3)
3. Cycle volume at 5 mL (level 3)
4. Number of cycles at 12 cycles (level 3)
5. Actuator push velocity at 40 mm/s (level 3)
6. Actuator pull velocity at 20 mm/s (level 1)
7. Duration of pause between cycles at 2 s (level 2)
8. Duration of pause during cycles at 2 or 3 s (level 2 or 3)

[2]Using Minitab release 15.

TABLE 20.4 Response Table for Signal-to-Noise Ratios

Level	Dilutent Temp.	Air Volume	Cycle Volume	Number of Cycles	Push Velocity	Pull Velocity	Pause Between Cycles	Pause During Cycle
1	50.75	52.14	50.66	47.70	50.83	55.06	50.97	52.23
2	53.57	52.88	53.18	54.71	52.74	54.75	53.89	51.29
3	53.95	53.44	54.41	55.48	54.71	48.99	53.81	54.42
Delta	3.20	1.29	3.75	7.78	3.88	6.06	2.92	3.13
Rank	5	8	4	1	3	2	7	6

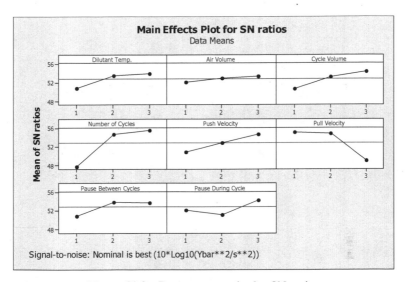

Figure 20.9 Response graphs for SN ratios.

The conductivity optimum SN ratio transfer function predicted is given by

$$SN_{G|preducted, optimum} = 52.757 + \sum_{i=1}^{8}\left(\overline{factor_i} - 52.757\right)$$
$$= 66.061\,dB$$

(20.3)

where $\overline{factor_i}$ is the average SN value at the significant factorial level.

The mean analysis indicates that there are a group of factors that are statistically significant (i.e., have a large delta gain in Table 20.5). The rank of each factor and the delta gains are listed in Table 20.5 and depicted graphically in Figure 20.10. The number of cycles is the most significant factor, with a gain of 8.5 µS. Table 20.6 exhibits ANOVA for the mean conductivity. From mean

TABLE 20.5   Response Table for Means

Level	Dilutent Temp.	Air Volume	Cycle Volume	Number of Cycles	Push Velocity	Pull Velocity	Pause Between Cycles	Pause During Cycle
1	437.7	437.8	433.7	433.1	434.6	438.4	439.1	435.6
2	439.2	438.3	439.9	440.8	439.6	438.6	437.9	440.2
3	438.5	439.3	441.8	441.6	441.2	438.4	438.4	439.6
Delta	1.5	1.4	8.1	8.5	6.6	0.1	1.2	4.6
Rank	5	6	2	1	3	8	7	4

TABLE 20.6   Analysis of Variance for Means

Source	DF	Seq SS	Adj SS	Adj MS	F	P
Dilutent temp.	2	41.765	10.266	5.133	3.56	0.096
Air volume	2	32.761	12.765	6.383	4.43	0.066
Cycle volume	2	190.025	206.867	103.433	71.73	0.000
Number of cycles	2	259.107	229.942	114.971	79.73	0.000
Push velocity	2	111.338	122.835	61.417	42.59	0.000
Pull velocity	2	8.392	1.141	0.571	0.40	0.690
Pause between cycles	2	2.508	4.736	2.368	1.64	0.270
Pause during cycle	2	68.560	68.560	34.280	23.77	0.001
Residual error	6	8.652	8.652	1.442		
Total	22	723.109				

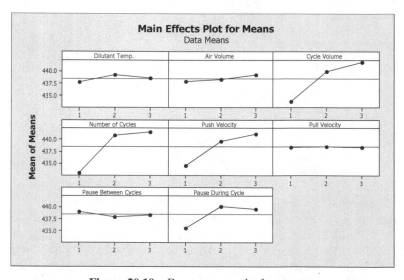

Figure 20.10   Response graphs for means.

perspective, the following factors are statistically significant and listed with the level that maximizes conductivity (G):

1. Cycle volume at 5 mL (level 3)
2. Number of cycles at 12 cycles (level 3)
3. Actuator push velocity at 40 mm/s (level 3)
4. Duration of pause during cycles at 2 s (level 2)

The conductivity optimum mean transfer function predicted is given by

$$
\begin{aligned}
\text{Mean}_G|_{\text{preducted, optimum}} &= 438.467 + \sum_{i-1}^{4} \left(\overline{\text{factor}_i} - 438.467 \right) \\
&= 449.399\,\mu\text{S}
\end{aligned}
\tag{20.4}
$$

where $\overline{\text{factor}_i}$ is the average mean at the significant factorial level. The current design performance is given as

$$
\begin{aligned}
\text{SN}_G|_{\text{preducted, current}} &= 52.757 + \sum_{i=1}^{8} \left(\overline{\text{factor}_i} - 52.757 \right) \\
&= 41.041\,\text{dB}
\end{aligned}
\tag{20.5}
$$

$$
\begin{aligned}
\text{Mean}_G|_{\text{preducted, current}} &= 438.467 + \sum_{i=1}^{4} \left(\overline{\text{factor}_i} - 438.467 \right) \\
&= 425.399\,\mu\text{S}
\end{aligned}
\tag{20.6}
$$

The current design SN ratio is 41.517 dB and the mean is = 425.399 μS. The SN delta gain (ΔSN) predicted = 66.061 − 41.517 = 24.544 dB. The mean delta gain (Δmean) predicted = 24 μS.

20.4.3 DOE Confirmation Run

Next, the robustness of this parameter optimization can be verified experimentally. This requires prediction and confirmation runs of both the optimum condition and one of the current design factors. Each treatment combination was predicted, and then two runs at these combinations were measured using the same experimental setup. These confirmation runs were performed at both levels of noise. The results of these confirmation runs, including the mean and the SN ratio, are shown in Table 20.7.

The current design SN ratio is 41.517 dB, and the mean is = 421 μS. The SN delta gain (ΔSN) predicted = 61.983 − 41.517 = 20.467 dB. The mean delta gain predicted (Δmean) = 23.25 μS. In other words, the DFSS team again predicted 24.544 dB, but they were able to confirm only 20.467 dB. This amounts to a 90%

TABLE 20.7 Confirmation Run Results

Design	N_1	N_2	Mean	σ	SN
Optimum	444.500	444.000	444.250	0.354	61.983
Current	418.500	423.500	421.000	3.536	41.517

reduction in variability. They also predicted a mean gain of 24 μS, but they were only able to confirm 23.24 μS. The confirmation run gave very excellent results.

20.5 DFSS VERIFY/VALIDATE PHASE

Like the others in this chapter, this section is intended to give a flavor of the Auto 3D DFSS project rather than to document every step and tool application. Design verification and validation are critical steps in the DFSS road map and needs to be thought out well in advance of final production of Auto 3D. Verification often requires prototypes that need to be close to the final design but are often subject to trade-offs in scope and completeness due to cost or availability. Assessing the components and subsystems of Auto 3D device against the type of design risk helps in determining when a prototype is required and what configuration must be available. Once prototypes are available, a comprehensive test plan was followed in order to capture any special event and go/no go decision was based on statistically significant criteria.

For verification and validation, a top-down approach from assembly to components was used to track APQP deliverables. The project champion decided to implement APQP deliverables on critical components such as the actuator assembly. The actuator assembly APQP deliverables follow the procedures outlined in Chapter 17. The strategy is as follows:

1. Define the actuator assembly critical components (Figure 20.11) as obtained from design mapping in the DFSS characterize phase.
2. Complete a quality of event checklist for each APQP deliverable for each critical component in the actuator assembly (an example is given in Table 20.8).
3. Track APQP deliverables as appropriate with an APQP tracking matrix for critical components in the actuator assembly

The device development verification plan and report is depicted in Figure 20.12. The QFD and the risk analysis tool Process FMEA (Table 20.9) were used as the bases for Auto 3D device verification and validation. All critical-to-quality (CTQ) device requirements defined in the QFD were verified using productionlike prototypes, and a customer validation evaluation was conducted and confirmed that customer needs were fulfilled.

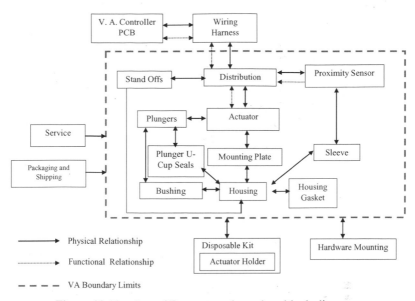

Physical Relationship

Functional Relationship

VA Boundary Limits

Figure 20.11 Auto 3D actuator boundary block diagram.

Design Verification Plan and Report (DVP&R)										
System: Auto 3D	Project: DFSS Project Number 1		DVP&R Revision Level: 0.0					Design Engineer: John Doe		
Subsystem: Actuator Assembly	Component: N/A		Latest Design Level: DL 0.0					DVP&R Number: 1		

Test No.	Test Name/Source	Acceptance Criteria	Design Level Tested	Sample Size		Statistical Test Acceptance Criteria		Timing		Test Results
				Required	Tested	Required	Tested	Sched.	Actual	
1	**Assembly functional test**	Pass a **1000 Cycles** under full load. Components must pass functional requirements	DL 0.0	6						
2	Actuator push force test	20 to 25 lb	DL 0.0	6						
3	Actuator load sensing capability test	7 to 10 lb	DL 0.0	6						
4	Actuator stroke accuracy test	0.750" ± 0.01"	DL 0.0	6						
5	Actuator repeatability test	± 0.005"	DL 0.0	6						
6	Proximity Sensor functional test	**TBD**	DL 0.0	6						
7	Assembly calibration test	TBD	DL 0.0	TBD						
8	Auto 3D system Functional Test (interaction)	**TBD**	DL 0.0	TBD						
	Environmental Testing									
9	Auto 3D HALT testing	**TBD**	DL 0.1	TBD						
10	Assembly test A	**TBD**	DL 0.0	TBD						
11	Assembly compatibility with blood and cleaning agents (fluid ingress)	**TBD**	DL 0.0	TBD						
12	Assembly extreme temp. & humidity	**TBD**	DL 0.0	TBD						
13	Assembly audible noise test	**TBD**	DL 0.0	TBD						
14	Assembly drop test	**TBD**	DL 0.0	TBD						
15	Assembly dust/contaminants test	**TBD**	DL 0.0	TBD						
	Reliability/ Life Testing									
16	Actuator Assembly Life cycle test	Pass a **400,000 Cycles** under full load. Assembly must pass functional requirements	DL 0.0	6						
17	Actuator degradation/ wear out test	**TBD**	DL 0.0	6						
18	O-rings degradation test	**TBD**	DL 0.0	6						
19	Bushing degradation	**TBD**	DL 0.0	6						
20	Plungers degradation	**TBD**	DL 0.0	6						

Figure 20.12 Actuator design verification plan and Report.

TABLE 20.8 Sourcing APQP Quality of Event Checklist

Item	Project Timing			Due Dates		Expectations	G/Y/R	Comments
	Start	Target		Program Timing	Supplier Timing			
1	2/6/2007	7/23/2007		9/15/2007		Ensure that the supplier's quality history is factored into the planning and sourcing decision	G	John Doe to provide plant 1 quality history
2	2/6/2007	7/23/2007		9/15/2007		Ensure that the company's supplier quality, purchasing, and supplier technical assistance group is aware of all supplier selected in the DFSS optimize phase and that a supplier evaluation request generated for all new suppliers	G	Cross-functional DFSS team met in plant 1 on 2/19/2007
3	2/6/2007	7/23/2007		9/15/2007		Complete and communicate the sourcing decisions to all affected suppliers and subsuppliers in the DFSS optimize phase.	G	Auto 3D instrument will be build in the plant 1 manufacturing plant

#				Description		Comments
4	2/6/2007	7/23/2007	9/15/2007	Ensure that appropriate suppliers and subsuppliers are on-board and involved with the program team early enough to understand all requirements.	G	Jean Doe manufacturing lead has been involved in the project since 12/2005
5	2/6/2007	7/23/2007	9/15/2007	Ensure that all company manufacturing plants are aware of all suppliers selected (see the APQP element "customer input")	G	Plant 1 is the only manufacturing plant
6	2/6/2007	7/23/2007	9/15/2007	Ensure that all applicable confidentiality agreements, supplier quality agreement, purchasing contract, supplier notice of change, and all the other related documents, have been signed by quality, purchasing, product development and the supplier and reviewed by quality.	G	Plant 1 is a company manufacturing plant; a supplier quality agreement was signed 12/19/07
Other						
Overall				Team's overall rating of this element (G/Y/R)	G	

TABLE 20.9 Actuator Assembly PFMEA (Shown Partially)

Item/Function	Potential Failure Mode	Potential Effect(s) of Failure	SEV	Class	Potential Causes(s) or Mechanism(s) of Failure	OCC	Current Design Controls Prevention and Detection	DET	RPN	Recommended Actions	Responsibility and Target Completion Date
1 Actuator assembly: actuator extends and retracts a precise distance	Does not extend or retract	Disposable kit loss	8	SC	Defective actuator	3	Implement APQP process on actuator manufacture; design/mfg reviews	5	120	Define as a critical product: characteristics in drawings and key product characteristics sheet, prototype control plan check, initiate assembly DVP&R, initiate process FMEA and control plan, continue APQP process, continue design/mfg reviews	Team and plant 1 mfg 9/8/07
		Procedure time delays (operation)			Defective distribution PCB	3	Implement APQP process on PCB manufacture; design/mfg reviews	5	120	Define as a critical product: characteristics in drawings and key product characteristics sheet, prototype control plan check, initiate assembly DVP&R, initiate process FEMA and control plan, continue APQP process, continue design/mfg reviews	Team and plant 1 mfg 9/8/07

Reduction in PI RBC suite production throughput	Defective proximity sensor	3	Design/mfg reviews	6	144	Define as a critical product: characteristics in drawings and key product characteristics sheet, implement APQP process on sensors manufacturer, prototype control plan check, initiate assembly DVP&R, initiate process FMEA and control plan, continue APQP process, continue design/mfg reviews	Team and plant 1 mfg 9/8/07
Customer dissatisfaction	Defective plunger bushing	2	Design/mfg reviews	6	96	Define as a critical product: characteristics in drawings and key product characteristics sheet, prototype control plan check, initiate Assembly DVP&R, initiate process FEMA and control plan, continue design/mfg reviews	Team and plant 1 mfg 9/8/07

TABLE 20.9 *Continued*

Item/ Function	Potential Failure Mode	Potential Effect(s) of Failure	SEV	Class	Potential Causes(s) or Mechanism(s) of Failure	OCC	Current Design Controls Prevention and Detection	DET	RPN	Recommended Actions	Responsibility and Target Completion Date
		Requires field service			Defective U-cup seal	3	Design/mfg reviews	6	144	Define as a critical product: characteristics in drawings and key product characteristics sheet, prototype control plan check, initiate assembly DVP&R, initiate process FMEA and control plan, continue design/mfg reviews	Team and plant 1 mfg 9/8/07

20.6 SUMMARY

In this chapter we show an application of DFSS on a medical device, Auto 3D, depicted in Figure 20.1. The intention here is to provide a high-level understanding of the project rather than to document every step and tool application.

GLOSSARY

DFSS TERMINOLOGY

2k full factorial   a specific type of design of experiments where two or more (k number of) factors, each with two levels, with all possible combinations between the factor levels, are studied. (Chapter 14)

Affinity diagram   a management tool to organize information gathered from brainstorming or survey activities. (Chapter 9)

Alignment   the condition in which processes and activities support organizational strategy, objectives, and goals. (Chapter 6)

Alpha risk   the risk of concluding that two characteristics are different when they are actually the same. (Chapters 3 and 14)

Analysis of variance (ANOVA)   a statistical method to determine the significant effects of variation in an experiment. (Chapter 14)

APQP   advanced product quality planning; the segment of the QS-9000 process that uses tools to offer the opportunity to get ahead of problems and solve them before the problems affect the customer. (Chapter 18)

Axiomatic design   a theoretical foundation based on logical and rational thought processes (axioms) as well as tools to aid design process and design improvements. (Chapter 9)

Benchmarking   a process in which a team measures its performance against that of best in class with respect to strategies, operations, processes, and procedures. (Chapter 7)

Medical Device Design for Six Sigma: A Road Map for Safety and Effectiveness,
By Basem S. El-Haik and Khalid S. Mekki
Copyright © 2008 John Wiley & Sons, Inc.

Beta risk   the risk of concluding that two characteristics are the same when they are actually different. (Chapters 3 and 14)

Block diagram   a visual representation of operations, interrelationships, and interdependencies of components in a system. (Chapter 9)

Blocking   a statistical technique to increase the precision of an experiment by separating the experimental space into blocks, each having homogeneous behavior, and comparing the conditions of interest within and across blocks. (Chapter 14)

Capability flow-up   the compilation of subsystem and component performance levels to estimate capabilities at supersystem and customer levels. *See also* Requirements flow-down. (Chapter 7)

Cascading   the continuing flow of quality requirements down to the next level until it reaches subsystems and components. (Chapter 9)

Center points   an additional data collection and analysis performed in design of experiments to test if the response is linear or nonlinear between two levels of a factor. (Chapter 14)

Central composite design   a common design of experiment matrix used to establish a valid second-order model for a response by superimposing additional points for data collection and analysis on a design matrix used for a linear model. (Chapter 14)

Central limit theorem   a probabilistic concept that postulates the properties of means of samples from a population; a fundamental basis of several statistical tools. Roughly, the central limit theorem states that the distribution of the sum of a large number of independent, identically distributed variables will be approximately normal, regardless of the underlying distribution. (Chapter 3)

Change management   the planned effective implementation of new methods and systems in an ongoing organization. (Chapter 6)

Change management tools   a philosophy and set of tools to initiate, sustain, and accelerate the desired change in an organization. (Chapter 6)

Chi-square analysis   a hypothesis test used in testing the goodness of fit between a sample and a hypothesized distribution, or the association of two or more variables. (Chapter 3)

Communication plan   a deliberate process of formulating the message, identifying the audience, selecting the channels, and scheduling of disseminating the message to attain the desired results. (Chapter 6)

Concurrent engineering   a collaborative product and process design using cross-functional teams to develop customer-focused new products and solve design problems. The activities of the team become parallel in nature to reduce product development time and increase team effectiveness. (Chapter 7)

Confidence interval   a range of numbers in which population parameters are likely to fall. (Chapter 3)

Configuration management a detailed and systematic approach to document, maintain, update, and add or delete parts or elements of a system. (Chapter 9)

Continuous flow production the means by which items are produced and moved from one processing step to the next, one piece at a time.

Control chart a graphical display with a central line and upper and lower control limits on which observed values for a series of samples and subgroups are plotted so as to detect trends and unstable conditions. (Chapter 18)

Control plan a document outlining critical process parameters, their intended behavior, and requisite activities to sustain the process performance at acceptable levels. (Chapters 17 and 18)

Correlation data identified as having a causal, complementary, parallel, or reciprocal relationship. (Chapter 3)

Critical to quality (CTQ) a product or process metric that determines quality as perceived by the customer. (Chapters 3 to 5)

Critical to satisfaction (CTS) those parameters of quality, delivery, and cost that are critical to customer satisfaction. (Chapters 6 and 8)

CTS tree a structure to represent factors critical to satisfaction (CTS) for a customer is defined by critical to quality (CTQ), critical to delivery (CTD), and critical to cost (CTC). These CTXs can, in turn, be subdivided further, depending on the problem.

Delighter a feature of a product or service that a customer does not expect but that gives pleasure to the customer when received. (Chapter 8)

Deliverable the resulting output of a task or series of tasks. Usually required as evidence of progress at an established milestone or tollgate. (Chapter 7)

Descriptive statistics used to describe the basic features of the data in a study. They provide simple summaries about the sample and the measures. Together with simple graphics analysis, they form the basis of virtually every quantitative analysis of data. (Chapter 3)

Design failure modes and effects analysis (DFMEA) a risk management tool to evaluate and mitigate risks for a designed product or service by assessing how a design might fail, what the modes will be of such failure, how often the failure will occur, how severe the impact would be, and how well such a failure can be detected and controlled. (Chapter 11)

Design for manufacturability/assembly (DFM/A) a systematic process for product design that enables simplification through component reduction and use of standardized methods, components, and materials. (Chapter 12)

Design for reliability a design methodology used to assure that the designed product or service will perform the desired function, without failure, for a stated period of time. (Chapter 12)

Design for six sigma (DFSS) designing products, services, and processes that satisfy both client and business needs at six sigma quality. (Chapters 5 to 7 and 8 to 19)

Design for X a catch-all term encompassing the primary and secondary goals of design, such as design for manufacturability, design for reliability, design for six sigma, and design for serviceability.

Design of experiments a formal methodology to explore the causal relationship between input factors and response variables effectively and efficiently. A deliberate planning, arrangement, and testing of various levels of input variables to reach valid and relevant conclusions on how the input variables affect output (response) variables. (Chapters 14 and 15)

Design project management planning and execution of a design project by tracking schedules, resources, and deliverables and balancing the resulting competing demands. Project management is critical to DFSS success—more so than for DMAIC. (Chapter 7)

Design scorecard a tool to help understand how well proposed designs meet customer requirements. (Chapter 13)

Design transfer a written document prepared by the design team to smoothly transfer the product and service responsibilities to the team responsible for ongoing operations. (Chapter 18)

DMAIC a six sigma methodology to define processes and metrics, measure critical parameters, analyze root causes, improve processes, and control them so as to produce consistent results continuously. (Chapter 4)

Experimental design *see* design of experiments.

Failure modes and effects analysis (FMEA) a systematized group of activities intended to recognize and evaluate the potential failure of a product or process and its effect; identify actions that could eliminate or reduce the chance of the potential failure occurring; and document the process. (Chapter 11)

Fractional factorial design experimental design where only a partial set of all possible combinations of factor levels are tested to identify important factors more efficiently. (Chapter 14)

Full factorial design experimental design where all possible combinations of factor levels are tested to study main and interaction effects of factors on the responses. (Chapter 14)

Function structure development an interrelated set of functions generated in the concept generation phase to fulfill the functional requirements identified in the earlier phases of DFSS. (Chapter 9)

Functional analysis a systematic scientific approach to define how product and service functions relate to one another. (Chapter 9)

House of quality (HOQ) a planning matrix, developed during various phases of quality function deployment (QFD), that shows the relationship between what needs to be accomplished (e.g., customer needs) and how (the means) to achieve them. (Chapter 8)

Hypothesis testing   a procedure by which a statement about a population parameter (usually, mean, standard deviation, or proportion) can be inferred using a sample data from the population. (Chapter 3)

ICOV   identify, characterize, optimize, and verify/validate. These are the four phases of DFSS. These stages are further decomposed into stages and toll-gates. (Chapter 7)

Ideal final result (IFR)   a fundamental TRIZ concept that defines an outcome in the absence of any constraints. (Chapter 10)

Interface management   in assessing design interfaces, all inputs can affect all outputs (coupled), with no obvious design sequence; inputs may affect multiple outputs in some sequence that decouples the design (decoupled); and one input may affect one output (uncoupled). Design sequence reveals how to approach design to eliminate/reduce harmful interfaces. That is, interface management helps to minimize the impact of coupling in design. (Chapter 9)

Kano analysis   a systematic methodology to collect customer data that enables classifying customer needs and wants into three categories: must-bes, satis-fiers, and delighters. (Chapter 8)

Lean methodology   a systematic way to reduce confusion and increase clarity in the existing processes using value stream mapping, streamlined work flow, reduction of waste in all its forms, output pull, and continuous process improvement. (Chapter 4)

Measurement systems analysis (MSA)   Quantitative evaluation of tools and processes used in a measurement system that makes discrete or variable observations. MSA is established, documented, and carried out continu-ously so as to ensure that a measurement system maintains an acceptable status. MSA is not just calibration or just gauge repeatability and reproduc-ibility. (Chapter 4)

Mistake-proofing   improving processes or designs to prevent mistakes from being made or to make a mistake obvious at a glance. (Chapter 12)

Monte Carlo simulation   a statistical method to generate approximate solu-tions by performing repeating randomly generated trials on a model repre-senting the problem. (Chapter 13)

Multigenerational plan   a systematic strategy to incorporate new features sequentially—features that cannot be accommodated at a certain genera-tion of the product or service will be set aside to be included in later gen-erations. (Chapter 6)

Multiple regression   estimation of output variable (y) from two or more continuous input variables (x_1, x_2, x_3, etc.) using a linear or nonlinear relationship (f) between the output and input variables [i.e., $y = f(x_1, x_2, x_3, \ldots)$].

Noise factor *see* Noise variable. (Chapter 15)

Noise management designing to minimize the effects of controllable and uncontrollable input variables. (Chapters 15 and 16)

Noise variable variable that affects product and service performance but is too expensive or outside the control of the designer [e.g., weather, buying patterns, S&P index]. (Chapters 15 and 16)

Operational definition a clear, understandable description of what is to be observed and measured, such that different people taking or interpreting the data will do so consistently. (Chapters 8 and 9)

Optimization the process of desensitizing a design to affect noise factors. (Chapters 15 and 16)

Optimized design a product, service, or process design that performs at the desired level while being affecting minimally by noise factors. (Chapters 15 and 16)

Parameter design the process of discovering the best combination of control variables and design configurations so that the product or service performs at the desired level while being affected minimally by noise factors. (Chapter 15)

Parameter diagram (P-diagram) a schematic showing outputs of a process, factors affecting the output, input variables, and noise variables. (Chapters 11, 15, and 16)

P-diagram *see* Parameter diagram.

Phase of ICOV a span of time during which several specific activities are managed and executed, resulting in a set of deliverables. These deliverables are instrumental to the continued progress of the project.

Piloting a small-scale real-life representation of an actual product or process built using the resources, methods, and materials that would be used for a full-scale implementation so as to test if the intended results are achieved and to improve the solution as necessary. (Chapters 17 and 18)

Plan–do–check–act a four-step process for quality improvement.

Poka–yoke *see* Mistake-proofing.

Probabilistic design a design philosophy that takes into account the randomness involved in inputs, functions, and components, thus producing nondeterministic responses in a product or a process, as opposed to deterministic design where the random nature of inputs, components, and responses are ignored.

Process capability a measure to determine how a process consistently produces a result that meets customer specifications. (Chapter 18)

Process design a systematic arrangement of a set of interrelated activities and specification of input variables and tasks that defines them in order to produce a desired outcome. (Chapters 7, 17, and 18)

Process mapping   a general visual representation of the important activities of a work flow and their inputs and outputs at each step. (Chapter 4)

Process validation   the stage in which a process is evaluated to test whether it is producing the desired outcome according to customer or design requirements in a statistically stable fashion. (Chapter 17)

Product/service technology road map   a high-level visual summary of potential technology options that can be used in the product/service development and design, ensuring multigenerational product/service plans leveraging these key technologies. (Chapters 6 and 7)

Program   a group of projects managed in a coordinated way to obtain benefits not available from managing them individually. Coordination is required if projects are interdependent or if they share limited resources. (Chapters 3 and 4)

Project   a finite endeavor undertaken to create or improve a product, process, or service resulting in measurable business value, such as to eliminate waste, reduce variability, innovate, or grow. (Chapter 7)

Project charter   a written commitment approved by management stating the scope, duration, resources, and goals for a project. (Chapter 7)

Project plan (Gantt chart)   a visual display of planned and finished work with respect to time. (Chapter 7)

Project scoping   an act of setting bounds of a project objective, scale, and timing. (Chapter 6)

Proportion   the relation of one part to another or to the whole with respect to magnitude, quantity, or degree: *ratio*. A fraction of the number of occurrences of a certain outcome to the number of all possible outcomes. (Chapter 4)

Prototyping   an act of building a mathematical or physical model of an intended solution to verify the feasibility and effectiveness of design concepts on which later developments are based. (Chapters 17 and 18)

Pugh concept selection   a matrix to compare different design concepts and to arrive at a newer concept by combining the best elements of each. (Chapter 8)

Quality function deployment (QFD)   a systematic methodology that aligns customer needs (voice of the customer) with the design process, which is executed by a multifunctional design team. It is used to prioritize customer needs and translate (flow down) these needs into technical characteristics and specifications for the product/service to be delivered. (Chapter 8)

Regression   a statistical technique used to investigate relationships between an output variable and one or more input variables.

Requirements flow-down   a systematic way of translating customer needs into functional requirements and all the way to subsystem and component-level characteristics. (Chapters 8 and 9)

Response surface method   the empirical study of relationships between one or more responses and input variables and factors, used to determine the best set of input variables to gain a better understanding of the process and to arrive at an optimal response condition. (Chapter 13)

Response variable   an output variable that depends on input factors in a designed experiment. The response is the function of input variables. (Chapters 13 to 16)

Risk management   a structured, formal, and disciplined approach, focused on appropriate steps and planning actions to contain risks within acceptable limits. It defines the sources of various types of risk in the life cycle of a product or a service and how to address and minimize the risk. (Chapter 11)

Robust design   the state in which the product or service performance is least susceptible and minimally sensitive to variables and factors that could potentially cause performance degradation. (Chapters 15 and 16)

Robust parameter design   *see* Parameter design.

Simulation   a disciplined process of building a model of an existing or proposed real system and performing experiments with this model to analyze and understand the behavior of selected characteristics of a real system so as to evaluate various operational strategies to manage real system.

SIPOC   a high-level view of a process that provides at a glance suppliers, inputs, process, outputs, and customers. (Chapter 4)

Statistical process control   a technique for collecting and studying process data to monitor and improve process performance using statistical signals. (Chapter 18)

Supply chain design   the strategy and planning of internal and external supplier requirements, sourcing, and supply management (includes management of suppliers, logistics, and inventory).

Supply chain readiness   an assessment of the capability of the supply chain design and its ability to integrate a new product, process, or service.

Survey design   development of a questionnaire that enables data collection and analysis about a process, product, or service from a sample set of individuals.

Technology assessment   an assessment of the availability and maturity of technologies required to meet anticipated or confirmed customer needs, desires, and delighters. It includes assessment of the impact of early adoption of a technology or technologies on customer satisfaction, warranty costs, and costs of maintaining, operating, or upgrading technology. (Chapter 5)

Theory of inventive problem solving   *see* TRIZ.

Tolerance design   the process of determining the specification limits for critical design parameters to increase the effectiveness of design while minimizing cost. (Chapter 16)

Tollgate   an event in time where a project is evaluated for completion of the prior phase deliverables. The evaluation will help determine the potential of the project to proceed, recycle, or cancel. (Chapter 7)

Training plan   documentation describing required training associated with a process or the use of a product or service, as well as to ensure that proper training is documented and administered to the appropriate stakeholders in the long term. (Chapter 6)

Transfer function   the relationship between the input and the output of a system, subsystem, or equipment in terms of the transfer characteristics. (Chapter 13)

TRIZ   a system of inventive problem solving to innovate new concepts systematically. *Analogy* is an example of one of the TRIZ tools:

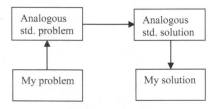

Variation reduction   *see* DMAIC.

Voice of the customer   the gathering of customer needs and desires, transferal to functional and design requirements, and assessment of the success of the final design in meeting customer expectations. (Chapter 8)

Waste elimination   *see* Lean methodology.

APPENDIX

STATISTICAL TABLES

TABLE A.1   Standard Cumulative Normal Distribution

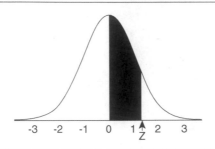

z	0.00	0.01	0.02	0.03	0.04	0.05	0.06	0.07	0.08	0.09
0.0	0.0000	0.0040	0.0080	0.0120	0.0160	0.0199	0.0239	0.0279	0.0319	0.0359
0.1	0.0398	0.0438	0.0478	0.0517	0.0557	0.0596	0.0636	0.0675	0.0714	0.0753
0.2	0.0793	0.0832	0.0871	0.0910	0.0948	0.0987	0.1026	0.1064	0.1103	0.1141
0.3	0.1179	0.1217	0.1255	0.1293	0.1331	0.1368	0.1406	0.1443	0.1480	0.1517
0.4	0.1554	0.1591	0.1628	0.1664	0.1700	0.1736	0.1772	0.1808	0.1844	0.1879
0.5	0.1915	0.1950	0.1985	0.2019	0.2054	0.2088	0.2123	0.2157	0.2190	0.2224
0.6	0.2257	0.2291	0.2324	0.2357	0.2389	0.2422	0.2454	0.2486	0.2517	0.2549
0.7	0.2580	0.2611	0.2642	0.2673	0.2704	0.2734	0.2764	0.2794	0.2823	0.2852
0.8	0.2881	0.2910	0.2939	0.2967	0.2995	0.3023	0.3051	0.3078	0.3106	0.3133
0.9	0.3159	0.3186	0.3212	0.3238	0.3264	0.3289	0.3315	0.3340	0.3365	0.3389
1.0	0.3413	0.3438	0.3461	0.3485	0.3508	0.3531	0.3554	0.3577	0.3599	0.3621
1.1	0.3643	0.3665	0.3686	0.3708	0.3729	0.3749	0.3770	0.3790	0.3810	0.3830
1.2	0.3849	0.3869	0.3888	0.3907	0.3925	0.3944	0.3962	0.3980	0.3997	0.4015
1.3	0.4032	0.4049	0.4066	0.4082	0.4099	0.4115	0.4131	0.4147	0.4162	0.4177
1.4	0.4192	0.4207	0.4222	0.4236	0.4251	0.4265	0.4279	0.4292	0.4306	0.4319
1.5	0.4332	0.4345	0.4357	0.4370	0.4382	0.4394	0.4406	0.4418	0.4429	0.4441
1.6	0.4452	0.4463	0.4474	0.4484	0.4495	0.4505	0.4515	0.4525	0.4535	0.4545
1.7	0.4554	0.4564	0.4573	0.4582	0.4591	0.4599	0.4608	0.4616	0.4625	0.4633
1.8	0.4641	0.4649	0.4656	0.4664	0.4671	0.4678	0.4686	0.4693	0.4699	0.4706
1.9	0.4713	0.4719	0.4726	0.4732	0.4738	0.4744	0.4750	0.4756	0.4761	0.4767
2.0	0.4772	0.4778	0.4783	0.4788	0.4793	0.4798	0.4803	0.4808	0.4812	0.4817
2.1	0.4821	0.4826	0.4830	0.4834	0.4838	0.4842	0.4846	0.4850	0.4854	0.4857
2.2	0.4861	0.4864	0.4868	0.4871	0.4875	0.4878	0.4881	0.4884	0.4887	0.4890
2.3	0.4893	0.4896	0.4898	0.4901	0.4904	0.4906	0.4909	0.4911	0.4913	0.4916
2.4	0.4918	0.4920	0.4922	0.4925	0.4927	0.4929	0.4931	0.4932	0.4934	0.4936
2.5	0.4938	0.4940	0.4941	0.4943	0.4945	0.4946	0.4948	0.4949	0.4951	0.4952
2.6	0.4953	0.4955	0.4956	0.4957	0.4959	0.4960	0.4961	0.4962	0.4963	0.4964
2.7	0.4965	0.4966	0.4967	0.4968	0.4969	0.4970	0.4971	0.4972	0.4973	0.4974
2.8	0.4974	0.4975	0.4976	0.4977	0.4977	0.4978	0.4979	0.4979	0.4980	0.4981
2.9	0.4981	0.4982	0.4982	0.4983	0.4984	0.4984	0.4985	0.4985	0.4986	0.4986
3.0	0.4987	0.4987	0.4987	0.4988	0.4988	0.4989	0.4989	0.4989	0.4990	0.4990
3.1	0.4990	0.4991	0.4991	0.4991	0.4992	0.4992	0.4992	0.4992	0.4993	0.4993
3.2	0.4993	0.4993	0.4994	0.4994	0.4994	0.4994	0.4994	0.4995	0.4995	0.4995
3.3	0.4995	0.4995	0.4995	0.4996	0.4996	0.4996	0.4996	0.4996	0.4996	0.4997
3.4	0.4997	0.4997	0.4997	0.4997	0.4997	0.4997	0.4997	0.4997	0.4997	0.4998

TABLE A.2 $t_{\alpha,df}$ **Table with Right-Tail Probabilities**

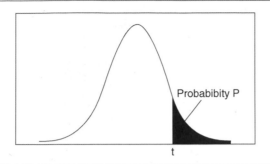

α df	0.40	0.25	0.10	0.05	0.025	0.01	0.005	0.0005
1	0.324920	1.000000	3.077684	6.313752	12.70620	31.82052	63.65674	636.6192
2	0.288675	0.816497	1.885618	2.919986	4.30265	6.96456	9.92484	31.5991
3	0.276671	0.764892	1.637744	2.353363	3.18245	4.54070	5.84091	12.9240
4	0.270722	0.740697	1.533206	2.131847	2.77645	3.74695	4.60409	8.6103
5	0.267181	0.726687	1.475884	2.015048	2.57058	3.36493	4.03214	6.8688
6	0.264835	0.717558	1.439756	1.943180	2.44691	3.14267	3.70743	5.9588
7	0.263167	0.711142	1.414924	1.894579	2.36462	2.99795	3.49948	5.4079
8	0.261921	0.706387	1.396815	1.859548	2.30600	2.89646	3.35539	5.0413
9	0.260955	0.702722	1.383029	1.833113	2.26216	2.82144	3.24984	4.7809
10	0.260185	0.699812	1.372184	1.812461	2.22814	2.76377	3.16927	4.5869
11	0.259556	0.697445	1.363040	1.795885	2.20099	2.71808	3.10581	4.4370
12	0.259033	0.695483	1.356217	1.782288	2.17881	2.68100	3.05454	4.3178
13	0.258591	0.693829	1.350171	1.770933	2.16037	2.65031	3.01228	4.2208
14	0.258213	0.692417	1.345030	1.761310	2.14479	2.62449	2.97684	4.1405
15	0.257885	0.691197	1.340606	1.753050	2.13145	2.60248	2.94671	4.0728
16	0.257599	0.690132	1.336757	1.745884	2.11991	2.58349	2.92078	4.0150
17	0.257347	0.689195	1.333379	1.739607	2.10982	2.56693	2.89823	3.9651
18	0.257123	0.688364	1.330391	1.734064	2.10092	2.55238	2.87844	3.9216
19	0.256923	0.687621	1.327728	1.729133	2.09302	2.53948	2.86093	3.8834
20	0.256743	0.686954	1.325341	1.724718	2.08596	2.52798	2.84534	3.8495
21	0.256580	0.686352	1.323188	1.720743	2.07961	2.51765	2.83136	3.8193
22	0.256432	0.685805	1.321237	1.717144	2.07387	2.50832	2.81876	3.7921
23	0.256297	0.685306	1.319460	1.713872	2.06866	2.49987	2.80734	3.7676
24	0.256173	0.684850	1.317836	1.710882	2.06390	2.49216	2.79694	3.7454
25	0.256060	0.684430	1.316345	1.708141	2.05954	2.48511	2.78744	3.7251
26	0255955	0.684043	1.314972	1.705618	2.05553	2.47863	2.77871	3.7066
27	0.255858	0.683685	1.313703	1.703288	2.05183	2.47266	2.77068	3.6896
28	0.255768	0.683353	1.312527	1.701131	2.04841	2.46714	2.76326	3.6739
29	0.255684	0.683044	1.311434	1.699127	2.04523	2.46202	2.75639	3.6594
30	0.255605	0.682756	1.310415	1.697261	2.04227	2.45726	2.75000	3.6460
∞	0.253347	0.674490	1.281552	1.644854	1.95996	2.32635	2.57583	3.2905

TABLE A.3 Right Tail Areas for the Chi-Square($\chi^2_{\alpha,df}$) Distribution

df \ α	0.995	0.990	0.975	0.950	0.900	0.750
1	0.00004	0.00016	0.00098	0.00393	0.01579	0.10153
2	0.01003	0.02010	0.05064	0.10259	0.21072	0.57536
3	0.07172	0.11483	0.21580	0.35185	0.58437	1.21253
4	0.20699	0.29711	0.48442	0.71072	1.06362	1.92256
5	0.41174	0.55430	0.83121	1.14548	1.61031	2.67460
6	0.67573	0.87209	1.23734	1.63538	2.20413	3.45460
7	0.98926	1.23904	1.68987	2.16735	2.83311	4.25485
8	1.34441	1.64650	2.17973	2.73264	3.48954	5.07064
9	1.73493	2.08790	2.70039	3.32511	4.16816	5.89883
10	2.15586	2.55821	3.24697	3.94030	4.86518	6.73720
11	2.60322	3.05348	3.81575	4.57481	5.57778	7.58414
12	3.07382	3.57057	4.40379	5.22603	6.30380	8.43842
13	3.56503	4.10692	5.00875	5.89186	7.04150	9.29907
14	4.07467	4.66043	5.62873	6.57063	7.78953	10.16531
15	4.60092	5.22935	6.26214	7.26094	8.54676	11.03654
16	5.14221	5.81221	6.90766	7.96165	9.31224	11.91222
17	5.69722	6.40776	7.56419	8.67176	10.08519	12.79193
18	6.26480	7.01491	8.23075	9.39046	10.86494	13.67529
19	6.84397	7.63273	8.90652	10.11701	11.65091	14.56200
20	7.43384	8.26040	9.59078	10.85081	12.44261	15.45177
21	8.03365	8.89720	10.28290	11.59131	13.23960	16.34438
22	8.64272	9.54249	10.98232	12.33801	14.04149	17.23962
23	93.6042	10.19572	11.68855	13.09051	14.84796	18.13730
24	9.88623	10.85636	12.40115	13.84843	15.65868	19.03725
25	10.51965	11.52398	13.11972	14.61141	16.47341	19.93934
26	11.16024	12.19815	13.84390	15.37916	17.29188	20.84343
27	11.80759	12.87850	14.57338	16.15140	18.11390	21.74940
28	12.46134	13.56471	15.30786	16.92788	18.93924	22.65716
29	13.12115	14.25645	16.04707	17.70837	19.76774	23.56659
30	13.78672	14.95346	16.79077	18.49262	20.59923	24.47761

0.500	0.250	0.100	0.050	0.025	0.010	0.005
0.45494	1.32330	2.70554	3.84146	5.02389	6.63490	7.87944
1.38629	2.77259	4.60517	5.99146	7.37776	9.21034	10.59663
2.36597	4.10834	6.25139	7.81473	9.34840	11.34487	12.83816
3.35669	5.38527	7.77944	9.48773	11.14329	13.27670	14.86026
4.35146	6.62568	9.23636	11.07050	12.83250	15.08627	16.74960
5.34812	7.84080	10.64464	12.59159	14.44938	16.81189	18.54758
6.34581	9.03715	12.01704	14.06714	16.01276	18.47531	20.27774
7.34412	10.21885	13.36157	15.50731	17.53455	20.09024	21.95495
8.34283	11.38875	14.68366	16.91898	19.02277	21.66599	23.58935
9.34182	12.54886	15.98718	18.30704	20.48318	23.20925	25.18818
10.34100	13.70069	17.27501	19.67514	21.92005	24.72497	26.75685
11.34032	14.84540	18.54935	21.02607	23.33666	26.21697	28.29952
12.33976	15.98391	19.81193	22.36203	24.73560	27.68825	29.81947
13.33927	17.11693	21.06414	23.68479	26.11895	29.14124	31.31935
14.33886	18.24509	22.30713	24.99579	27.48839	30.57791	32.80132
15.33850	19.36886	23.54183	26.29623	28.84535	31.99993	34.26719
16.33818	20.48868	24.76904	27.58711	30.19101	33.40866	35.71847
17.33790	21.60489	25.98942	28.86930	31.52638	34.80531	37.15645
18.33765	22.71781	27.20357	30.14353	32.85233	36.19087	38.58226
19.33743	23.82769	28.41198	31.41043	34.16961	37.56623	39.99685
20.33723	24.93478	29.61509	32.867057	35.47888	38.93217	41.40106
21.33704	26.03927	30.81328	33.92444	36.78071	40.28936	42.79565
22.33688	27.14134	32.00690	35.17246	38.07563	41.63840	44.18128
23.33673	28.24115	33.19624	36.41503	39.36408	42.97982	45.55851
24.33659	29.33885	34.38159	37.65248	40.64647	44.31410	46.92789
25.33646	30.43457	35.56317	38.88514	41.92317	45.64168	48.28988
26.33634	31.52841	36.74122	40.11327	43.19451	46.96294	49.64492
27.33623	32.62049	37.91592	41.33714	44.46079	48.27824	50.99338
28.33613	33.71091	39.08747	42.55697	45.72229	49.58788	52.33562
29.33603	34.79974	40.25602	43.77297	46.97924	50.89218	53.67196

TABLE A.4   F-Distribution Tables

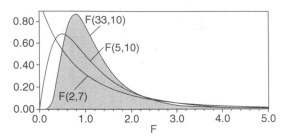

For α = 0.10

df1 df2	1	2	3	4	5	6	7	8	9
1	39.86346	49.50000	53.59324	55.83296	57.24008	58.20442	58.90595	59.43898	59.85759
2	8.52632	9.00000	9.16179	9.24342	9.29263	9.32553	9.34908	9.36677	9.38054
3	5.53832	5.46238	5.39077	5.34264	5.30916	5.28473	5.26619	5.25167	5.24000
4	4.54477	4.32456	4.19086	4.10725	4.05058	4.00975	3.97897	3.95494	3.93567
5	4.06042	3.77972	3.61948	3.52020	3.45298	3.40451	3.36790	3.33928	3.31628
6	3.77595	3.46330	3.28876	3.18076	3.10751	3.05455	3.01446	2.98304	2.95774
7	3.58943	3.25744	3.07407	2.96053	2.88334	2.82739	2.78493	2.75158	2.72468
8	3.45792	3.11312	2.92380	2.80643	2.72645	2.66833	2.62413	2.58935	2.56124
9	3.36030	3.00645	2.81286	2.69268	2.61061	2.55086	2.50531	2.46941	2.44034
10	3.28502	2.92447	2.72767	2.60534	2.52164	2.46058	2.41397	2.37715	2.34731
11	3.22520	2.85951	2.66023	2.53619	2.45118	2.38907	2.34157	2.30400	2.27350
12	3.17655	2.80680	2.60552	2.48010	2.39402	2.33102	2.28278	2.24457	2.21352
13	3.13621	2.76317	2.56027	2.43371	2.34672	2.28298	2.23410	2.19535	2.16382
14	3.10221	2.72647	2.52222	2.39469	2.30694	2.24256	2.19313	2.15390	2.12195
15	3.07319	2.69517	2.48979	2.36143	2.27302	2.20808	2.15818	2.11853	2.08621
16	3.04811	2.66817	2.46181	2.33274	2.24376	2.17833	2.12800	2.08798	2.05533
17	3.02623	2.64464	2.43743	2.30775	2.21825	2.15239	2.10169	2.06134	2.02839
18	3.00698	2.62395	2.41601	2.28577	2.19583	2.12958	2.07854	2.03789	2.00467
19	2.98990	2.60561	2.39702	2.26630	2.17596	2.10936	2.05802	2.01710	1.98364
20	2.97465	2.58925	2.38009	2.24893	2.15823	2.09132	2.03970	1.99853	1.96485
21	2.96096	2.57457	2.36489	2.23334	2.14231	2.07512	2.02325	1.98186	1.94797
22	2.94858	2.56131	2.35117	2.21927	2.12794	2.06050	2.00840	1.96680	1.93273
23	2.93736	2.54929	2.33873	2.20651	2.11491	2.04723	1.99492	1.95312	1.91888
24	2.92712	2.53833	2.32739	2.19488	2.10303	2.03513	1.98263	1.94066	1.90625
25	2.91774	2.52831	2.31702	2.18424	2.09216	2.02406	1.97138	1.92925	1.89469
26	2.90913	2.51910	2.30749	2.17447	2.08218	2.01389	1.96104	1.91876	1.88407
27	2.90119	2.51061	2.29871	2.16546	2.07298	2.00452	1.95151	1.90909	1.87427
28	2.89385	2.50276	2.29060	2.15714	2.06447	1.99585	1.94270	1.90014	1.86520
29	2.88703	2.49548	2.28307	2.14941	2.05658	1.98781	1.93452	1.89184	1.85679
30	2.88069	2.48872	2.27607	2.14223	2.04925	1.98033	1.92692	1.88412	1.84896
40	2.83535	2.44037	2.22609	2.09095	1.99682	1.92688	1.87252	1.82886	1.79290
60	2.79107	2.39325	2.17741	2.04099	1.94571	1.87472	1.81939	1.77483	1.73802
120	2.74781	2.34734	2.12999	1.99230	1.89587	1.82381	1.76748	1.72196	1.68425
∞	2.70554	2.30259	2.08380	1.94486	1.84727	1.77411	1.71672	1.67020	1.63152

10	12	15	20	24	30	40	60	120	∞
60.19498	60.70521	61.22034	61.74029	62.00205	62.26497	62.52905	62.79428	63.06064	63.32812
9.39157	9.40813	9.42471	9.44131	9.44962	9.45793	9.46624	9.47456	9.48289	9.49122
5.23041	5.21562	5.20031	5.18448	5.17636	5.16811	5.15972	5.15119	5.14251	5.13370
3.91988	3.89553	3.87036	3.84434	3.83099	3.81742	3.80361	3.78957	3.77527	3.76073
3.29740	3.26824	3.23801	3.20665	3.19052	3.17408	3.15732	3.14023	3.12279	3.10500
2.93693	2.90472	2.87122	2.83634	2.81834	2.79996	2.78117	2.76195	2.74229	2.72216
2.70251	2.66811	2.63223	2.59473	2.57533	2.55546	2.53510	2.51422	2.49279	2.47079
2.53804	2.50196	2.46422	2.42464	2.40410	2.38302	2.36136	2.33910	2.31618	2.29257
2.41632	2.37888	2.33962	2.29832	2.27683	2.25472	2.23196	2.20849	2.18427	2.15923
2.32260	2.28405	2.24351	2.20074	2.17843	2.15543	2.13169	2.10716	2.08176	2.05542
2.24823	2.20873	2.16709	2.12305	2.10001	2.07621	2.05161	2.02612	1.99965	1.97211
2.18776	2.14744	2.10485	2.05968	2.03599	2.01149	1.98610	1.95973	1.93228	1.90361
2.13763	2.09659	2.05316	2.00698	1.98272	1.95757	1.93147	1.90429	1.87591	1.84620
2.09540	2.05371	2.00953	1.96245	1.93766	1.91193	1.88516	1.85723	1.82800	1.79728
2.05932	2.01707	1.97222	1.92431	1.89904	1.87277	1.84539	1.81676	1.78672	1.75505
2.02815	1.98539	1.93992	1.89127	1.86556	1.83879	1.81084	1.78156	1.75075	1.71817
2.00094	1.95772	1.91169	1.86236	1.83624	1.80901	1.78053	1.75063	1.71909	1.68564
1.97698	1.93334	1.88681	1.83685	1.81035	1.78269	1.75371	1.72322	1.69099	1.65671
1.95573	1.91170	1.86471	1.81416	1.78731	1.75924	1.72979	1.69876	1.66587	1.63077
1.93674	1.89236	1.84494	1.79384	1.76667	1.73822	1.70833	1.67678	1.64326	1.60738
1.91967	1.87497	1.82715	1.77555	1.74807	1.71927	1.68896	1.65691	1.62278	1.58615
1.90425	1.85925	1.81106	1.75899	1.73122	1.70208	1.67138	1.63885	1.60415	1.56678
1.89025	1.84497	1.79643	1.74392	1.71588	1.68643	1.65535	1.62237	1.58711	1.54903
1.87748	1.83194	1.78308	1.73015	1.70185	1.67210	1.64067	1.60726	1.57146	1.53270
1.86578	1.82000	1.77083	1.71752	1.68898	1.65895	1.62718	1.59335	1.55703	1.51760
1.85503	1.80902	1.75957	1.70589	1.67712	1.64682	1.61472	1.58050	1.54368	1.50360
1.84511	1.79889	1.74917	1.69514	1.66616	1.63560	1.60320	1.56859	1.53129	1.49057
1.83593	1.78951	1.73954	1.68519	1.65600	1.62519	1.59250	1.55753	1.51976	1.47841
1.82741	1.78081	1.73060	1.67593	1.64655	1.61551	1.58253	1.54721	1.50899	1.46704
1.81949	1.77270	1.72227	1.66731	1.63774	1.60648	1.57323	1.53757	1.49891	1.45636
1.76269	1.71456	1.66241	1.60515	1.57411	1.54108	1.50562	1.46716	1.42476	1.37691
1.70701	1.65743	1.60337	1.54349	1.51072	1.47554	1.43734	1.39520	1.34757	1.29146
1.65238	1.60120	1.54500	1.48207	1.44723	1.40938	1.36760	1.32034	1.26457	1.19256
1.59872	1.54578	1.48714	1.42060	1.38318	1.34187	1.29513	1.23995	1.16860	1.00000

TABLE A.4 *Continued*

For α = 0.05

df2 \ df1	1	2	3	4	5	6	7	8	9
1	161.4476	199.5000	215.7073	224.5832	230.1619	233.9860	236.7684	238.8827	240.5433
2	18.5128	19.0000	19.1643	19.2468	19.2964	19.3295	19.3532	19.3710	19.3848
3	10.1280	9.5521	9.2766	9.1172	9.0135	8.9406	8.8867	8.8452	8.8123
4	7.7086	6.9443	6.5914	6.3882	6.2561	6.1631	6.0942	6.0410	5.9988
5	6.6079	5.7861	5.4095	5.1922	5.0503	4.9503	4.8759	4.8183	4.7725
6	5.9874	5.1433	4.7571	4.5337	4.3874	4.2839	4.2067	4.1468	4.0990
7	5.5914	4.7374	4.3468	4.1203	3.9715	3.8660	3.7870	3.7257	3.6767
8	5.3177	4.4590	4.0662	3.8379	3.6875	3.5806	3.5005	3.4381	3.3881
9	5.1174	4.2565	3.8625	3.6331	3.4817	3.3738	3.2927	3.2296	3.1789
10	4.9646	4.1028	3.7083	3.4780	3.3258	3.2172	3.1355	3.0717	3.0204
11	4.8443	3.9823	3.5874	3.3567	3.2039	3.0946	3.0123	2.9480	2.8962
12	4.7472	3.8853	3.4903	3.2592	3.1059	2.9961	2.9134	2.8486	2.7964
13	4.6672	3.8056	3.4105	3.1791	3.0254	2.9153	2.8321	2.76769	2.7144
14	4.6001	3.7389	3.3439	3.1122	2.9582	2.8477	2.7642	2.6987	2.6458
15	4.5431	3.6823	2.2874	3.0556	2.9013	2.7905	2.7066	2.6408	2.5876
16	4.4940	3.6337	3.2389	3.0069	2.8524	2.7413	2.6572	2.5911	2.5377
17	4.4513	3.5915	3.1968	2.9647	2.8100	2.6987	2.6143	2.5480	2.4943
18	4.4139	3.5546	3.1599	2.9277	2.7729	2.6613	2.5767	2.5102	2.4563
19	4.3807	3.5219	3.1274	2.8951	2.7401	2.6283	2.5435	2.4768	2.4227
20	4.3512	3.4928	3.0984	2.8661	2.7109	2.5990	2.5140	2.4471	2.3928
21	4.3248	3.4668	3.0725	2.8401	2.6848	2.5727	2.4876	2.4205	2.3660
22	4.3009	3.4434	3.0491	2.8167	2.6613	2.5491	2.4638	2.3965	2.3419
23	4.2793	3.4221	3.0280	2.7955	2.6400	2.5277	2.4422	2.3748	2.3201
24	4.2597	3.4028	3.0088	2.7763	2.6207	2.5082	2.4226	2.3551	2.3002
25	4.2417	3.3852	2.9912	2.7587	2.6030	2.4904	2.4047	2.3371	2.2821
26	4.2252	3.3690	2.9752	2.7426	2.5868	2.4741	2.3883	2.3205	2.2655
27	4.2100	3.3541	2.9604	2.7278	2.5719	2.4591	2.3732	2.3053	2.2501
28	4.1960	3.3404	2.9467	2.7141	2.5581	2.4453	2.3593	2.2913	2.2360
29	4.1830	3.3277	2.9340	2.7014	2.5454	2.4324	2.3463	2.2783	2.2229
30	4.1709	3.3158	2.9223	2.6896	2.5336	2.4205	2.3343	2.2662	2.2107
40	4.0847	3.2317	2.8387	2.6060	2.4495	2.3359	2.2490	2.1802	2.1240
60	4.0012	3.1504	2.7581	2.5252	2.3683	2.2541	2.1665	2.0970	2.0401
120	3.9201	3.0718	2.6802	2.4472	2.2899	2.1750	2.0868	2.0164	1.9588
∞	3.8415	2.9957	2.6049	2.3719	2.2141	2.0986	2.0096	1.9384	1.8799

For α = 0.025

df2 \ df1	1	2	3	4	5	6	7	8	9
1	647.7890	799.5000	864.1630	899.5833	921.8479	937.1111	948.2169	956.6562	963.2846
2	38.5063	39.0000	39.1655	39.2484	39.2982	39.3315	39.3552	39.3730	39.3869
3	17.4434	16.0441	15.4392	15.1010	14.8848	14.7347	14.6244	14.5399	14.4731
4	12.2179	10.6491	9.9792	9.6045	9.3645	9.1973	9.0741	8.9796	8.9047
5	10.0070	8.4336	7.7636	7.3879	7.1464	6.9777	6.8531	6.7572	6.6811
6	8.8131	7.2599	6.5988	6.2272	5.9876	5.8198	5.6955	5.5996	5.5234
7	8.0727	6.5415	5.8898	5.5226	5.2852	5.1186	4.9949	4.8993	4.8232
8	7.5709	6.0595	5.4160	5.0526	4.8173	4.6517	4.5286	4.4333	4.3572
9	9.2093	5.7147	5.0781	4.7181	4.4844	4.3197	4.1970	4.1020	4.0260
10	6.9367	5.4564	4.8256	4.4683	4.2361	4.0721	3.9498	3.8549	3.7790
11	6.7241	5.2559	4.6300	4.2751	4.0440	3.8807	3.7586	3.6638	3.5879
12	6.5538	5.0959	4.4742	4.1212	3.8911	3.7283	3.6065	3.5118	3.4358
13	6.4143	4.9653	4.3472	3.9959	3.7667	3.6043	3.4827	3.3880	3.3120

10	12	15	20	24	30	40	60	120	∞
241.8817	243.9060	245.9499	248.0131	249.0518	250.0951	251.1432	252.1957	253.2529	254.3144
19.3959	19.4125	19.4291	19.4458	19.4541	19.4624	19.4707	19.4791	19.4874	19.4957
8.7855	8.7446	8.7029	8.6602	8.6385	8.6166	8.5944	8.5720	8.5494	8.5264
5.9644	5.9117	5.8578	5.8025	5.7744	5.7459	5.7170	5.6877	5.6581	5.6281
4.7351	4.6777	4.6188	4.5581	4.5272	4.4957	4.4638	4.4314	4.3985	4.3650
4.0600	3.9999	3.9381	3.8742	3.8415	3.8082	3.7743	3.7398	3.7047	3.6689
3.6365	3.5747	3.5107	3.4445	3.4105	3.3758	3.3404	3.3043	3.2674	3.2298
3.3472	3.2839	3.2184	3.1503	3.1152	3.0794	3.0428	3.0053	2.9669	2.9276
3.1373	3.0729	3.0061	2.9365	2.9005	2.8637	2.8259	2.7872	2.7475	2.7067
2.9782	2.9130	2.8450	2.7740	2.7372	2.6996	2.6609	2.6211	2.5801	2.5379
2.8536	2.7876	2.7186	2.6464	2.6090	2.5705	2.5309	2.4901	2.4480	2.4045
2.7534	2.6866	2.6169	2.5436	2.5055	2.4663	2.4259	2.3842	2.3410	2.2962
2.6710	2.6037	2.5331	2.4589	2.4202	2.3803	2.3392	2.2966	2.2524	2.2064
2.6022	2.5342	2.4630	2.3879	2.3487	2.3082	2.2664	2.2229	2.1778	2.1307
2.5437	2.4753	2.4034	2.3275	2.2878	2.2468	2.2043	2.1601	2.1141	2.0658
2.4935	2.4247	2.3522	2.2756	2.2354	2.1938	2.1507	2.1058	2.0589	2.0096
2.4499	2.3807	2.3077	2.2304	2.1898	2.1477	2.1040	2.0584	2.0107	1.9604
2.4117	2.3421	2.2686	2.1906	2.1497	2.1071	2.0629	2.0166	1.9681	1.9168
2.3779	2.3080	2.2341	2.1555	2.1141	2.0712	2.0264	1.9795	1.9302	1.8780
2.3479	2.2776	2.2033	2.1242	2.0825	2.0391	1.9938	1.9464	1.8963	1.8432
2.3210	2.2504	2.1757	2.0960	2.0540	2.0102	1.9645	1.9165	1.8657	1.8117
2.2967	2.2258	2.1508	2.0707	2.0283	1.9842	1.9380	1.8894	1.8380	1.7831
2.2747	2.2036	2.1282	2.0476	2.0050	1.9605	1.9139	1.8648	1.8128	1.7570
2.2547	2.1834	2.1077	2.0267	1.9838	1.9390	1.8920	1.8424	1.7896	1.7330
2.2365	2.1649	2.0889	2.0075	1.9643	1.9192	1.8718	1.8217	1.7684	1.7110
2.2197	2.1479	2.0716	1.9898	1.9464	1.9010	1.8533	1.8027	1.7488	1.6906
2.2043	2.1323	2.0558	1.9736	1.9299	1.8842	1.8361	1.7851	1.7306	1.6717
2.1900	2.1179	2.0411	1.9586	1.9147	1.8687	1.8203	1.7689	1.7138	1.6541
2.1768	2.1045	2.0275	1.9446	1.9005	1.8543	1.8055	1.7537	1.6981	1.6376
2.1646	2.0921	2.0148	1.9317	1.8874	1.8409	1.7918	1.7396	1.6835	1.6223
2.0772	2.0035	1.9245	1.8389	1.7929	1.7444	1.6928	1.6373	1.5766	1.5089
1.9926	1.9174	1.8364	1.7480	1.7001	1.6491	1.5943	1.5343	1.4673	1.3893
1.9105	1.8337	1.7505	1.6587	1.6084	1.5543	1.4952	1.4290	1.3519	1.2539
1.8307	1.7522	1.6664	1.5705	1.5173	1.4591	1.3940	1.3180	1.2214	1.0000

10	12	15	20	24	30	40	60	120	∞
968.6274	976.7079	984.8668	993.1028	997.2492	1001.414	1005.598	1009.800	1014.020	1018.258
39.3980	39.4146	39.4313	39.4479	39.4562	39.465	39.473	39.481	39.490	39.498
14.4189	14.3366	14.2527	14.1674	14.1241	14.081	14.037	13.992	13.947	13.902
8.8439	8.7512	8.6565	8.5599	8.5109	8.461	8.411	8.360	8.309	8.257
6.6192	6.5245	6.4277	6.3286	6.2780	6.227	6.175	6.123	6.069	6.015
5.4613	5.3662	5.2687	5.1684	5.1172	5.065	5.012	4.959	4.904	4.849
4.7611	4.6658	4.5678	4.4667	4.4150	4.362	4.309	4.254	4.199	4.142
4.2951	4.1997	4.1012	3.9995	3.9472	3.894	3.840	3.784	3.728	3.670
3.9639	3.8682	3.7694	3.6669	3.6142	3.560	3.505	3.449	3.392	3.333
3.7168	3.6209	3.5217	3.4185	3.3654	3.311	3.255	3.198	3.140	3.080
3.5257	3.4296	3.3299	3.2261	3.1725	3.118	3.061	3.004	2.944	2.883
3.3736	3.2773	3.1772	3.0728	3.0187	2.963	2.906	2.848	2.787	2.725
3.2497	3.1532	3.0527	2.9477	2.8932	2.837	2.780	2.720	2.659	2.595

TABLE A.4 *Continued*

For α = 0.025

df2 \ df1	1	2	3	4	5	6	7	8	9
14	6.2979	4.8567	4.2417	3.8919	3.6634	3.5014	3.3799	3.2853	3.2093
15	6.1995	4.7650	4.1528	3.8043	3.5764	3.4147	3.2934	3.1987	3.1227
16	6.1151	4.6867	4.0768	3.7294	3.5021	3.3406	3.2194	3.1248	3.0488
17	6.0420	4.6189	4.0112	3.6648	3.4379	3.2767	3.1556	3.0610	2.9849
18	5.9781	4.5597	3.9539	3.6083	3.3820	3.2209	3.0999	3.0053	2.9291
19	5.9216	4.5075	3.9034	3.5587	3.3327	3.1718	3.0509	2.9563	2.8801
20	5.8715	4.4613	3.8587	3.5147	3.2891	3.1283	3.0074	2.9128	2.8365
21	5.8266	4.4199	3.8188	3.4754	3.2501	3.0895	2.9686	2.8740	2.7977
22	5.7863	4.3828	3.7829	3.4401	3.2151	3.0546	2.9338	2.8392	2.7628
23	5.7498	4.3492	3.7505	3.4083	3.1835	3.0232	2.9023	2.8077	2.7313
24	5.7166	4.3187	3.7211	3.3794	3.1548	2.9946	2.8738	2.7791	2.7027
25	5.6864	4.2909	3.6943	3.3530	3.1287	2.9685	2.8478	2.7531	2.6766
26	5.6586	4.2655	3.6697	3.3289	3.1048	2.9447	2.8240	2.7293	2.6528
27	5.6331	4.2421	3.6472	3.3067	3.0828	2.9228	2.8021	2.7074	2.6309
28	5.6096	4.2205	3.6264	3.2863	3.0626	2.9027	2.7820	2.6872	2.6106
29	5.5878	4.2006	3.6072	3.2674	3.0438	2.8840	2.7633	2.6686	2.5919
30	5.5675	4.1821	3.5894	3.2499	3.0265	2.8667	2.7460	2.6513	2.5746
40	5.4239	4.0510	3.4633	3.1261	2.9037	2.7444	2.6238	2.5289	2.4519
60	5.2856	3.9253	3.3425	3.0077	2.7863	2.6274	2.5068	2.4117	2.3344
120	5.1523	3.8046	3.2269	2.8943	2.6740	2.5154	2.3948	2.2994	2.2217
∞	5.0239	3.6889	3.1161	2.7858	2.5665	2.4082	2.2875	2.1918	2.1136

For α = 0.01

df2 \ df1	1	2	3	4	5	6	7	8	9
1	4052.181	4999.500	5403.352	5624.583	5763.650	5858.986	5928.356	5981.070	6022.473
2	98.503	99.000	99.166	99.249	99.299	99.333	99.356	99.374	99.388
3	34.116	30.817	29.457	28.710	28.237	27.911	27.672	27.489	27.345
4	21.198	18.000	16.694	15.977	15.522	15.207	14.976	14.799	14.659
5	16.285	13.274	12.060	11.392	10.967	10.672	10.456	10.289	10.158
6	13.745	10.925	9.780	9.148	8.746	8.466	8.260	8.102	7.976
7	12.246	9.547	8.451	7.847	7.460	7.191	6.993	6.840	6.719
8	11.259	8.649	7.591	7.006	6.632	6.371	6.178	6.029	5.911
9	10.561	8.022	6.992	6.422	6.057	5.802	5.613	5.467	5.351
10	10.044	7.559	6.552	5.994	5.636	5.386	5.200	5.057	4.942
11	9.646	7.206	6.217	5.668	5.316	5.069	4.886	4.744	4.632
12	9.330	6.927	5.953	5.412	5.064	4.821	4.640	4.499	4.388
13	9.074	6.701	5.739	5.205	4.862	4.620	4.441	4.302	4.191
14	8.862	6.515	5.564	5.035	4.695	4.456	4.278	4.140	4.030
15	8.683	6.359	5.417	4.893	4.556	4.318	4.142	4.004	3.895
16	8.531	6.226	5.292	4.773	4.437	4.202	4.026	3.890	3.780
17	8.400	6.112	5.185	4.669	4.336	4.102	3.927	3.791	3.682
18	8.285	6.013	5.092	4.579	4.248	4.015	3.841	3.705	3.597
19	8.185	5.926	5.010	4.500	4.171	3.939	3.765	3.631	3.523
20	8.096	5.849	4.938	4.431	4.103	3.871	3.699	3.564	3.457
21	8.017	5.780	4.874	4.369	4.042	3.812	3.640	3.506	3.398
22	7.945	5.719	4.817	4.313	3.988	3.758	3.587	3.453	3.346

10	12	15	20	24	30	40	60	120	∞
3.1469	3.0502	2.9493	2.8437	2.7888	2.732	2.674	2.614	2.552	2.487
3.0602	2.9633	2.8621	2.7559	2.7006	2.644	2.585	2.524	2.461	2.395
2.9862	2.8890	2.7875	2.6808	2.6252	2.568	2.509	2.447	2.383	2.316
2.9222	2.8249	2.7230	2.6158	2.5598	2.502	2.442	2.380	2.315	2.247
2.8664	2.7689	2.6667	2.5590	2.5027	2.445	2.384	2.321	2.256	2.187
2.8172	2.7196	2.6171	2.5089	2.4523	2.394	2.333	2.270	2.203	2.133
2.7737	2.6758	2.5731	2.4645	2.4076	2.349	2.287	2.223	2.156	2.085
2.7348	2.6368	2.5338	2.4247	2.3675	2.308	2.246	2.182	2.114	2.042
2.6998	2.6017	2.4984	2.3890	2.3315	2.272	2.210	2.145	2.076	2.003
2.6682	2.5699	2.4665	2.3567	2.2989	2.239	2.176	2.111	2.041	1.968
2.6396	2.5411	2.4374	2.3273	2.2693	2.209	2.146	2.080	2.010	1.935
2.6135	2.5149	2.4110	2.3005	2.2422	2.182	2.118	2.052	1.981	1.906
2.5896	2.4908	2.3867	2.2759	2.2174	2.157	2.093	2.026	1.954	1.878
2.5676	2.4688	2.3644	2.2533	2.1946	2.133	2.069	2.002	1.930	1.853
2.5473	2.4484	2.3438	2.2324	2.1735	2.112	2.048	1.980	1.907	1.829
2.5286	2.4295	2.3248	2.2131	2.1540	2.092	2.028	1.959	1.886	1.807
2.5112	2.4120	2.3072	2.1952	2.1359	2.074	2.009	1.940	1.866	1.787
2.3882	2.2882	2.1819	2.0677	2.0069	1.943	1.875	1.803	1.724	1.637
2.2702	2.1692	2.0613	1.9445	1.8817	1.815	1.744	1.667	1.581	1.482
2.1570	2.0548	1.9450	1.8249	1.7597	1.690	1.614	1.530	1.433	1.310
2.0483	1.9447	1.8326	1.7085	1.6402	1.566	1.484	1.388	1.268	1.000

10	12	15	20	24	30	40	60	120	∞
6055.847	6106.321	6157.285	6208.730	6234.631	6260.649	6286.782	6313.030	6339.391	6365.864
99.399	99.416	99.433	99.449	99.458	99.466	99.474	99.482	99.491	99.499
27.229	27.052	26.872	26.690	26.598	26.505	26.411	26.316	26.221	26.125
14.546	14.374	14.198	14.020	13.929	13.838	13.745	13.652	13.558	13.463
10.051	9.888	9.722	9.553	9.466	9.379	9.291	9.202	9.112	9.020
7.874	7.718	7.559	7.396	7.313	7.229	7.143	7.057	6.969	6.880
6.620	6.469	6.314	6.155	6.074	5.992	5.908	5.824	5.737	5.650
5.814	5.667	5.515	5.359	5.279	5.198	5.116	5.032	4.964	4.859
5.257	5.111	4.962	4.808	4.729	4.649	4.567	4.483	4.398	4.311
4.849	4.706	4.558	4.405	4.327	4.247	4.165	4.082	3.996	3.909
4.539	4.397	4.251	4.099	4.021	3.941	3.860	3.776	3.690	3.602
4.296	4.155	4.010	3.858	3.780	3.701	3.619	3.535	3.449	3.361
4.100	3.960	3.815	3.665	3.587	3.507	3.425	3.341	3.255	3.165
3.939	3.800	3.656	3.505	3.427	3.348	3.266	3.181	3.094	3.004
3.805	3.666	3.522	3.372	3.294	3.214	3.132	3.047	2.959	2.868
3.691	3.553	3.409	3.259	3.181	3.101	3.018	2.933	2.845	2.753
3.593	3.455	3.312	3.162	3.084	3.003	2.920	2.835	2.746	2.653
3.508	3.371	3.227	3.077	2.999	2.919	2.835	2.749	2.660	2.566
3.434	3.297	3.153	3.003	2.925	2.844	2.761	2.674	2.584	2.489
3.368	3.231	3.088	2.938	2.859	2.778	2.695	2.608	2.517	2.421
3.310	3.173	3.030	2.880	2.801	2.720	2.636	2.548	2.457	2.360
3.258	3.121	2.978	2.827	2.749	2.667	2.583	2.495	2.403	2.305

TABLE A.4 *Continued*

For $\alpha = 0.01$

df2 \ df1	1	2	3	4	5	6	7	8	9
23	7.881	5.664	4.765	4.264	3.939	3.710	3.539	3.406	3.299
24	7.823	5.614	4.718	4.218	3.895	3.667	3.496	3.363	3.256
25	7.770	5.568	4.675	4.177	3.855	3.627	3.457	3.324	3.217
26	7.721	5.526	4.637	4.140	3.818	3.591	3.421	3.288	3.182
27	7.677	5.488	4.601	4.106	3.785	3.558	3.388	3.256	3.149
28	7.636	5.453	4.568	4.074	3.754	3.528	3.358	3.226	3.120
29	7.598	5.420	4.538	4.045	3.725	3.499	3.330	3.198	3.092
30	7.562	5.390	4.510	4.018	3.699	3.473	3.304	3.173	3.067
40	7.314	5.179	4.313	3.828	3.514	3.291	3.124	2.993	2.888
60	7.077	4.977	4.126	3.649	3.339	3.119	2.953	2.823	2.718
120	6.851	4.787	3.949	3.480	3.174	2.956	2.792	2.663	2.559
∞	6.635	4.605	3.782	3.319	3.017	2.802	2.639	2.511	2.407

10	12	15	20	24	30	40	60	120	∞
3.211	3.074	2.931	2.781	2.702	2.620	2.535	2.447	2.354	2.256
3.168	3.032	2.889	2.738	2.659	2.577	2.492	2.403	2.310	2.211
3.129	2.993	2.850	2.699	2.620	2.538	2.453	2.364	2.270	2.169
3.094	2.958	2.815	2.664	2.585	2.503	2.417	2.327	2.223	2.131
3.062	2.926	2.783	2.632	2.552	2.470	2.384	2.294	2.198	2.097
3.032	2.896	2.753	2.602	2.522	2.440	2.354	2.263	2.167	2.064
3.005	2.868	2.726	2.574	2.495	2.412	2.325	2.234	2.138	2.034
2.979	2.843	2.700	2.549	2.469	2.386	2.299	2.208	2.111	2.006
2.801	2.665	2.522	2.369	2.288	2.203	2.114	2.019	1.917	1.805
2.632	2.496	2.352	2.198	2.115	2.028	1.936	1.836	1.726	1.601
2.472	2.336	2.192	2.035	1.950	1.860	1.763	1.656	1.533	1.381
2.321	2.185	2.039	1.878	1.791	1.696	1.592	1.473	1.325	1.000

REFERENCES

Abbatiello, N. (1995). Development of Design for Service Strategy, M.S. thesis, University of Rhode Island, Kingston, RI.

Akao, Y. (1972). New Product Development and Quality Assurance: Quality Deployment System (in Japanese), *Standardization and Quality Control*, Vol. 25, No. 4, pp. 7–14.

Akao, Y. (1997). QFD: Past, Present, and Future, *Proceedings of the 3rd Annual International QFD Conference*, Linköping, Sweden, October, http://www.qfdi.org/qfd_history.pdf.

Alabano, L. D., Conner, J. J., and Suh, N. P. (1993). A Framework for Performance-Based Design, *Journal of Research in Engineering Design*, Vol. 5, pp. 105–119.

Altshuller, G. S. (1988). *Creativity as Exact Science*, Gordon and Breach, New York.

Altshuller, G. S. (1990). On the Theory of Solving Inventive Problems, *Design Methods and Theories*, Vol. 24, No. 2, pp. 1216–1222.

Arcidiacono, G., Campatelli, G., and Citti, P. (2002). Axiomatic Design for Six Sigma, *Proceedings of the 2nd International Conference on Axiomatic Design*, MIT, Cambridge, MA, June.

Arciszewsky, T. (1988). ARIZ 77: An Innovative Design Method, *Design Methods and Theories*, Vol. 22, No. 2, pp. 796–820.

Arimoto, S., Ohashi, T., Ikeda, M., and Miyakawa, S. (1993). Development of Machining Productivity Evaluation Method (MEM), *Annals of CIRP*, Vol. 42, No. 1, pp. 119–1222.

Ashby, W. R. (1973). Some Peculiarities of Complex Systems, *Cybernetic Medicine Journal*, No. 9, pp. 1–7.

Babic, B. (1999). Axiomatic Design of Flexible Manufacturing Systems, *International Journal of Production Research*, Vol. 37, No. 5, pp. 1159–1173.

Beitz, W. (1990). Design for Ease of Recycling (Guidelines VDI 2243), *ICED Proceedings*, Heurista, Zurich, Switzerland.

Bhattacharya, A. (1996). Reliability Evaluation of Systems with Dependent Failures, *International Journal of Systems Science*, Vol. 27, No. 9, pp. 881–885.

Birnbaum, Z. W. (1969). On the Importance of Different Components in a Multicomponent System, *Proceedings of the 2nd International Symposium on Multivariate Analysis, in Multivariate Analysis II*, P. Krishnaiah, eds., Academic Press, New York.

Boothroyd, G., and Dewhurst, P. (1983). *Product Design for Assembly Handbook*, Boothroyd-Dewhurst Inc., Wakefield, RI.

Boothroyd, G., and Dewhurst, P. (1990). *Product Design for Assembly Handbook*, 2nd ed., Boothroyd-Dewhurst Inc., Wakefield, RI.

Boothroyd, G., Dewhurst, P., and Knight, W. (1994). *Product Design for Manufacture and Assembly*, Marcel Dekker, New York.

Bowker, A. H., and Lieberman, G. J. (1959). *Engineering Statistics*, Prentice-Hall, Englewood Cliffs, NJ.

Box, G. E. P., and Draper, N. R. (1987). *Empirical Model Building and Response Surfaces*, Wiley, New York.

Box, G. E. P., Hunter, W. G., and Hunter, J. S. (1978). *Statistics for Experiments*, Wiley, New York.

Brandt, D. R. (1988). How Service Marketers Can Identify Value-Enhancing Service Elements, *Journal of Services Marketing*, Vol. 2, No. 3, pp. 35–41.

Brandt, D. R., and Scharioth, J. (1998). Attribute Life Cycle Analysis: Alternatives to the Kanomethod, *Proceedings of the 51st Esomar Congress*, pp. 413–429.

Brejcha, M. F. (1982). *Automatic Transmission*, 2nd ed., Prentice-Hall, Englewood Cliffs, NJ.

Breyfogle, F. W. (1999). *Implementing Six Sigma: Smarter Solutions Using Statistical Methods*, Wiley, New York.

Brunnelle, R. D., and Kapur, K. C. (1997). Customer-Centered Reliability Methodology, *Proceedings of the Annual Reliability and Maintainability Symposium*, pp. 286–292.

Burchill, G., and Brodie, C. H. (1997). *Voices into Choices: Acting on the Voice of the Customer*, Joiner Associates, Madison, WI.

Cadotte, E. R., and Turgeon, N. (1988). Dissatisfiers and Satisfiers: Suggestions from Consumer Complaints and Compliments, Journal of Consumer Satisfaction, *Dissatisfaction and Complaining Behavior*, Vol. 1, pp. 74–79.

Carnap, R. (1977). *Two Essays on Entropy*, University of California Press, Berkeley, CA.

CCPS (1992). Guidelines for Hazard Evaluation Procedures, with Worked Examples, 2nd ed., Center for Chemical Process Safety, New York.

Cekecek, E., and Yang, K. (2004). Design Vulnerability Analysis and Design Improvement by Using Warranty Data, *Quality and Reliability Engineering International*, Vol. 20, pp. 121–133.

Chase, K. W., and Greenwood, W. H. (1988). Design Issues in Mechanical Tolerance Analysis, *Manufacturing Review*, Vol. 1, No. 1, pp. 50–59.

Chen, S. J., and Hwang, C. L. (1992). *Fuzzy Multiple Attributes Decision Making*, Spring-Verlag, New York.

Chen, G., and Kapur, K. C. (1989). Quality Evaluation Using Loss Function, International Industrial Engineering Conference and Societies' Manufacturing and Productivity Symposium Proceedings.

Clausing, D. P. (1994). *Total Quality Development: A Step by Step Guide to World-Class Concurrent Engineering*, ASME Press, New York.

Cohen, L. (1988). Quality Function Deployment and Application Perspective from Digital Equipment Corporation, *National Productivity Review Journal*, Vol. 7, No. 3, pp. 197–208.

Cohen, L. (1995). *Quality Function Deployment: How to Make QFD Work for You*, Addison-Wesley, Reading, MA.

Cook, D. L. (1990). Evolution of VLSI Reliability Engineering, *Proceedings of the International Reliability Physics Symposium*, pp. 2–11.

Creveling, C. M. (1997). *Tolerance Design: A Handbook for Developing Optimal Specifications*, Addison-Wesley, Reading, MA.

Dewhurst, P. (1988). Cutting Costs with Molded Parts, *Machine Design*.

Dewhurst, P., and Blum, C. (1989). Supporting Analyses for the Economic Assessment of Due Casting in Product Design, *Annals of the CIRP*, Vol. 28, No. 1, p. 161.

Dovoino, I. (1993). Forecasting Additional Functions in Technical Systems, *Proceeding of ICED '93*, The Hague, The Netherlands, Vol. 1, pp. 247–277.

Dubois, D., and Prade, H. (1982). On Several Representations of an Uncertainty of Evidence, in *Fuzzy Information and Decision Processes*, M. M. Gupta and E. Sanches, eds., North-Holland, Amsterdam, pp. 167–182.

Dubois, D., and Prade, H. (1988). *Possibility Theory*, Wiley, New York.

Dubois, D., and Prade, H. (1997). Fuzzy Real Algebra: Some Results, *Fuzzy Sets and Systems Journal*, No. 2, pp. 327–348.

Durmusoglu, M. B., Kulak, O., and Tufecki, S. (2002). An Implementation Methodology for Transition from Traditional Manufacturing to Cellular Manufacturing Using Axiomatic Design, *Proceedings of the 2nd International Conference on Axiomatic Design*, MIT, Cambridge, MA, June.

Dutta, A. (1985). Reasoning with Imprecise Knowledge in Expert Systems, *Information Sciences Journal*, No. 37, pp. 2–24.

El-Haik, B. S. (2005). *Axiomatic Quality and Reliability*, Wiley, Hoboken, NJ.

El-Haik, B. (2007). *Encyclopedia of Statistics in Quality and Reliability*, Wiley, Hoboken, NJ.

El-Haik, B. S., and Alaomar, R. (2006). *Simulation-Based Lean Six Sigma and Design for Lean Six Sigma*, Wiley, Hoboken, NJ.

El-Haik, B. S., and Roy, D. (2005). *Service Design for Six Sigma: A Roadmap for Excellence*, Wiley, Hoboken, NJ.

El-Haik, B. S., and Yang, K. (1999). The Components of Complexity in Engineering Design, *IIE Transactions*, Vol. 31, No. 10, pp. 925–934.

El-Haik, B. S., Johnston, P., and Mohsen, H. (1995). A Framework to Integrate QFD, Pugh Concept Selection, and Value Engineering in Concept Design, *Proceedings of the Total Product Development Conference*, American Supplier Institute, Dearborn, MI, November 1–3.

El-Haik, B. S., Johnston, P., Slater, L., and Nolf, J. (1997). A Robust Design Optimization Study of Room Temperature Vulcanizing (RTV) Silicon Seal for a Generic Oil Pan System, *Proceedings of the American Supplier Institute Symposium*, Dearborn, MI, November 5–6.

Fey, V. R., Rivin, E. I., and Verkin, I. M. (1994). Application of the Theory of Inventive Problem Solving to Design and Manufacturing Systems, *Annals of the CIRP*, Vol. 43, No. 1, pp. 107–110.

Foo, G., Clancy, J. P., Kinney, L. E., and Lindemudler, C. R. (1990). Design for Material Logistics, *AT&T Technical Journal*, Vol. 69, No. 3, pp. 61–67.

Fowlkes, W. Y., and Creveling, C. M. (1995). *Engineering Methods for Robust Product Design: Using Taguchi Methods in Technology and Product Development*, Addison-Wesley, Reading, MA.

Fragole, J. R. (1993). Designing for Success: Reliability Technology in the Current Design Era, *Proceedings of the Annual Reliability and Maintainability Symposium*, pp. 77–82.

Fredrikson, B. (1994). Holistic Systems Engineering in Product Development, The Saab-Scania Griffin, November.

Gardner, S., and Sheldon, D. F. (1995). Maintainability as an Issue for Design, *Journal of Engineering Design*, Vol. 6, No. 2, pp. 75–89.

Garrett, R. (1990). Eight Steps to Simultaneous Engineering, Manufacturing Engineering, November, pp. 41–47.

Gebala, D. A., and Suh, N. P. (1992). An Application of Axiomatic Design, *Journal of Research in Engineering Design*, Vol. 3, pp. 149–162.

Gershenson, J., and Ishii, K. (1991). Life Cycle Serviceability Design, *Proceedings of the ASME Conference on Design Theory and Methodology*.

GHTF (Global Harmonization Task Force) (1999). Design Control Guidance for Medical Device Manufacturers, GHTF/FD: 99-9.

GHTF (Global Harmonization Task Force) (2004). Quality Management Systems: Process Validation Guidane, 2nd ed., GHTF/SG3/N99-10:2004.

Greig, G. L. (1993). Second Moment Reliability Analysis of Redundant Systems with Dependant Failures, *Reliability Engineering and Systems Safety*, Vol. 41, No. 1, pp. 57–70.

Gunst, R. F., Mason, R. L., and Hess, J. L. (1989). *Statistical Design and Analysis of Experiments*, Wiley, New York.

Harry, M. J. (1994). *The Vision of Six-Sigma: A Roadmap for Breakthrough*, Sigma Publishing Company, Phoenix, AZ.

Harry, M. J. (1998). Six Sigma: A Breakthrough Strategy for Profitability, Quality Progress, May, pp. 60–64.

Hartley, R. V. (1928). Transmission of Information, *The Bell Systems Technical Journal*, No. 7, pp. 535–563.

Hauser, J. R., and Clausing, D. (1988). The House of Quality, *Harvard Business Review*, Vol. 66, No. 3, pp. 63–73.

Hillstrom F. (1994). On Axiomatic Design in Modular Product Development, licentiate thesis, machine and vehicle design, Chalmers University of Technology, Göteborg, Sweden.

Hines, W. W., and Montgomery, D. C. (1990). *Probability and Statistics for Engineering and Management Science*, 2nd ed., Wiley, New York.

Hintersteiner, J. D. (1999). A Fractal Representation for Systems, Presented at the International CIRP Design Seminar, Enschede, The Netherlands, March 24–26.

Hintersteiner, J. D., and Nain, A. S. (1999). Integrating Software into Systems: An Axiomatic Design Approach, *Proceedings of the 3rd International Conference on Engineering Design and Automation*, Vancouver, Canada, August 1–4.

Hintersteiner, J. D., and Tate, D. (1998). Command and Control in Axiomatic Design Theory: Its Role and Placement in System Architecture, *Proceedings of the 2nd International Conference on Engineering Design and Automation*, Maui, HI, August, pp. 9–12.

Huang, G. Q., ed. (1996). *Design for X: Concurrent Engineering Imperatives*, Chapman & Hall, London.

Hubka, V. (1980). *Principles of Engineering Design*, Butterworth Scientific Publishing, London.

Igata, H. (1996). Application of Axiomatic Design to Rapid-Prototyping Support for Real-Time Control Software, S.M. thesis, Department of Mechanical Engineering, MIT, Cambridge, MA.

Jacobs, B. (2002). Were the Ancient Egyptians System Engineers? How the Building of Khufu's Great Pyramid Satisfies Systems Engineering Axioms, University of Maryland, College Park, MD, http://www.bandisoftware.com/Incose2002.pdf.

Jaynes, E. T. (1957a). Information Theory and Statistical Mechanics, I, *Physical Review Journal*, No. 106, pp. 620–630.

Jaynes, E. T. (1957b). Information Theory and Statistical Mechanics, II, *Physical Review Journal*, No. 108, pp. 171–190.

Kácker, R. N. (1985). Off-Line Quality Control, Parameter Design, and the Taguchi Method, *Journal of Quality Technology*, No. 17, pp. 176–188.

Kapur, K. C. (1988). An Approach for the Development of Specifications for Quality Improvement, *Quality Engineering*, Vol. 1, No. 1, pp. 63–77.

Kapur, K. C. (1991a). Quality Engineering and Tolerance Design, *Concurrent Engineering: Automation, Tools and Techniques*, 287–306.

Kapur, K. C. (1991b). Quality Improvement Through Robust Design, *International Institute of Industrial Engineering Conference Proceedings*.

Killander, A. J. (1995). Concurrent Development Requires Uncoupled Concepts and Projects, Presented at the International Conference on Concurrent Engineering, Reston, VA.

Kim, S. J., and Suh, N. P. (1987). Knowledge-Based Synthesis System for Injection Molding, *Robotics and Computer Integrated Manufacturing Journal*, Vol. 3, No. 2, pp. 181.

Kim, S. J., Suh, N. P., and Kim, S. (1991). Design of Software Systems Based on AD, *Annals of the CIRP*, Vol. 40, pp. 165–170.

Klir, J. G., and Folger, T. A. (1988). *Fuzzy Sets, Uncertainty, and Information*, Prentice-Hall, Englewood Cliffs, NJ.

Knight, W. A. (1991). Design for Manufacture Analysis: Early Estimates of Tool Costs for Sintered Parts, *Annals of the CIRP*, Vol. 40, No. 1.

Ku, H. H. (1966). Notes on the Use of Propagation of Error Formulas, *Journal of Research of the National Bureau of Standards, C: Engineering and Instrumentation*, Vol. 70, No. 4, pp. 263–273.

Lee, T. S. (1999). The System Architecture Concept in Axiomatic Design Theory: Hypotheses Generation and Case-Study Validation, S.M. thesis, Department of Mechanical Engineering, MIT, Cambridge, MA.

Lehner, M. (1997). *The Complete Pyramids*, Thames & Hudson, London.

Lentz, V. A., Lerner, B., and Whitecomb, C. (2002). The Validation of a Modular Commercial Product Architecture, *Proceedings of the 2nd International Conference on Axiomatic Design*, MIT, Cambridge, MA, June.

Leung, Y. (1980). Maximum Entropy Estimation with Inexact Information, in *Fuzzy Set Possibility Theory: Recent Developments*, Yager, R. R., eds., Pergamon Press, Elmsford, NY, pp. 32–37.

Lewis, E. E. (1987). *Introduction to Reliability Engineering*, Wiley, New York.

Luenberger, D. G. (1989). *Linear and Non-linear Programming*, 2nd ed., Addison-Wesley, Reading, MA.

Maskell, B. H. (1991). *Performance Measurement for World Class Manufacturing*, Productivity Press, New York.

Matousek, R. (1957). *Engineering Design: A Systematic Approach*, Lackie & Son, London.

Mazur, G. (1993). Quality Function Deployment for a Medical Device, presented at the 6th Annual IEEE Computer-Based Medical Systems Conference.

Mekki, K. S. (2006). Robust Design Failure Mode and Effects Analysis in Design for Six Sigma, *International Journal of Product Development*, Vol. 3, No. 3–4, pp. 292–304.

Miles, B. L. (1989). Design for Assembly: A Key Element Within Design for Manufacture, *Proceedings of IMechE, Part D, Journal of Automobile Engineering*, No. 203.

Mizuno, S., and Akao, Y., eds. (1978). *Quality Function Deployment: A Company Wide Quality Approach* (in Japanese), JUSE Press, Tokyo.

Mizuno, S., and Akao, Y., eds. (1994). *QFD: The Customer-Driven Approach to Quality Planning and Deployment*, translated by G. H. Mazur, Asian Productivity Organization, Tokyo.

Montgomery, D. (1991). *Design and Analysis of Experiments*, 3rd ed., Wiley, New York.

Montgomery, D. C. (1997). *Design and Analysis of Experiments*, 4th ed., Wiley, New York.

Mueller, G. (1999). Accurately and Rapidly Predicting Next-Generation Product Breakthroughs in the Medical-Devices, Disposable Shaving Systems, and Cosmetics Industries, TRIZ Journal, March.

Mughal, H., and Osborne, R. (1995). Design for Profit, *World Class Design to Manufacture*, Vol. 2, No. 5, pp. 160–126.

Murty, K. G. (1983). *Linear Programming*, Wiley, New York.

Nair, V. N. (1992). Taguchi's Parameter Design: A Panel Discussion, *Econometrics*, Vol. 34, No. 2.

Nakazawa, H., and Suh, N. P. (1984). Process Planning Based on Information Concept, *Journal of Robotics and Computer Integrated Manufacturing*, Vol. 1, pp. 115–123.

Navichandra, D. (1991). Design for Environmentality, *Proceedings of the ASME Conference on Design Theory and Methodology*, New York.

Neibel, G., and Baldwin, C. (1957). *Designing for Production*, Richard D. Irwin, Hornewood, IL.

Nolan, P. (2006). Treat the Packaging as an Accessory, *Medical Design Magazine*, http://www.medicaldesign.com/articles/ID/13015.

Nordlund, M. (1996). An Information Framework for Engineering Design Based on Axiomatic Design, doctoral dissertation, The Royal Institute of Technology (KTH), Department of Manufacturing Systems, Stockholm, Sweden.

Nordlund, M., Tate, D., and Suh, N. P. (1996). Growth of Axiomatic Design Through Industrial Practice, *Proceedings of the 3rd CIRP Workshop on Design and Implementation of Intelligent Manufacturing Systems*, Tokyo, June 19–21, pp. 77–84.

Novitskaya, E. (2002). Transformation of Structurally Similar Elements of Technical System, http//www.gnrtr.com/tools/en/a011.html.

O'Grady, P., and Oh, J. (1991). A Review of Approaches to Design for Assembly, *Concurrent Engineering*, Vol. 1, pp. 5–11.

Pahl, G., and Beitz, W. (1988). *Engineering Design: A Systematic Approach*, 2nd ed., Springer-Verlag, New York.

Pal, N. R., and Pal, S. K. (1992). Higher Order Fuzzy Entropy and Hybrid Entropy of a Set, *Information Science Journal*, Vol. 61, No. 3, pp. 211–231.

Palady, P. (1995). *Failure Mode and Effect Analysis*, PT Publication, Miami, FL.

Pech, H. (1973). *Designing for Manufacture*, Topics in Engineering Design Series, Pitman & Sons, London.

Pecht, M., et al. (1994). Reliability Predictions: Their Use and Misuse, *Proceedings of the Annual Reliability and Maintainability Symposium*, pp. 386–389.

Peters, T. J., and Waterman, R. H. (1980). *In Search of Excellence: Lessons from America's Best-Run Companies*, Collins Publishing, Cleveland, OH.

Phadke, M. S. (1989). *Quality Engineering Using Robust Design*, Prentice-Hall, Englewood Cliffs, NJ.

Plackett, R. L., and Burman, J. P. (1946). The Design of Optimum Multifactorial Experiment, *Biometrika*, Vol. 33, pp. 305–325.

Prazen, E. (1960). *Modern Probability Theory and Its Applications*, Wiley, New York.

Pressman, R. S. (2000). *Software Engineering: A Practitioner's Approach*, 5th ed., McGraw-Hill, New York.

Pugh, S. (1991). *Total Design*, Addison-Wesley, Reading, MA.

Pugh, S. (1996). *In Creating Innovative Products Using Total Design*, Clausing, D., and Andrade, R., eds., Addison-Wesley, Reading, MA.

Ramakumar, R. (1993). *Engineering Reliability: Fundamentals and Applications*, Prentice Hall, Englewood Cliffs, NJ.

Rantanen, K. (1988). Altshuller's Methodology in Solving Inventive Problems, presented at ICED-88, Budapest, Hungary, August 23–25.

Rinderle, J. R. (1982). Measures of Functional Coupling in Design, Ph.D. dissertation, MIT, Cambridge, MA.

Ross, P. (1988). *Taguchi Techniques for Quality Engineering*, McGraw-Hill, New York.

Rother, M., and Shook, J. (2000). *Learning to See: Value Stream Mapping to Create Value and Eliminate Muda*, Lean Enterprise Institute, Cambridge, MA.

Sackett, P., and Holbrook, A. (1988). DFA as a Primary Process Decreases Design Deficiencies, *Assembly Automation*, Vol. 12, No. 2, pp. 15–16.

Salkin, H. M., and Mathur, K. (1989). *Foundations of Integer Programming*, Elsevier Science, New York.

Shannon, C. E. (1948). The Mathematical Theory of Communication, *Bell System Technical Journal*, No. 27, pp. 379–423, 623–656.

Sheldon, D. F., Perks, R., Jackson, M., Miles, B. L., and Holland, J. (1990). Designing for Whole-Life Costs at the Concept Stage, *Proceedings of ICED*, Heurista, Zurich, Switzerland.

Shiba, S., Graham, A., Walden, D., and Asay, D. (1993). *A New American TQM: Four Practical Revolutions in Management*, Productivity Press, New York.

Shpakovsky, N., and Novitskaya, E. (2002a). Multifunctional Heel, http://www.gnrtr.com/solutions/en/s040.html.

Shpakovsky, N., and Novitskaya, E. (2002b). Frying Pan, http://www.gnrtr.com/solutions/en/s054.html.

Simon, H. A. (1981). *The Science of the Artificial*, 2nd ed., MIT Press, Cambridge, MA.

Sohlenius, G., Kjellberg, A., and Holmstedt, P. (1999). Productivity System Design and Competence Management, World 11th Productivity Congress, Edinburgh, Scotland.

Spotts, M. F. (1973). Allocation of Tolerance to Minimize Cost of Assembly, *Transactions of the ASME*, Vol. 95, pp. 762–764.

Stark, H., and Woods, W. W. (1986). *Probability, Random Processes, and Estimation Theory for Engineers*, Prentice-Hall, Englewood Cliffs, NJ.

Suh, N. P. (1984). Development of the Science Base for the Manufacturing Field Through the Axiomatic Approach, *Robotics and Computer Integrated Manufacturing Journal*, Vol. 1, No. 3–4.

Suh, N. P. (1990). *The Principles of Design*, Oxford University Press, New York.

Suh, N. P. (1995a). Design and Operation of Large Systems, *Journal of Manufacturing Systems*, Vol. 14, No. 3.

Suh, N. P. (1995b). Design and Operation of Large Systems, *Annals of the CIRP*, Vol. 14, No. 3, pp. 203–213.

Suh, N. P. (1996). Axiomatic Design Course, Ford Motor Co., Dearborn, MI, April.

Suh, N. P. (1997). Design of Systems, *Annals of the CIRP*, Vol. 46, No. 1, pp. 75–80.

Suh, N. P. (2001). *Axiomatic Design: Advances and Applications*, Oxford University Press, New York.

Suh, N. P., and Rinderle, J. R. (1982). Qualitative and Quantitative Use of Design and Manufacturing Axiom, *Annals of the CIRP*, Vol. 31, No. 1, pp. 333–338.

Suh, N. P., Cochran, D. S., and Lima, P. C. (1998). Manufacturing System Design, *Annals of the CIRP*, Vol. 47, No. 2, pp. 627–639.

Suskkov, V. V., Mars, N. J., and Wognum, P. M. (1995). Introduction to TIPS: A Theory for Creative Design, Artificial Intelligence in Engineering, Vol. 9, pp. 177–189.

Suzue, T., and Kohodate, A. (1988). *Variety Reduction Program: A Production Strategy for Product Diversification*, Productivity Press, Cambridge, MA.

Swartz, J. B. (1995). *The Hunters and the Hunted: A Non-linear Solution for Reengineering the Workplace*, Productivity Press, Cambridge, MA.

Swenson, A., and Nordlund, M. (1996). Axiomatic Design of a Water Faucet, published report, Saab, Linkoping, Sweden.

Tadikamalia, P. (1994). The Confusion About Six Sigma, Quality Progress, July.

Taguchi, G. (1986). *Introduction to Quality Engineering*, UNIPUB/Kraus International Publications, White Plains, NY; American Supplier Institute, Dearborn, MI; Nordica International, Hong Kong, China.

Taguchi, G. (1987). *System of Experimental Design*, Vols. 1 and 2, American Supplier Institute, Dearborn, MI.

Taguchi, G. (1993). *Taguchi on Robust Technology Development: Bring Quality Engineering Upstream*, American Society of Mechanical Engineers, New York.

Taguchi, G., and Wu, Y. (1980). *Introduction to Off-Line Quality Control*, Central Japan Quality Control Association, Nagoya, Japan.

Taguchi, G., and Wu, Y. (1986). *Introduction to Off-line Quality Control*, 2nd ed., Central Japan Quality Association, Nagoya, Japan.

Taguchi, G., Elsayed, E., and Hsiang, T. (1989). *Quality Engineering in Production Systems*, McGraw-Hill, New York.

Taguchi, G., Chowdhury, S., and Taguchi, S. (1999). *Robust Engineering: Learn How to Boost Quality While Reducing Costs and Time to Market*, McGraw-Hill, New York.

Tate, D., and Nordlund, M. (1998). A Design Process Roadmap as a General Tool for Structuring and Supporting Design Activities, *SDPS Journal of Integrated Design and Process Science*, Vol. 2, No. 3, pp. 11–19.

Tayyari, F. (1993). Design for Human Factors, in *Concurrent Engineering*, H. R. Parsaei and W. G. Sullivan, eds., Chapman & Hall, London, pp. 297–325.

Teng, S., and Ho, S. (1995). Reliability Analysis for the Design of an Inflator, *Quality and Reliability Engineering International*, Vol. 11, pp. 203–214.

Trewn, J. (1999). Functional Reliability Design and Evaluation Methodology: A Systems Approach, doctorate dissertation, Wayne State University, Detroit, MI.

Tribus, M. (1961). *Thermostatics and Thermodynamics*, Van Nostrand, Princeton, NJ.

Tsourikov, V. M. (1993). Inventive Machine: Second Generation, *Artificial Intelligence and Society*, No. 7, pp. 62–77.

Ulman, D. G. (1992). *The Mechanical Design Process*, McGraw-Hill, New York.

Ulrich, K. T., and Eppinger, S. D. (1995). *Product Design and Development*, McGraw-Hill, New York.

VDI (Verein Deutscher Ingenieure) (1986). *Systematic Approach to the Design of Technical Systems and Products*, VDI-2221, translation of the German edition, VDI-Verlag, Dusseldorf, Germany.

Venkitaraman, R. K., and Jaworski, C. (1993). Restructuring Customer Satisfaction Measurement for Better Resource Allocation Decisions: An Integrated Approach, presented at the 4th Annual Advanced Research Techniques Forum of the American Marketing Association, June.

Wang, J., and Ruxton, T. (1993). Design for Safety of Make-to-Order Products, presented at the National Design Engineering Conference of ASME, 93-DE-1.

Wasiloff, J., and El-Haik, B. S. (2004). Practical Application of DFSS with a Focus on Axiomatic Design: A Transmission Planetary Case Study, *Proceedings of the International Society of Automotive Engineers*, Detroit, MI, March.

Weaver, W. (1948). Science and Complexity, *American Scientist*, No. 36, pp. 536–544.

Wilson, A. G. (1970). *Entropy in Urban and Regional Modeling*, Pion Publishing, London.

Worona, T. (2006). A Product Design Approach to Developing Design Controls, *MDDI Magazine*, November; http://www.devicelink.com/mddi/archive/06/11/005.html.

Xie, W. X., and Bedrosian, S. D. (1984). An Information Measure for Fuzzy Sets, *IEEE Transactions on Systems, Man, and Cybernetics*, Vol. 14, pp. 151–156.

Yang, K., and El-Haik, B. (2003). *Design for Six Sigma: A Roadmap for Product Excellence*, McGraw-Hill, New York.

Zaccai, G. (1994). The New DFM: Design for Marketability, *World-Class Manufacture to Design*, Vol. 1, No. 6, pp. 5–11.

Zadeh, L. A. (1965). Fuzzy Sets, *Information and Control Journal*, No. 8, pp. 338–353.

Zadeh, L. A. (1968). Probability Measures of Fuzzy Events, *Journal of Mathematical Analysis and Applications*, Vol. 23, pp. 421–427.

Zadeh, L. A. (1975). The Concept of Linguistic Variable and Its Application to Approximate Reasoning, *Information Sciences Journal*, Vol. 8, Part I (pp. 199–249), II (pp. 301–357), and III (pp. 43–96).

Zadeh, L. A. (1978). Fuzzy Sets as a Basis for Theory of Possibility, *Fuzzy Sets and Systems*, No. 1, pp. 3–28.

Zenger, D., and Dewhurst, P. (1988). Early Assessment of Tooling Costs in the Design of Sheet Metal Parts, Report 29, Department of Industrial and Manufacturing Engineering, University of Rhode Island, Kingston, RI.

Zimmermann, H. J. (1985). *Fuzzy Set Theory and Its Applications*, Kluwer-Nijhoff, Baston, MA.

Zoltin, B., et al. (1996). TRIZ/Ideation Methodology for Customer Driven Innovation, *Proceedings of the 8th Symposium on Quality Function Qeployment*, Novi, MI, June, pp. 448–510.

Zwicky, F. (1948). *Morphological Analysis and Construction*, Wiley-Interscience, New York.

MEDICAL DEVICES REFERENCES

IEC 60601-1-6:2004, Medical Electrical Equipment, Part 6: General Requirements for Safety—Usability.

IEC 62366 Ed. 1, Medical Devices: General Requirements for Safety and Essential Performance—Usability.

ISO 13485:2003, Medical Devices: Quality Management Systems—Requirements for Regulatory Purposes.

ISO 14971:2007, Medical Devices: Application of Risk Management to Medical Devices.

ISO/TR 14969:2004, Medical Devices: Quality Management Systems—Guidance on the Application of ISO 13485:2003.

Design Control Guidance for Medical Device Manufacturers, Center for Devices and Radiological Health, Food and Drug Administration, March 1997.

Design Control Guidance for Medical Device Manufacturers, Global Harmonization Task Force, June 29, 1999, GHTF/FD: 99-9.

Do It by Design, An Introduction to Human Factors in Medical Devices, Center for Devices and Radiological Health, Food and Drug Administration, March 1997.

Electronic Records; Electronic Signatures Final Rule, 62 Federal Register 13430, March 20, 1997.

Glossary of Computerized System and Software Development Terminology, Division of Field Investigations, Office of Regional Operations, Office of Regulatory Affairs, Food and Drug Administration, August 1995.

Guideline on General Principles of Process Validation, Center for Drugs and Biologics, and Center for Devices and Radiological Health, Food and Drug Administration, May 1987.

Guide to Inspections of Quality Systems, August 1999, FDA, http://www.fda.gov/ora/inspect_ref/igs/qsit/qsitguide.htm.

Implementation of Risk Management Principles and Activities Within a Quality Management System, Global Harmonization Task Force, May 20, 2005, GHTF/SG3/N15R8.

Information Document Concerning the Definition of the Term "Medical Device" Global Harmonization Task Force, May 20, 2005, GHTF/SG1/N29R16.

Medical Device Regulations: Global Overview and Guiding Principles, World Health Organization, 2003, ISBN 92 4 154618 2.

Medical Devices; Current Good Manufacturing Practice (CGMP) Final Rule; Quality System Regulation, 61 Federal Register 52602, October 7, 1996.

Medical Device Use—Safety: Incorporating Human Factors Engineering into Risk Management, July 18, 2000.

Principles of Medical Devices Classification, Global Harmonization Task Force, August 31, 2006, GHTF/ SG1-N15-2006.

USEFUL WEB SITES

American National Standards Institute, www.ANSI.org.
Food and Drug Administration, www.fda.gov.
Global Harmonization Task Force, www.GHTF.org.
International Electrotechnical Commission, www.IEC.ch.
International Organization for Standardization, www.ISO.org.

INDEX